T0220706

Contraception and Modern Ireland

Contraception was the subject of intense controversy in twentieth-century Ireland. Banned in 1935 and stigmatised by the Catholic Church, it was the focus of some of the most polarised debates before and after its legalisation in 1979. This is the first comprehensive, dedicated history of contraception in Ireland from the establishment of the Irish Free State in 1922 to the 1990s. Drawing on the experiences of Irish citizens through a wide range of archival sources and oral history, Laura Kelly provides insights into the lived experiences of those negotiating family planning, alongside the memories of activists who campaigned for and against legalisation. She highlights the influence of the Catholic Church's teachings and legal structures on Irish life, showing how, for many, sex and contraception were obscured by shame. Yet, in spite of these constraints, many Irish women and men showed resistance in accessing contraceptive methods. This title is also available as open access.

Laura Kelly is Senior Lecturer in the History of Health and Medicine at the University of Strathclyde and Co-Director of the Centre for the Social History of Health and Healthcare.

Contraception and Modern Ireland

A Social History, c. 1922–92

Laura Kelly

University of Strathclyde

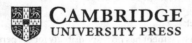

CAMBRIDGE
UNIVERSITY PRESS

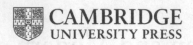

Shaftesbury Road, Cambridge CB2 8EA, United Kingdom

One Liberty Plaza, 20th Floor, New York, NY 10006, USA

477 Williamstown Road, Port Melbourne, VIC 3207, Australia

314–321, 3rd Floor, Plot 3, Splendor Forum, Jasola District Centre,
New Delhi – 110025, India

103 Penang Road, #05–06/07, Visioncrest Commercial, Singapore 238467

Cambridge University Press is part of Cambridge University Press & Assessment, a
department of the University of Cambridge.

We share the University's mission to contribute to society through the pursuit of education,
learning and research at the highest international levels of excellence.

www.cambridge.org
Information on this title: www.cambridge.org/9781108839105

DOI: 10.1017/9781108979740

When citing this work, please include a reference to the DOI 10.1017/9781108979740

First published 2023

A catalogue record for this publication is available from the British Library.

Library of Congress Cataloging-in-Publication Data
Names: Kelly, Laura, 1986- author.
Title: Contraception and modern Ireland : a social history, c.1922-92 / Laura Kelly,
   University of Strathclyde.
Description: Cambridge, United Kingdom ; New York, NY : Cambridge University Press,
   2023. | Includes bibliographical references and index.
Identifiers: LCCN 2022025732 (print) | LCCN 2022025733 (ebook) |
ISBN 9781108839105 (hardback) | ISBN 9781108969772 (paperback) |
ISBN 9781108979740 (epub)
Subjects: LCSH: Birth control–Ireland–History–20th century. | Family planning–Ireland–
   History–20th century. | Contraception–Social aspects–Ireland–History–20th century.
Classification: LCC HQ766.5.I735 K45 2023 (print) | LCC HQ766.5.I735 (ebook) |
   DDC 363.9/609417–dc23/eng/20220705
LC record available at https://lccn.loc.gov/2022025732
LC ebook record available at https://lccn.loc.gov/2022025733

ISBN 978-1-108-83910-5 Hardback
ISBN 978-1-108-96977-2 Paperback

For everyone who shared their experiences with me

Contents

Figures

Acknowledgements

This book is dedicated to all of my oral history respondents with enormous gratitude and respect. This project would not have been possible without their generosity in sharing their memories with me. I am very grateful to them all for speaking to me so openly about their lives and experiences – thank you.

I am also indebted to the Wellcome Trust for their support through a Research Fellowship (Grant Ref: 106593/Z/14/Z) from 20216 to 2021 and for open access funding which has made this book freely available online. I will always be grateful to the Wellcome Trust for their support of my work. In particular, I would like to thank Dan O'Connor, Jack Harrington, Tom Bray, Lauren Couch and Sophie Hutchison at the Wellcome Trust. My editor at Cambridge University Press, Lucy Rhymer, has been hugely supportive of the book from the beginning, and I am really grateful for her guidance and encouragement throughout. Sincere thanks also to the two anonymous reviewers for their useful feedback. I would also like to thank Conor Reidy for preparing the index and for his encouragement. Some sections of Chapter 4 and Chapter 7 have been published in the journals *Medical History* and *Irish Historical Studies*, respectively, and are reprinted with permission.[1]

A number of individuals have provided mentorship and excellent advice over the last few years. I would particularly like to thank Catherine Cox at UCD, who provided invaluable support to me during my time as a postdoctoral fellow there, and who was integral in helping me develop this project from its inception. I would also like to thank former colleagues from my time at the School of History at UCD, and Máire Coyle of the UCD Research Office for all of her help with grant

---

[1] See: Laura Kelly, 'The contraceptive pill in Ireland c.1964–79: activism, women and patient–doctor relationships', *Medical History*, 64:2, (April 2020), pp. 195–218 and 'Irishwomen United, The Contraception Action Programme and the feminist campaign for free, legal, contraception in Ireland, c.1975–1981', *Irish Historical Studies*, 43:164, (November 2019), pp. 269–97.

applications for this project. In 2016–17, I was lucky enough to spend an academic year at the Section for the History of Medicine at Yale University, and I am grateful to Naomi Rogers for her input and inspiration. I would also like to thank Matt Smith and Jim Mills at the University of Strathclyde, who have both been wonderful mentors and always generous with their time and support. I am also thankful to Greta Jones for her support and interest over the years. Thanks also to former mentors and lecturers from my time as a student at NUI Galway, including Catriona Clear, Barry Crosbie, Steven Ellis, Aileen Fyfe and Enda Leaney.

The archival research for this project was conducted at a number of libraries and archives. I am grateful to the staff at the National Archives of Ireland, National Library of Ireland, New York Academy of Medicine, UL Special Collections, UCC Special Collections and Wellcome Collection. I would especially like to thank Noelle Dowling at the Dublin Diocesan Archives for all of her help and support.

A number of individuals provided extra support during the research process. I am very grateful to all of the actively retired individuals and to the community groups I visited for allowing me to speak about my research. I would also like to give special thanks to Liam Bluett for his assistance with recruiting interviewees. Thanks also to Jon O'Brien for connecting me with the members of the IFPA youth group, for patiently answering my many questions and for sending me archival documents. I would also like to thank John O'Reilly for his kind assistance with my project and for his generosity in providing me with archival sources I would not have been able to access otherwise. Thanks also to Niall Meehan, Emer Nowlan, Susan Solomons and Evelyn Stevens for providing me with additional archival sources, and to Niall Behan for providing me with access to the IFPA archives.

I would also like to thank photographers Clodagh Boyd, Beth Lazroe, Joanne O'Brien and Derek Speirs for permission to use their wonderful photographs that enrich the book. Thanks also to Berni Metcalfe at the NLI for scans of images from the NLI collection.

I am grateful to a number of colleagues and friends who provided invaluable feedback and support at different stages of the writing process. Thank you to Jennifer Crane, Cara Delay, Catriona Ellis, Olivia Dee, Susan Grant, Jenna Healey, Agata Ignaciuk, Lauren MacIvor Thompson, Emma Newlands, Maeve O'Brien, Kelly O'Donnell, Jennifer Redmond, Naomi Rogers, Caroline Rusterholz, Maya Sandler, Niall Whelehan and David Wilson for helpful feedback on chapter drafts. Thanks also to the 'Catholicizing Reproduction, Reproducing Catholicism' research team and to fellow members of the 'KU Leuven Medicine and Catholicism since the Late 19th Century' network.

I would also like to thank Donna Drucker, Máiréad Enright, Lindsey Earner-Byrne, Phoebe Harkins and Ross MacFarlane for their support and encouragement throughout the project.

Thank you to my colleagues at the Centre for the Social History of Health and Healthcare (CSHHH) and the School of Humanities at the University of Strathclyde for their support. In particular, I would like to thank Patricia Barton, Tanja Bueltmann, Catriona Ellis, Mark Ellis, Janet Greenlees, Churnjeet Mahn, Yvonne McFadden, Arthur McIvor, Jim Mills, Kate Mitchell, David Murphy, Emma Newlands, Matt Smith, Angela Turner, Niall Whelehan, Manuela Williams and David Wilson. I am also thankful to the Central Support Team in the School for their administrative support. I would also like to thank my PhD students, Mara Dougall, Georgia Grainger, Kristin Hay, Jois Stansfield, Rory Stride and Jasmine Wood, who have each inspired me through our conversations over the last few years.

I am also so lucky to have had the friendship and support of many friends, both inside and outside academia. Thanks in particular to Rebecca Barr, Sarah-Anne Buckley, Elaine Farrell, Susan Grant, Yuliya Hilevych, Carole Holohan, Agata Ignaciuk, Rob Kirk, Wendy Kline, Sylwia Kuźma, Leanne McCormick, Emma Newlands, Neil Pemberton, Linsey Robb, Caroline Rusterholz, Christabelle Sethna and Niamh Wycherley for their kindness and encouragement and for inspiring me with their own work. I would also like to thank Kate Bluett, Nicola Carty, Gaelen Britton, Sarah Corbett, Breda Doherty, Lucy Fleming, Jennifer Goff, Maria Ní Fhlatharta, Emma O'Callaghan and Maeve O'Brien for their friendship and inspiring conversations, which often centred around some of the themes in this book. I would also like to especially thank MaryJo Kelly Novak and Richard and Gracia Elkin for always showing great interest in my work. Huge thanks also to Maeve O'Brien for encouraging me at every stage of this project.

Thanks, as always, to my family, in particular, my parents, John and Angela, and my brothers Seán and Ciaran, for supporting me throughout this project in immeasurable ways. Finally, a huge thank you, with all my love, to Chris Elkin for giving me endless encouragement and support throughout the research and writing process, as well as lots of joyful and happy times away from it.

Abbreviations

CAP	Contraception Action Programme
CFPC	Cork Family Planning Clinic
CLAA	Criminal Law Amendment Act
CMAC	Catholic Marriage Advisory Council
COSC	Council of Social Concern
FGC	Fertility Guidance Company
FPS	Family Planning Services
GFPA	Galway Family Planning Association
GFPC	Galway Family Planning Clinic
IFL	Irish Family League
IFPA	Irish Family Planning Association
IFPRA	Irish Family Planning Rights Association
IPPF	International Planned Parenthood Federation
IWLM	Irish Women's Liberation Movement
IWU	Irishwomen United
LFPC	Limerick Family Planning Clinic
NAOMI	National Association for the Ovulation Method Ireland
NFPC	Navan Family Planning Clinic
RTÉ	Raidió Teilifís Éireann
SPUC	Society for the Protection of Unborn Children
TCD	Trinity College Dublin
UCC	University College Cork
UCD	University College Dublin
UCG	University College Galway
WWC	Well Woman Centre

Archives

DDA	Dublin Diocesan Archives
NAI	National Archives of Ireland
RCAPA	Roisin Conroy/Attic Press Archive
WC	Wellcome Collection

Introduction

In the summer of 2019, I interviewed Deirdre (b.1936) in the kitchen of her suburban home. Deirdre had grown up in a city in the west of Ireland, one of six children, and after school she worked in the confectionary trade. In her late teens, she met her husband, and got married aged 23. She recalled what she knew about contraception and sex on her marriage in 1959:

We were awful innocent, we were innocent, we were awful innocent. I don't know, now today, I do often say they're going on their honeymoon, sure they've had their honeymoon, well over, by the time they go on honeymoons! We go on our honeymoons, we were innocent, what did we know, we didn't know anything about life. You didn't because you didn't talk about it. We never spoke about anything like that.

Deirdre's first child was born a year and seven months later. A year later, her second child died at birth. A year following this, she had her third child, and then three more children followed, explaining 'every 14 months for four years I had one'. Her seventh and final child was born when she was 38, after which she explained she told her husband '"That's it now", I said, "the last one I'm going to have", I said. "Whether you like it or not", you know. And it's just as it happened, that's the way it happened'.

Deirdre's testimony is revealing on many levels. It illustrates the lack of knowledge she felt she had in relation to sex and contraception, in contrast with younger generations, and the telling silences around the issue. Moreover, her testimony illustrates the stark reality of recurring pregnancy for many Irish women without access to contraception or information about fertility control. Yet, her account also illustrates her agency and resistance towards her husband when she ultimately decided not to have any more children.

The people like Deirdre who are at the heart of this study were coming of age, marrying and having children in a period of intense and lasting social change in modern Ireland. This book traces their experiences living without legal access to contraception in the 1950s, 1960s and

1970s in the Republic of Ireland, and how people resisted legal and religious restrictions. It also explores the experiences of activists who campaigned for and against changes in the law. The book begins around 1922 with the establishment of the Irish Free State and ends with the passing of the Health (Family Planning) Amendment Act in 1992. This amendment removed many of the restrictions regarding where condoms could be sold; it was amended in 1993 to remove the age restriction on the sale of condoms.[1] As such, the book spans roughly a 70-year period, allowing an examination of continuities and change over the course of the twentieth century.[2]

The Legal and Social Context

From 1922 with the foundation of the Irish Free State, the country gradually became more conservative as the Irish government worked to ensure that Catholic values were enshrined in the new state's concept of Irishness. This could be seen particularly with a range of laws that were passed during the 1920s and 1930s which reinforced moral codes as well as a series of official investigations which generated lengthy reports which often themselves led to legislation addressing moral and social issues.[3]

Of particular relevance to contraception was the 1926 Evil Literature Committee which went on to influence the 1929 Censorship of Publications Act.[4] Witnesses and delegates to the committee suggested that British birth control 'propaganda' was widely available, at least in Dublin and that literature relating to the use of contraceptives was obscene and would encourage sexual activity outside of marriage.[5] Sections 16 and 17 of the 1929 act banned the advertising of contraception or abortion as well as prohibiting the sale and distribution of 'indecent or

---

[1] Under the Health Family Planning Amendment Act (1992), contraceptives could be sold to persons aged 17 or over; the 1993 amendment removed this restriction. See: *Health (Family Planning) (Amendment) Act, 1992*, and *Health (Family Planning) (Amendment) Act, 1993*.

[2] On the benefits of long durée histories, see: Jo Guldi and David Armitage, *The History Manifesto* (Cambridge University Press, 2014), pp. 14–37.

[3] James M. Smith, 'The politics of sexual knowledge: The origins of Ireland's containment culture and the Carrigan Report (1931)', *Journal of the History of Sexuality*, 13:2, (April 2004), pp. 208–33, on pp. 208–9.

[4] Sandra McAvoy, '"A perpetual nightmare": Women, fertility control, the Irish State, and the 1935 ban on contraceptives' in Margaret Ó hÓgartaigh and Margaret Preston (eds.), *Gender and Medicine in Ireland, 1700–1950* (Syracuse University Press, 2014), pp.189–202, on p. 194.

[5] *Ibid.*, p. 195.

obscene' books.[6] The Committee on Evil Literature had recommended that the terms 'indecent' or 'obscene' should have a wide interpretation, 'so as to make the law applicable to matters intended to excite sensual passion'.[7] In practice, this meant that a wide range of books could be banned, including texts which provided basic information on fertility. Subsequently, the 1931 Carrigan Committee Report suggested that the use of contraceptives was prevalent in a lot of the country and linked access to contraceptives with sexual promiscuity.[8] It also drew attention to the circulation of advertisements relating to contraception and a cross-Channel trade of contraceptives between Ireland and Britain.[9] The Criminal Law Amendment Act (CLAA) of 1935, an Irish update to the British CLAA of 1885, thus dealt with a host of issues relating to sexuality and 'marked a break with a neighbouring British culture in which contraception was increasingly accepted'.[10] It raised the age of consent from 16 to 17 years and unlawful carnal knowledge of a girl between the age of 15 and 17, and 'attempted unlawful carnal knowledge' of a girl under 15, were now classed as misdemeanours, rather than felonies.[11] The CLAA abolished the 'reasonable cause to believe' clause of the 1885 act, meaning that 'no defence was possible for having sex with a girl under the age of 15 once her age and the act of sex were confirmed'.[12] In practice, this meant that a defence of not knowing the girl's age could be used in cases of rape and sexual assault. The act also increased the penalties for prostitution and had a section which related to public indecency.[13] Crucially, for our purposes, the CLAA criminalised the importation and sale of contraceptives. The ban, as historian Sandra McAvoy has pointed out, arguably 'delayed the emancipation of Irish women – not least by subordinating their rights to life and health to their reproductive functions'.[14] Ultimately, the combination of the CLAA and Censorship of Publications Act meant that both contraceptives and

---

[6] Una Crowley and Rob Kitchin, 'Producing "decent girls": governmentality and the moral geographies of sexual conduct in Ireland, (1922–1937)', *Gender, Place and Culture*, 15:4, (August 2008), pp. 355–72, on p.356.

[7] Michael Adams, *Censorship: The Irish Experience* (University of Alabama Press, 1968), p. 35.

[8] McAvoy, 'A perpetual nightmare', p. 199.

[9] Maryann Gialanella Valiulis, 'Virtuous mothers and dutiful wives: the politics of sexuality in the Irish Free State' in M.G. Valiulus, (ed.), *Gender and Power*, pp. 100–114, on p. 106.

[10] McAvoy, 'A perpetual nightmare', p. 289.

[11] Diarmaid Ferriter, *Occasions of Sin: Sex and Society in Modern Ireland* (London: Profile Books, 2009), p. 145.

[12] Ferriter, *Occasions of Sin*, p. 145.

[13] Crowley and Kitchin, 'Producing "decent girls"', p. 3.

[14] McAvoy, 'A perpetual nightmare', p. 202.

information about birth control were being suppressed. Working-class women and men were, undoubtedly, the most affected by this legislation.

However, the Irish government was not unique in its preoccupation with the sexual health and behaviour of its population, but perhaps what characterised Ireland was the extent to which Catholic ethos influenced its legislation. Similar bans on birth control were implemented in France, Belgium and Italy, but in these countries, this was owing to concerns about depopulation after the First World War.[15] As Senia Pašeta has argued in relation to legislation around censorship of birth control information in Ireland, 'the moral argument remained imperative: birth control was a sin against God, nature and Catholicism'.[16] Ireland could therefore be said to have more in common with Franco's Spain where a ban on the sale, usage and advertisement of contraception was introduced in 1941 and not decriminalised until 1978.[17]

Motherhood and family were elevated in status under the Irish Free State with the dominant religious discourse backing this.[18] Women, in particular, were 'critical to the Free State's definition of itself as a pure and virtuous nation'. While women had played a crucial role in the struggle for Irish independence, in the Irish Free State, they 'needed to be returned to the home' through the enaction of gender legislation which tried to block women from political and economic involvement in the State.[19] Contraception was abhorred by the Catholic hierarchy in Ireland, and by extension the Irish Free State government.[20] Members of other churches, such as the Church of Ireland, were unjustly impacted by this sectarian legislation; Protestants were 'encouraged to keep a low, even a cringing profile'.[21] More broadly, while the Church of Ireland was also concerned with moral issues, as Jennifer Redmond has argued 'there does not seem to be the same volubility and panic over a perceived decline in moral standards as existed in the Catholic Church and expressed in Lenten pastorals and newspaper articles'.[22] Indeed, more widely, the Lambeth conferences of 1930 and 1958 indicated an acceptance of contraception in the Anglican Church. As Maryann Valiulis has shown, in the

---

[15] Senia Pašeta, 'Censorship and Its Critics in the Irish Free State 1922–1932', *Past and Present*, 181, (November 2003), pp. 193–218, p. 217.

[16] *Ibid.*, p. 217.   [17] Ferriter, *Occasions of Sin*, pp. 118–19.

[18] Valiulis, 'Virtuous mothers', pp. 101–2.   [19] *Ibid.*, p.101.   [20] *Ibid.*, p.107.

[21] Ian d'Alton, '"No country"? Protestant "belongings" in independent Ireland, 1922–49' in Ian d'Alton and Ida Milne (eds.), *Protestant and Irish: The Minority's Search for Place in Independent Ireland* (Cork University Press, 2019), pp. 19–33, on p.22.

[22] Jennifer Redmond, 'The politics of emigrant bodies: Irish women's sexual practice in question' in Jennifer Redmond, Sonja Tiernan, Sandra McAvoy, and Mary McAuliffe, (eds.), *Sexual Politics in Modern Ireland* (Dublin: Irish Academic Press, 2015), pp. 73–89, on p. 74.

Irish context, birth control was equated with race suicide and became construed as 'the attempt by the forces of the former colonial power to exert a negative influence on a virtuous Irish population'.[23]

Recent important work by Sandra McAvoy, Lindsey Earner-Byrne and Deirdre Foley, has explored the role of the Catholic Church hierarchy, Irish government and the medical profession in shaping debates on contraception.[24] Lindsey Earner-Byrne has shown that in the early twentieth century many members of the medical profession framed the contraception debate as a moral issue rather than a medical one.[25] In particular, the Irish Guild of Saint Luke, SS Cosmas and Damian was active in the anti-birth control movement and the campaign against a free maternity service in Ireland in the late 1940s and early 1950s.[26] Members of organisations like the Irish Guild of Saint Luke, SS Cosmas and Damian overlapped with other Catholic action groups such as the Knights of Saint Columbanus.[27] It is also important to note that the majority of Irish maternity hospitals had a Catholic atmosphere; for example, in Dublin, two of the three largest maternity hospitals 'operated with a Catholic ethos, and the Archbishop of Dublin, John Charles McQuaid, was particularly mindful of how medics operated within these hospitals with regard to birth control'.[28] From the 1960s, the topic of contraception began to be more widely discussed in the media. Yet, the Catholic Church maintained its stance in relation to contraception being morally wrong with the publication of *Humanae Vitae* in 1968. As Deirdre Foley has shown, in the wake of *Humanae Vitae*, 'a strong, patriarchal network of authority, made up of the Irish Catholic hierarchy and an obeisant section of the medical profession, sought to reaffirm control over Catholic women's bodies'.[29] Similarly, in Northern Ireland,

[23] Valulius, 'Virtuous mothers', p. 108.
[24] Sandra McAvoy, 'The Regulation of Sexuality in the Irish Free State, 1929–1935' in Elizabeth Malcolm and Greta Jones (eds.), *Medicine, Disease and the State in Ireland, 1650–1940* (Cork: Cork University Press, 1999), pp. 253–6; Sandra McAvoy, 'Its effect on public morality is vicious in the extreme: defining birth control as obscene and unethical, 1926–32' in Elaine Farrell (ed.), *She Said She Was in the Family Way: Pregnancy and Infancy in Modern Ireland* (London: Institute of Historical Research, 2012), pp. 35–52; McAvoy, 'A perpetual nightmare'.
[25] Lindsey Earner-Byrne, 'Moral prescription: the Irish medical profession, the Roman Catholic Church and the prohibition of birth control in twentieth-century Ireland' in Catherine Cox and Maria Luddy (eds.), *Cultures of Care in Irish Medical History, 1750–1950* (Palgrave, 2010), pp. 207–28.
[26] Earner-Byrne, 'Moral prescription', pp. 209–10.   [27] *Ibid.*, p. 221.
[28] Deirdre Foley, 'Too many children?' Family planning and *Humanae Vitae* in Dublin, 1960–72', *Irish Economic and Social History*, 43:1, (December 2019), pp. 142–160, on p. 144.
[29] *Ibid.*, p. 144.

artificial birth control was unavailable and largely condemned until the 1960s and there was significant opposition from the Catholic Church and politicians there to the establishment of family planning services.[30] Yet, we know from valuable scholarship by gender historians that both north and south, some Irish women in the twentieth century were resisting and rejecting traditional notions of motherhood.[31]

Ireland's population history has been characterised by long-term population decline, high rates of emigration as well as low rates of marriage and late age of marriage, high marital fertility and a late transition to smaller families.[32] The birth rate in Ireland fell steadily from the 1870s up until the Second World War, rising sharply during the 1940s.[33] Between 1911 and 1946, family size fell by approximately 20 per cent; in 1946, as Mary E. Daly has shown, couples who had been married for 30–34 years had an average of 4.94 children compared with 6.77 children for couples with marriages of a similar duration in 1911.[34] Nevertheless, when compared with British couples who had been married for a similar duration, Irish couples with marriages of 20 years duration in 1946 had twice as many children as their counterparts in Britain, 4.39 compared to 2.16.[35] In the 1950s, the Irish birth rate was close to the Western European average, however, as Daly has posited, this was due to the combination of a low marriage rate and a very high marital fertility rate.[36]

---

[30] See: Lindsey Earner-Byrne and Diane Urquhart, *The Irish Abortion Journey, 1920–2018* (Basingstoke: Palgrave, 2019), pp. 51–68; Leanne McCormick, '"The scarlet woman in person": the establishment of a Family Planning Service in Northern Ireland, 1950–1974' in *Social History of Medicine*, 21:2, (August 2008), pp. 345–60; Leanne McCormick, *Regulating Sexuality: Women in Twentieth-Century Northern Ireland* (Manchester, 2009); Greta Jones, 'Marie Stopes in Ireland: The Mother's Clinic in Belfast, 1936-47' in *Social History of Medicine*, 5:2, (August 1992), pp. 255–77.

[31] See: Cara Delay, 'Pills, potions, and purgatives: Women and abortion methods in Ireland, 1900–1950.' *Women's History Review*, 28:3, (2019), pp. 479–99 and Cara Delay, 'Kitchens and kettles: Domestic spaces, ordinary things, and female networks in Irish abortion history, 1922–1949', On illegal abortion in Northern Ireland, see Leanne McCormick, '"No sense of wrongdoing": Abortion in Belfast 1917–1967, *Journal of Social History*, 49:1, (Fall 2015), pp. 125–48.

[32] Mary E. Daly, *The Slow Failure: Population Decline and Independent Ireland, 1920–1973* (University of Wisconsin Press, 2003), p. 4.

[33] Finola Kennedy, *Cottage to Creche: Family Change in Ireland* (Dublin: Institute of Public Administration, 2001), p. 30. We know little about individuals' personal birth control experiences in the nineteenth century; one of the few Irish proponents of birth control was Thomas Haslam, who published an anonymous pamphlet on the safe period in 1868. See: Carmel Quinlan, *Genteel Revolutionaries: Anna and Thomas Haslam and the Irish Women's Movement* (Cork University Press, 2002), pp. 25–52.

[34] Daly, *The Slow Failure*, p. 122.   [35] *Ibid.*, p. 122.

[36] Mary E. Daly, *Sixties Ireland: Reshaping the Economy, State and Society, 1957–1973* (Cambridge University Press, 2016), p. 144.

In 1961, for instance, the Irish statistic for the number of legitimate births per married woman was 195.5 per thousand, which was almost double the figure in England and Wales (108.3).[37]

From the 1960s, it is clear that some couples were trying to limit the number of children they had. For example, between 1966 and 1968, the number of births fell by almost 3 per cent, amounting to a 7 per cent decrease in fertility in two years.[38] However, Daly warns caution against exaggerating this transformation, pointing to the fact that in 1967, 23 per cent of women who gave birth in Dublin's National Maternity Hospital were having their fifth child, and the number of births peaked in 1980, with marital fertility in Ireland remaining 'seriously out of line with any other country in the Western world, and remained so because fertility elsewhere was falling sharply.'[39] Yet, the introduction of contraception arguably had a significant impact. During the 1960s and 1970s, the average number of children per family in Ireland was usually above 3, before declining quickly in the 1980s, hitting a low of 1.85 in 1995, and then beginning to rise again during the period of economic growth.[40] After a slight increase in the marriage rate in the spurt of economic expansion in the 1970s, marriage began to lose popularity into the 1980s and there was a sharp fall in marriage rates and a rise in births outside marriage.[41] And, by 1993, 19 per cent of births were outside marriage (compared to 2 per cent in the 1960s), rising to over 31 per cent in 2003.[42]

From the early 1970s, some Irish politicians, in particular Senator Mary Robinson, began to try to have the law relating to contraception changed. The political and legal debates around the contraception issue have been well-documented.[43] Meanwhile, activists began to challenge the law through the establishment of family planning clinics, such as the Fertility Guidance Company in Dublin in 1969. Chrystel Hug rightly argues that 1971 was a 'crucial year in the fight for the right to contraception', pointing to the Irish Women's Liberation Movement's Contraceptive Train, the seizure of a packet of spermicide jelly sent to Mary (May) McGee in Co. Dublin, and Senator Mary Robinson's seven

---

[37] Robert E. Kennedy, *The Irish, Emigration, Marriage and Fertility* (Berkeley: University of California Press, 1973), p. 75 cited in Daly, p. 144.

[38] Daly, *Sixties Ireland*, p. 144.   [39] *Ibid.*, p. 145.   [40] Ferriter, *Occasions of Sin*, p. 427.

[41] Kennedy, *Cottage to Creche*, p. 24.   [42] Ferriter, *Occasions of Sin*, p. 427.

[43] See for example: Chrystel Hug, *The Politics of Sexual Morality in Ireland* (Basingstoke: Palgrave Macmillan, 1999), pp. 76–140; Brian Girvin, 'Contraception, moral panic and social change in Ireland, 1969–79', *Irish Political Studies*, 23:4, (December, 2008), pp. 555–76 and 'An Irish solution to an Irish problem: Catholicism, contraception and change, 1922–1979', *Contemporary European History*, 27:1, (2018), pp. 1–22; Aidan Beatty, 'Irish modernity and the politics of contraception, 1979–1993', *New Hibernia Review*, 17:3, (Autumn, 2013), pp. 100–118.

attempts to have her bills on contraception read in the Seanad, as important moments.[44] Indeed, the 1970s was a critical period for activism around the contraception issue and several studies have illuminated the campaigns of feminist and activist groups to legalise contraception.[45] In her 2012 memoir, Robinson explained the hypocrisy of the ban of contraception in that 'it was legal to use contraceptives, but not to buy or sell them' while the contraceptive pill could be prescribed as a cycle regulator.[46] In October 1970, Robinson announced her intention to introduce a private members' bill to repeal the CLAA of 1935.[47] The Irish government refused to put her bill on the agenda six times between March and June 1971.[48] With the support of John Horgan and Trevor West, a second bill was put on the agenda on 7 July 1971; it would have allowed the limited sale of contraceptives in hospitals, chemists and other licensed settings, and would have enabled the publication of information about family planning.[49] Reflecting on this bill, Robinson remarked:

One of the points we tried to make in the Senate was that everyone in the country seemed to be debating the issue except the legislators. There was an Irish tendency to dodge sexual and moral issues by upholding in the law Catholic principles while in practice, doing otherwise. I was offending this fudge by wanting the law to reflect the need for openness and diversity in Irish society. Access to contraception, I argued, was a matter of private morality.[50]

Robinson faced significant backlash from the Catholic Church, stating that the Church hierarchy 'rose up against the bill, condemning it from the pulpit and denouncing me, personally.'[51] The bill was opposed by a majority of senators (25 to 14) in its first reading.[52] The following year, Labour TDs Noel Browne and John O'Connell attempted to have the same bill read in the Dail but its first reading was opposed by a majority of government TDs.[53]

In the meantime, 27-year-old Mary (May) McGee took on a crucial legal challenge in 1972. McGee had left school at 16 and had lost most of her hearing as a result of childhood illness.[54] She and her husband

---

[44] Hug, *The Politics of Sexual Morality*, p. 94.

[45] Hug, *The Politics of Sexual Morality*, (particularly chapters 3 and 4); Emilie Cloatre and Máiréad Enright, '"On the perimeter of the lawful": Enduring illegality in the Irish Family Planning Movement, 1972–1985', *Journal of Law and Society*, 44:4, (December, 2017), pp. 471–500; Linda Connolly, *The Irish Women's Movement*.

[46] Mary Robinson, *Everybody Matters: A Memoir* (London: Hodder & Stoughton, 2012), p. 64.

[47] *Ibid.*, p. 65.   [48] Hug, *The Politics of Sexual Morality*, p. 95.   [49] *Ibid.*

[50] Robinson, *Everybody Matters*, p. 72,   [51] *Ibid.*

[52] Hug, *The Politics of Sexual Morality*, p. 95.   [53] *Ibid.*

[54] Emilie Cloatre and Máiréad Enright. 'Commentary on *McGee v Attorney General*' in Máiréad Enright, Julie McCandless and Aoife O'Donoghue, *Northern/Irish Feminist*

Seamus, a fisherman, lived in a mobile home at her mother's house in Skerries with three of their four children; the eldest son lived with his grandmother due to the lack of space.[55] In spite of efforts at family planning, the McGees had four children (including a set of twins) in less than two years, and May had experienced significant health issues during her pregnancies, including toxaemia during her first pregnancy, a stroke at the end of her second pregnancy, and toxaemia again in her third pregnancy, with her twins arriving prematurely after serious complications.[56] Dr. James Loughran (a founding member of the Fertility Guidance Company) advised her not to have any more children believing that further pregnancies would place her life at risk.[57] She was fitted with a cap by Loughran and ordered spermicide jelly by post from England; this was seized by customs. McGee was encouraged to go to court by Loughran and his lawyer because the seizure of the package meant that her life was being put at risk by another potential pregnancy and this contravened the Constitution's articles on the citizens' personal rights (40.3.1) and the authority of the family (41.1.2).[58]

The McGee case was heard by the High Court in July 1972; Judge O'Keeffe rejected the case arguing that 'the personal rights of the citizen did not include a right to the protection of privacy, and the 1935 law was not inconsistent with the authority of the family'. In an interview with scholars Emilie Cloatre and Máiréad Enright, McGee recalled of the judgement:

[He] just threw it out, didn't want to know … He didn't even listen, didn't even try five minutes and I couldn't believe it and I said to myself 'Is that the way women are really treated?' sort of thing …I have to say that it was only then I realised just how badly women were really treated in the way we were seen but not heard. Our opinion didn't count.[59]

May McGee appealed to the Supreme Court and in December 1973, four out of the five judges ruled in her favour, arguing that the ban on contraception was an invasion of her personal rights and that she was entitled to the 'protection of the privacy of her marital relations'.[60] It is important to note that the judgement was in favour of marital privacy, rather than contraception. As a result of this decision, the importation of contraceptives for one's own personal use was now allowed, however, the

---

Judgments: Judges' Troubles and the Gendered Politics of Identity (Oxford: Hart Publishing, 2017), pp. 95–116, on p.107.

[55] *Ibid.*, p. 107.   [56] *Ibid.*   [57] *Ibid.*, p. 107.
[58] Hug, *The Politics of Sexual Morality*, pp. 96–97.
[59] Cloatre and Enright. 'Commentary on *McGee v Attorney General*', p. 96.
[60] Hug, *The Politics of Sexual Morality*, p. 97.

ban on the importation of contraceptives for sale, as well as the ban on the proliferation of information on birth control, were maintained.[61] Meanwhile, in 1973, Mary Robinson had won the vote in the Seanad to have a revised version of her 1971 bill read.[62] On the same day that senators were due to vote on Mary Robinson's bill, they also received a draft of a government bill introduced by Patrick Cooney, Minister for Justice, on the same issue; Cooney's bill dealt with the regulation of the import of contraceptives and authorisation of their sale.[63] Robinson's bill was defeated in the Seanad on 24 March 1974 with 32 votes against and 10 votes in favour.[64] Cooney's bill was defeated on 16 July 1974 with 75 votes against and 61 in favour, with the Taoiseach Liam Cosgrave famously voting against his own minister's bill.[65] Robinson made one more attempt to have a bill introduced; her Family Planning Bill of 1974 was, in Hug's words 'a compromise between her relatively liberal bill of 1973 and the more conservative Cooney bill' and would have enabled anyone to import contraceptives for their personal use but for a licence to be required for their importation for sale. It also classed contraceptives as medical appliances which implied that individuals from low-income groups who held medical cards could have obtained contraception for free.[66] 23 senators voted in favour of a second reading of the bill in December 1974, with 16 against, and when the bill eventually receive its second reading in December, 1976, it was narrowly defeated and prevented from reaching the committee stage with 23 votes against and 20 in favour.[67]

In June 1977, the Fianna Fáil government regained power, and Taoiseach Jack Lynch assigned the task of introducing a law on family planning to then Minister for Health, Charles Haughey. In Girvin's view, 'When legislation was finally passed in 1979 it reflected the dominant conservative moral values in every way short of prohibition. Moreover, for over a decade after 1979, Ireland continued to diverge from its European neighbours on moral questions'.[68] The Family Planning Act closely reflected the position of the Catholic hierarchy on the issue of contraception, with Haughey taking their concerns relating to the young and unmarried, prescribing of condoms and advertising into account with the legislation, as well as providing state finance for the provision of natural family planning advice and research into this method.[69] The only concern of the bishops that Haughey could not address was their

---

[61] *Ibid.*, p. 98.   [62] *Ibid..*   [63] *Ibid.*, p. 102.
[64] Family Planning Bill, 1973: second stage (resumed), Seanad Éireann debate, March 27, 1974. Accessed: www.oireachtas.ie/en/debates/debate/seanad/1974-03-27/4/
[65] Hug, *The Politics of Sexual Morality*, p. 107.   [66] *Ibid.*   [67] *Ibid.*, p. 108.
[68] Girvin, 'An Irish solution', p. 3.   [69] *Ibid.*, p. 20.

desire for contraception to be restricted 'primarily to married couples', instead, the act worded that contraception would be available for *bona fide* family planning purposes only.[70] Yet, as Chrystel Hug has suggested, the phrase '*bona fide* family planning' was likely 'inserted to keep good Catholics and Fianna Fáil backbenchers happy, who wanted birth control practised in a family context'.[71] The Health (Family Planning) Act was passed on 26 June 1979 with 58 votes in favour and 36 against.[72]

This legislation, which was famously referred to by Haughey as an 'Irish solution to an Irish problem', came into operation on 1 November 1980. It allowed contraception on prescription for *bona fide* family planning purposes only, with this stipulation widely interpreted as meaning that contraceptives were only available to married couples. Under this legislation, a prescription from a doctor was required for all contraceptives, including condoms. As Brian Girvin has recently argued, the Family Planning Act of 1979 should not be viewed as 'a turning point or as a liberal point of departure for a progressive future'.[73] Indeed, it was followed by a divisive referendum over abortion (1983), resulting in the introduction of the eighth amendment of the constitution.[74] As this book will show, access to contraceptives remained restrictive into the 1980s and early 1990s, and the act essentially handed power to the medical profession and pharmacists. As journalist Stephen O'Byrnes astutely surmised in the *Irish Independent* in 1985:

To an extent the problem did go away after 1979 because the problem was largely resolved in the Dublin area and especially for the middle-classes, and media people in general and middle-class letter writers to the papers were no longer personally motivated by the subject. But if we are honest with ourselves we will see that the unhappy Kerry Tribunal hearing is removing the veil on the tragic and traumatic reality of sexually active adults, ignorant of, or unable to avail of contraceptives.[75]

The Family Planning Act was amended in 1985 under the Minister for Health, Barry Desmond, during a Fine Gael-Labour coalition government which had been formed in November 1982, with Taoiseach Garret FitzGerald, in the face of significant opposition from Fianna Fáil, the

---

[70] *Ibid.*   [71] Hug, *The Politics of Sexual Morality*, p. 113.   [72] *Ibid.*, p. 114.
[73] Girvin, 'An Irish solution', p. 3.
[74] On the legal impact of the eighth amendment, see: Fiona de Londras, 'Constitutionalizing fetal rights: a salutary tale from Ireland', *Michigan Journal of Gender & Law*, 22:2, (2015), pp. 243–289; J. Schweppe (ed.), *The Unborn Child, Article 40.3.3 and Abortion in Ireland: Twenty Five Years of Protection?* (Dublin: Liffey Press, 2008).
[75] 'Family plan bill debate', *Irish Independent*, 7 February 1985, p. 8.

Catholic Church and conservative campaigners.[76] The 1985 Health (Family Planning) (Amendment) Bill intended to allow the sale of non-medical contraceptives such as condoms and spermicides which could be sold without a prescription to anyone over the age of 18 at outlets which included chemists, family planning clinics, VD clinics and maternity hospitals.[77] In contrast to Charles Haughey, Barry Desmond did not consult with the Catholic Church hierarchy when devising the amendment.[78] The discussion over the Act took five days of parliamentary time and narrowly passed with 83 votes in favour and 80 against.[79] However, while the amendment to the law meant that non-medical contraceptives such as condoms and spermicides no longer required a prescription and could be bought in a chemist, access remained restrictive, with many chemists and GPs refusing to prescribe and stock contraceptives for moral reasons. During the early 1990s, direct action campaigns such as the Irish Family Planning Association's selling of condoms in the Virgin Megastore in Dublin ('the case of the Virgin condom'), and the Condom Sense campaign, where activists illegally installed condom vending machines in bars and nightclubs, were crucial in helping to further change the law around the sale of condoms in Ireland.[80]

Using Oral History

In a 2003 article on the possibilities for oral history in Ireland, Guy Beiner and Anna Bryson suggested that 'the social history of twentieth-century Ireland needs to be re-written and the standard archival sources currently open to researchers are inadequate for such an undertaking'.[81] Since then, there have been several important studies which have used oral history to help uncover 'hidden' histories, on topics as diverse as the Spanish Flu of 1918, Irish women's experiences during the Second World War, the lives of Irish religious sisters, women's experiences of work, and the impact of the Northern Irish Troubles on healthcare provision and medical practice.[82] Oral history has also been used

[76] Hug, *The Politics of Sexual Morality*, p. 115.   [77] *Ibid.*, p. 118.
[78] Girvin, 'An Irish solution', p. 22.
[79] Health (Family Planning) (Amendment) Bill, 1985: Second Stage (Resumed), 20 February 1985. www.oireachtas.ie/en/debates/debate/dail/1985-02-20/15/
[80] Emilie Cloatre and Máiréad Enright, 'Transformative illegality: How condoms 'became legal' in Ireland, 1991–1993', *Feminist Legal Studies*, 26, (2018), pp. 261–84, on p. 262.
[81] Guy Beiner and Anna Bryson, 'Listening to the past and talking to each other: problems and possibilities facing oral history in Ireland', *Irish Economic and Social History*, 30, (2003), pp. 71–8, on p. 77.
[82] Ida Milne, *Stacking the Coffins: Influenza, War and Revolution in Ireland, 1918–19*, (Manchester University Press, 2018); Elizabeth Kiely and Máire Leane, *Irish Women at*

effectively and respectfully to uncover the lived experiences of women in Magdalene laundries and mother and baby homes through the Clann Project and Justice for Magdalene Research as well as more recently, the Northern Irish Mother and Baby Homes and Magdalen Laundries Report.[83]

The case for oral history, since it developed as a field in the 1970s, has always been that it allows scholars 'to rescue for the historical record the lives of social groups for whom other kinds of records were sparse or non-existent, or in which the angle of vision was only that of those in power'.[84] Put simply, oral history provided me with a unique opportunity to ask individuals, activists and medical practitioners directly about their experiences, how it felt at the time, and what it means to them now.[85] Or, as Paul Thompson puts it, 'Oral history, by transforming the 'objects' of study into 'subjects', makes for a history which is not just richer, more vivid, and heart-rending, but *truer*'.[86] In addition, when utilised in research in gender history, an oral history methodology can allow a means of 'integrating women into historical scholarship'.[87] As Kathryn Anderson and Dana Jack have argued, oral history interviews 'provide an invaluable means of generating new insights about women's experiences of themselves in their worlds'.[88]

To date, there have been limited studies which have used oral history as a means of understanding reproductive and sexual health in Ireland.[89]

Work 1930–1960: An Oral History (Irish Academic Press, 2012); Yvonne McKenna, *Made Holy: Irish Women Religious at Home and Abroad* (Irish Academic Press, 2006); Mary Muldowney, *The Second World War and Irish Women: An Oral History* (Irish Academic Press, 2007); Ruth Coon, *The Impact of The Northern Ireland Troubles on Healthcare Provision and Medical Practice* (PhD thesis, Ulster University, 2021).

[83] See: Clann Project (http://clannproject.org/) and Justice for Magdalenes Research (http://jfmresearch.com). Leanne McCormick, Sean O'Connell, Olivia Dee and John Privilege, *Mother and Baby Homes and Magdalene Laundries in Northern Ireland, 1922–1990, Report for the Inter Departmental Working Group on Mother and Baby Homes, Magdalene Laundries and Historical Clerical Child Abuse*, (January 2021). On the Tuam Oral History project, see www.nuigalway.ie/tuam-oral-history/

[84] Penny Summerfield, 'Culture and composure: creating narratives of the gendered self in oral history interviews', *Cultural and Social History*, 1:1, (2004), pp. 65–93, on p. 66

[85] Alessandro Portelli, 'What makes oral history different' in Robert Perks and Alistair Thomson (eds.), *The Oral History Reader* (Routledge, 2003 edition), p. 67.

[86] Paul Thompson, *The Voice of the Past: Oral History*, 3rd edition (Oxford University Press, 2000), p. 117.

[87] Joanne Sangster, 'Telling our stories: feminist debates and the use of oral history', *Women's History Review*, 3:1,(1994), p. 5.

[88] Kathryn Anderson and Dana C. Jack, 'Learning to listen: interview techniques and analyses' in Sherna Berger Gluck and Daphne Patai (eds.), *Women's Words: The Feminist Practice of Oral History* (London, Routledge, 1991), pp. 11–26, on p.11.

[89] Important exceptions include Betty Hilliard, 'The Catholic Church and married women's sexuality: Habitus change in late 20th century Ireland', *Irish Journal of*

My aim, with this project, was to explore the experiences of Irish men and women in navigating access to contraception and trying to plan their families in a period of tremendous social change, but also to illuminate the experiences of activists involved in campaigns related to the contraception issue. A major problem within the historiography of contraception has been the question of how to explore what has been traditionally seen as a very private facet of everyday life. My methodology has been adapted from successful studies of birth control practices and sexuality in the UK which have utilised oral history as a means of gaining access to attitudes towards contraception. I have been particularly inspired by Kate Fisher's ground-breaking work on birth control practices in England and Wales in the early twentieth century, and her follow-up book with Simon Szreter on sex before the sexual revolution.[90] These studies also showed me the importance of interviewing both men and women about birth control practices. Recent valuable studies by Caroline Rusterholz and David Geiringer have also highlighted the power of oral history to shed light on individuals' birth control practices.[91] In addition, I utilised a range of more traditional documentary sources, including women's magazines, newspaper sources, government records, contemporary literature, feminist archives and memoirs. The combination of these sources provides us with a rich, multi-faceted account that includes the voices of those who have previously been left out of the historical narrative.

For this project, I conducted interviews with 103 men and women who were born in Ireland before 1955[92] and 42 interviews with individuals involved in activism related to the contraception issue in the period from the 1970s to the 1990s, as well as some members of the medical profession and priesthood. Activists were, for the most part, identified through archival sources and traced online, or through snowballing. In order to recruit interviewees to talk about their birth control practices, I gave short

Sociology, 12:2, (2003), pp. 28–49; Máire Leane, 'Embodied sexualities: Exploring accounts of Irish women's sexual knowledge and sexual experiences, 1920–1970', in M. Leane and E. Kiely (eds.) *Sexualities and Irish Society: A Reader* (Dublin: Orpen Press, 2014), pp. 29–56; and Hazel Lyder, '"Silence and Secrecy": Exploring Female Sexuality During Childhood in 1930s and 1940s Dublin', *Irish Journal of Feminist Studies*, 5:1&2, (2003), pp. 77–88.

90 Kate Fisher, *Birth Control, Sex and Marriage in Britain, 1918–1960* (Oxford University Press, 2006) and Kate Fisher and Simon Szreter, *Sex Before the Sexual Revolution: Intimate Life in England, 1918–1963* (Cambridge University Press, 2010).

91 Caroline Rusterholz, 'Reproductive behavior and contraceptive practices in comparative perspective, Switzerland (1955–1970)', *The History of the Family*, 20:1, (2015), pp. 41–68 and *'Deux enfants c'est déjà pas mal', Famille et fécondité en Suisse, 1955–1970* (Lausanne: Editions Antipodes, 2017); David Geiringer, *The Pope and the Pill: Sex, Catholicism and Women in Post-War England* (Manchester University Press, 2019).

92 With three exceptions who were born in 1956, 1957 and 1961, respectively.

talks about my research project at fourteen community groups aimed at older people across the country in a range of locations which included urban and rural areas. I then invited individuals to sign up for a one-to-one interview if they were interested in being involved in the project. Individuals were also recruited by word-of-mouth, snowballing, and I also interviewed some friends' parents. In total, I interviewed 30 men and 73 women from a range of socioeconomic backgrounds. All respondents were white, perhaps reflecting much of the population born in the country before 1955. Undoubtedly, people of colour and Irish Travellers would have experienced particular challenges in relation to birth control in the period of this study, and their experiences are worthy of a separate project. None of my interviewees reported a disability, although this was not directly asked in the interview.[93]

The majority of these individuals were interviewed on their own, but in five cases I interviewed married couples together. Most participants had been or were still married; only five individuals had not been married. Participants were provided with an information sheet in advance of the interview and signed off on a consent form. Following the interview, they could decide whether they wanted their interview to be archived at the Scottish Oral History Centre and the conditions of access through signing a recording agreement form. In line with best oral history practice, the interview transcript was returned to participants, and they had the opportunity to correct any errors so as to ensure they were happy with their written testimony.[94] All respondents were assigned pseudonyms unless they requested otherwise.[95] In cases where participants mentioned the name of a partner or family member, this name has been changed in the text.

As Srigley, Zembrzycki and Iacovetta have asserted in their recent collection on feminist approaches to oral history, 'Feminists who work with oral history methods want to tell stories that matter. They know, too, that the telling of those stories—the processes by which they are generated and recorded, and the contexts in which they are shared and interpreted—also matters—a lot.'[96] In my case, intersubjectivity was crucial, and my positionality as an Irish woman in her early thirties at the time of the interviews, undoubtedly had a bearing on the ways that interviewees

---

[93] On Irish deaf women's experiences, see: Grainne Meehan, *Flourishing at the Margins: An Exploration of Deaf and Hard-of-Hearing Women's Stories of Their Intimate Lives in Ireland* (PhD thesis, NUI Maynooth, 2019). Important ongoing work by the Re(al) productive Justice project at NUI Galway is exploring the experiences of disabled people in Ireland seeking reproductive justice.

[94] Lynn Abrams, *Oral History Theory*, 2nd ed. (Abingdon: Routledge, 2016), p. 165.

[95] I have chosen not to indicate where individuals requested a pseudonym or not.

[96] 'Introduction', in K. Srigley, S. Zembrzycki, F. Iacovetta, *Beyond Women's Words: Feminisms and the Practices of Oral History in the Twenty-First Century* (London: Routledge, 2018), p. 1.

related to me. For example, my respondents often compared their experiences of sex education and wider attitudes to sex with attitudes today, and this may have been in part because of our intersubjectivity, as I would have been close in age to their granddaughters or daughters.[97] For instance, in relation to single mothers, Mary Ellen (b.1944) compared the stigma of unmarried motherhood in the past with attitudes today, stating 'That wouldn't happen today because they're allowed to have their babies today'. Similarly, with regard to sex education, Noreen (b.1954) explained that young people 'pick it up from the internet, only it's not magazines, it's the internet you know? Only they do it much younger, and they're more savvy, in one way they're more savvy and in another way they're not. I think ... the real sex education doesn't occur'.

Before beginning the project, I would regularly get asked about whether I thought people would be open in sharing their personal experiences. For the most part, people were remarkably candid about their lives. It is also important to note that the majority of interviews took place during 2018–19 when there was increased discussion about Irish mother and baby homes in the news. In May 2018 there was a referendum to repeal the eighth amendment and in May 2015 there had been a referendum on same-sex marriage. This perhaps meant that issues relating to sexual morality were to the front of people's minds. Moreover, being an Irish woman meant that I benefited from shared experiences of culture and the Catholic religion in some cases, and meant that I could empathise with some of the experiences individuals recalled, based on my own experiences and family history, which perhaps made people feel comfortable telling their stories to me. Yet, with regard to the male respondents, the fact that I was young and female meant that in some cases, men were perhaps not as open with me as they might have been with a male interviewer, although no male respondents raised this issue directly.

The power of oral history is evident in these interviews. Following a life story approach meant that individuals talked not only about their experiences of contraception and family planning, but that they also discussed related issues such as sex education, courtship and marriage, single motherhood, attitudes to sexuality more broadly, as well as traumatic events such as miscarriage or the loss of a child.[98] Oral histories also provided me with access to 'emotions which are not evident in paper

---

[97] Angela Davis reported similar findings in her study. Davis, 'Generation and memories of sex and reproduction in mid-twentieth-century Britain', *The Oral History Review*, 45:2, pp. 249–64, on p. 260.

[98] On unexpected trauma in oral history interviewing, see: Emma Vickers, 'Unexpected trauma in oral interviewing', *The Oral History Review*, 46:1, (2019), pp. 134–41. For an excellent example of a life story approach to oral history, see: Judy Yung, 'Giving voice to Chinese American women', *Frontiers: A Journal of Women's Studies*, 19:3, (1998), pp. 130–156.

documents'.[99] In the telling of their experiences, individuals laughed, joked, expressed sadness, regret, and in some instances, became emotional. I am indebted to my interviewees for trusting me with their memories. Their accounts have enabled a clearer picture of people's experiences relating to contraception than would have been possible through a reliance on archival evidence.

Why is This Book Important?

This book broadly examines the experiences of two groups of people: Irish men and women born in Ireland in the period before 1955, and activists who campaigned for the legalisation of contraception and/or provided access to contraception through family planning clinics as well as conservative campaigners who were against the legalisation of contraception. Neither of these groups' experiences have been captured on this scale before. The first five chapters are predominantly focused on the experiences of Irish men and women who were of fertile age during the 1950s, 60s, 70s and 80s. Chapters 6, 7, and 8 explore activists' experiences. Chapter 9 looks at both.

My study provides, for the first time, an insight into the experiences of and attitudes to birth control of Irish citizens living in this period of rapid social change, assessing how these were shaped by Ireland's social and cultural context while also illuminating related facets of everyday life such as sexuality, gender relations, marriage and pregnancy. In spite of the ban on contraception, declining family sizes in the period prior to legalisation suggest that many Irish men and women were practising fertility control measures. This book seeks to explain how and why through the use of a 'bottom-up' approach which centres the voices of men and women who lived through this period.[100] It is not concerned

---

[99] Katie Holmes, 'Does it matter if she cried? Recording emotion and the Australian generations Oral History Project', *The Oral History Review*, 44:1, (2017), pp. 56–76, on p.75.

[100] For works which have greatly expanded our knowledge of women's experiences in relation to sex, maternal health and welfare, see: Elaine Farrell, *A Most Diabolical Deed: Infanticide and Irish Society, 1850–1900* (Manchester University Press, 2013); Maria Luddy, *Prostitution and Irish Society, 1800–1940* (Cambridge University Press, 2007); Cliona Rattigan, *What Else Could I Do?: Single Mothers and Infanticide, Ireland 1900–1950* (Irish Academic Press, 2011), Lindsey Earner-Byrne, *Mother and Child: Maternity and Child Welfare in Ireland, 1920s–1960s* (Manchester: Manchester University Press, 2007). Related to this, valuable work by Lindsey Earner-Byrne, Cara Diver and Linda Connolly has also uncovered women's experiences of sexual and marital violence: Lindsey Earner-Byrne, 'The rape of Mary M.: A microhistory of sexual violence and moral redemption in 1920s Ireland', *Journal of the History of Sexuality*, 24:1, (January 2015), 75–98; Cara Diver, *Marital Violence in Post-Independence Ireland, 1922–6: 'A Living Tomb for Women'* (Manchester University

with the legislators and politicians involved in debates around contraception, but with the experiences of 'ordinary' people and activists. However, it is crucial to note the problem with the use of the term 'ordinary'.[101] These individuals' accounts of resilience and resistance when barriers including societal, medical and legal structures as well as Church teachings were stacked against them, were deeply inspiring, and in many cases, extraordinary. As such, the book also seeks to contribute to the history of sexuality in Ireland, which, to date, has tended to focus on the darker side of sexuality.[102] Crucially, the book seeks to highlight the agency of Irish people in gaining access to contraception illegally and in going against the traditional teachings of the Catholic Church, as well as suggesting the continuing reliance on 'natural' methods of birth control such as the 'withdrawal method', Billings method and abstinence. Moreover, the stories of activists who campaigned both for and against the legalisation of contraception, and who have previously received limited attention from scholars, are also explored.

As well as implicitly making a case for the value of oral history as a methodology to understand individuals' personal experiences of reproductive and sexual health, this book also makes a number of key arguments. Firstly, it illustrates the impact of Church teachings and State laws on both attitudes to sexuality and on individuals' family planning practices, and in particular how Church and State laws essentially meant that members of the medical profession and Church representatives were allocated significant power and authority over individuals' reproductive health choices. However, in spite of this, it is clear that many Irish men and women were beginning to resist this power and authority and through a focus on men and women's experiences, this book seeks to highlight individuals' agency in family planning. It also shows how responsibility for family planning tended to lie with women in this period, and how women's resistance in this area helped to drive significant change. Yet, as a result of lack of access to artificial methods, combined with the impact of Church teaching, natural methods of family planning remained one of the few options for the majority of men and women. Class and location were clearly important in relation to who had the option to engage in effective family planning. Second, significant work by

Press, 2019); Linda Connolly, 'Sexual violence in the Irish Civil War: a forgotten war crime?', *Women's History Review*, 30:1, (2021), pp. 126–43. Sarah-Anne Buckley's important work has illuminated hidden histories of child abuse and welfare. See: Sarah-Anne Buckley, *The Cruelty Man: Child Welfare, the NSPCC and the State in Ireland, 1889–1956* (Manchester University Press, 2013).

[101] Claire Langhamer, '"Who the hell are ordinary people?" Ordinariness as a category of historical analysis', *Transactions of the Royal Historical Society*, 28, (2018), pp. 175–195.

[102] Diarmaid Ferriter's *Occasions of Sin* touched on the debates surrounding contraception in Ireland, however, the main focus of the study was what he terms more 'clandestine and illicit sexual behaviour'.

Earner-Byrne, Rossiter, Delay, and Earner-Byrne and Urquhart, has illuminated the consequences of lack of contraceptive and abortion options in Ireland, and in particular highlighted the pattern of travel to England for reproductive healthcare.[103] Mary Gilmartin and Sinéad Kennedy have devised the term 'reproductive mobility' to refer to travel for the purposes of accessing reproductive health services.[104] This book further emphasises the impact of lack of access to contraception on individuals but also shows the hypocrisy of the Irish situation which meant that while Britain was routinely invoked as a 'heathen' or permissive society, Ireland's proximity to Britain meant that the UK market was relied upon as a provider of contraceptives such as condoms, as well as female sterilisation. Third, through the use of oral history interviews with activists involved in campaigns for and against the legalisation of contraception, this book shows the importance of activists in generating debate, challenging the law and in some cases providing services, but also emphasises the personal impact that this work had on these individuals. Through discussion of the experiences of activists on both sides, I aim to show how the issue was one of the most polarised debates in Irish society in the twentieth century, and contribute to the growing history of activism in Ireland.[105] In the case of anti-contraception campaigners, it is clear that their activism around contraception was a key foundation for the pro-life campaigns of the 1980s and beyond.[106] More broadly, this book seeks to contribute to the history of contraception internationally; a growing field of research, which in recent years has begun to focus on the

---

[103] See: Earner-Byrne and Urquhart, *The Irish Abortion Journey*; Ann Rossiter, *Ireland's Hidden Diaspora: The Abortion Trail and the Making of a London-Irish Underground, 1980–2000* (IASC publishing, 2009); Cara Delay, 'From the backstreet to Britain: Women and abortion travel in Modern Ireland', in Charlotte Beyer, Janet MacLennan, Dorsía Smith Silva, and Marjorie Tesser (eds.), *Travellin' Mama: Mothers, Mothering, and Travel* (Demeter Press, 2019).

[104] Mary Gilmartin and Sinéad Kennedy, 'A double movement: the politics of reproductive mobility in Ireland', in Christabelle Sethna and Gayle Davis (eds.), *Abortion Across Borders: Transnational Travel and Access to Abortion Services* (Baltimore: Johns Hopkins Press, 2019), pp.123–43.

[105] See for example: Cloatre and Enright, 'Transformative illegality' and 'On the perimeter of the lawful'; Mary Muldowney, 'Breaking the silence: pro-choice activism in Ireland since 1983' in Jennifer Redmond, Sonja Tiernan, Sandra McAvoy and Sonja Tiernan (eds.), *Sexual Politics in Ireland* (Irish Academic Press, 2015), pp. 127–53; Patrick McDonagh, *Gay and Lesbian Activism in the Republic of Ireland, 1973–93* (Bloomsbury, 2021); David Kilgannon, '"Responsible, effective and caring": Gay Health Action, AIDS Activism and Sexual Health in the Republic of Ireland, 1985–1989', *Irish Economic and Social History*, (online, August 2021).

[106] The terms 'pro-life' and 'pro-choice' are, of course, highly politicised but I have chosen to use these terms in the book out of a preference to refer to campaigners by the terms they wish to be called.

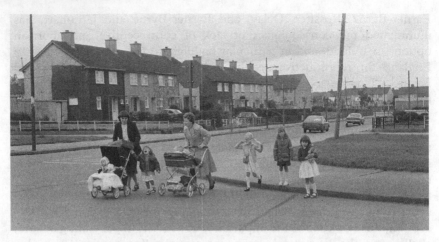

I.1 *Heavy Traffic (2)*, Ballyfermot, Dublin, June 1981. Photograph by Beth Lazroe.

personal experiences of individuals and activists.[107] It aims to illustrate that the Irish history of contraception was not exceptional, but that Irish men and women had much in common with the experiences of individuals in other predominantly Catholic European countries, such as Italy, Spain and Switzerland, as well as the experiences of individuals in regions which did not have the same legal restrictions on contraception such as Quebec, England and the United States.[108] Finally, the book argues that unlike other countries, Ireland did not experience a sexual revolution until at least the 1990s. I argue that the Family Planning Act of 1979 was not a turning point, and that restricted access to contraception, and shame and stigma around sexual matters more generally, persisted until at least the 1990s, if not beyond.

---

[107] For example: Hera Cook, *The Long Sexual Revolution: English Women, Sex, and Contraception: 1800–1975* (Oxford University Press, 2004); Elizabeth Siegel Watkins, *On the Pill: A Social History of Oral Contraceptives 1950–1970* (Baltimore: Johns Hopkins University Press, 1998); Raúl Necochea López, *A History of Family Planning in Twentieth-Century Peru* (Chapel Hill, NC: University of North Carolina Press, 2014); Susanne M. Klausen, *Race, Maternity, and the Politics of Birth Control on South Africa* (Houndmills, UK: Palgrave MacMillan, 2004); Nicole C. Bourbonnais, *Birth Control in the Decolonizing Caribbean: Reproductive Politics and Practice on Four Islands, 1930–1970* (Cambridge University Press, 2016); Caroline Rusterholz, *Women's Medicine: Sex, Family Planning and British Female Doctors in Transnational Perspective*, (Manchester University Press, 2020).

[108] See for instance: Alana Harris (ed.), *The schism of '68: Catholics, Contraception and Humanae Vitae in Europe, 1945–1975* (London: Palgrave McMillan, 2018); Teresa Ortiz-Gómez, and Agata Ignaciuk, 'The family planning movement in Spain during the democratic transition', *Journal of Women's History* (2018); Diane Gervais and Danielle Gauvreau, 'Women, priests, and physicians: family limitation in Quebec, 1940–1970', *Journal of Interdisciplinary History*, 34:2 (2003), pp. 293–314; Leslie W. Tentler, *Catholics and Contraception: An American History* (Cornell University Press, 2008).

1 Access to Contraception and Family Planning Information in Ireland from the 1920s to the 1950s

In a letter to British birth control campaigner, Marie Stopes in February 1923, a 28-year-old woman from Limerick wrote:

> I have read for the first time off the paper about your good work and your book about birth control. I am just twenty eight years old married nine years today and the mother of six children so I feel I have done my bit and only wish I could be in London to go to your clinic. I am too poor to afford a maid and have to (sic) all my own sewing washing and scrubbing and the thought of having any more children would drive me mad. Wishing you all success and hoping I may get your book.

On the top of the letter the woman wrote 'Please accept my apology for my impertinence in asking for a book or how I may obtain one but I really feel it's a Godsend to people like us and shall always be grateful'.[1] This Irish woman, like many who wrote in desperation to Marie Stopes in the 1920s and 1930s, (and many who did not), was subject to Ireland's laws relating to sexual morality. For much of the twentieth century, it was difficult for Irish men and women to obtain information on birth control, including publications by Marie Stopes, as a result of the 1929 Censorship of Publications Act. As mentioned in the introduction, under this act, there was a wide interpretation of what constituted 'indecent and obscene'. In 1931, Marie Stopes wrote to two members of the Irish censorship board, William B. Joyce and P.J. Keawell to complain that her book *Radiant Motherhood*, which had been written 'to give specific help to pregnant women, rules of health for the nine months of their pregnancy, in order that they may bring to birth healthy and happy children' had been unfairly banned on 'the ground of "advocating unnatural methods of contraception"'. No reply to her letter exists in the archive so we do not know Joyce's response, however, Keawell replied to state that it was not usual practice to enter into correspondence with authors but that he would bring her letter

---

[1] Letters to Marie Stopes concerning *Married Love* [Wellcome Collection (WC), PP/MCS/ A/182].

to the meeting of the next board.[2] Nevertheless, Stopes' request appears to have had no effect. A 1936 list of books prohibited in the Irish Free State included all of her publications.[3]

In the early decades of post-independent Ireland, perceived threats to the Irish family were othered as foreign influences. George L. Mosse's work on nationalism, sexuality, and respectability in twentieth-century Europe is pertinent here; in linking racism and sexuality, he has argued that 'sexuality was not just one more attribute of the racist stereotype, but by its attack upon respectability threatened the very foundations of bourgeois society'.[4] For instance, Cara Delay and Annika Liger have shown how abortionists in post-independent Ireland were perceived to be 'a corrupting and possibly contagious force, harming Irish women and Irish society and threatening the very fabric of the nation in a key post-colonial moment'.[5] Similarly, in debates around the Censorship Act, as Senia Pašeta has shown, 'anti-birth control propaganda became increasingly entwined with anti-Protestantism'.[6] More broadly, and as outlined in the introduction, concerns about sexual morality were expressed in other legislative initiatives around censorship, restrictions on dance halls, as well as the efforts of the Church hierarchy through Lenten pastorals, and voluntary efforts to eradicate sex work by religious groups such as the Legion of Mary.[7]

However, in spite of the legislative ban, we know that individuals found ways to access contraception. Andrea Tone's pioneering work on the black market for contraceptives in the United States in the late nineteenth century has highlighted the value in exploring illegal trades in contraception, in particular showing how such a study can 'call into question assumptions of draconian enforcement of birth control restrictions and tell us new things about law, commerce and everyday sexual practice'.[8] Similarly, as I will show through the evidence of newspaper

---

[2] [WC, PP/MCS/A/147].

[3] *Books Prohibited in the Irish Free State under the Censorship of Publications Act, 1929 (as on 30 April 1936)* (Dublin: Eason & Son Ltd., 1936).

[4] George L. Mosse, *Nationalism and Sexuality: Respectability and Abnormal Sexuality in Modern Europe* (New York: Howard Fertig, 1985), p. 151.

[5] Cara Delay and Annika Liger, 'Bad mothers and dirty lousers: Representing abortionists in postindependence Ireland', *Journal of Social History*, 54:1, (Fall 2020), pp. 286–305, on p. 300.

[6] Pašeta, 'Censorship and Its Critics', pp. 211–212.   [7] Ferriter, *Occasions of Sin*, p. 102.

[8] Andrea Tone, 'Black market birth control: Contraceptive entrepreneurship and criminality in the Gilded Age', *The Journal of American History*, 87:2, (September 2000), pp. 435–59, on p. 437. See also: Tone, *Devices and Desires: A History of Contraceptives in America* (Hill and Wang, 2002).

accounts of court cases, Ireland also had a flourishing black market for contraceptives in the early decades of the twentieth century.

As outlined in the introduction, it is men and women's everyday experiences which are at the heart of this study. As a result of recent scholarship by Cara Delay, Elaine Farrell, and Cliona Rattigan on illegal abortion and infanticide, we know the impact that legal and moral restrictions had on individuals' reproductive health choices in early twentieth-century Ireland.[9] Beginning with recollections from oral history respondents about their parents' experiences and building on this work, this chapter seeks to highlight the profound influence of the legal context on individuals' choices around family planning in the early twentieth century. As a result of the legal barriers and effects of religious and moral condemnation, it was difficult for Irish men and women to access contraception. Individuals' accounts suggest that their parents lacked knowledge of contraception and complied with Church teachings. Yet, the documentation of court cases relating to contraception in the Irish press, and letters from Irish men and women to Marie Stopes complicates this picture and suggests a tension between what oral history interviewees think about their parents' reproductive health experiences and the lived realities of men and women of fertile age in early post-independent Ireland. This chapter provides clear evidence of resistance and attempts at resistance. In addition, the letters from Irish men and women to Marie Stopes and published accounts in Stopes' newspaper *Birth Control News*, suggest that many Irish men and women perceived a lack of access to birth control as having a negative impact on both maternal and infant health, and that this was what motivated their desire for access to effective contraception.

1.1   Oral Histories

As outlined in the introduction, the oral histories conducted as part of this project were primarily with men and women born before 1955. As such, it is difficult to trace the experiences of individuals in the previous generations and we lack personal accounts of family planning from the early twentieth century. One of the few studies to address family limitation was Alexander Humphrey's 1966 book *New Dubliners* which explored the impact of urbanisation on the family. Humphreys conducted interviews with eleven couples from the artisan class in Dublin

---

[9] On abortion in Ireland, see Cara Delay, 'Pills, potions, and purgatives' and 'Kitchens and kettles' On infanticide see: Rattigan, *What Else Could I Do?* On infanticide in the nineteenth century see: Farrell, *A Most Diabolical Deed.*

and his book detailed some of these individuals' attitudes to sex. One 'typical' couple was the Dunns who had married in 1923, both at the age of 29, and had six children. According to Humphreys:

Despite this positive orientation towards having children, Joan and John entered marriage with a rather remarkable ignorance of the sexual and birth processes. Neither of them had received instructions in these matters from their parents, nor did they seek such instructions from a physician prior to their marriage. They had to make shift with the haphazard knowledge of marriage which they picked up from their contemporaries at work.[10]

Moreover, Humphreys noted that 'one cannot escape the strong impression that towards sex John and Joan have a sense of danger and even evil' and reflected on their embarrassment around the issue.[11] Humphreys wrote that in general among the eleven couples he interviewed, there was a complete ignorance of sexual matters on marriage as a result of a lack of parental instruction. One woman interviewed by Humphreys for instance stated:

I think that it was really sinful that I was allowed to marry as ignorant and as innocent as I was about the whole matter. At that time the only way you learned was from with girls you worked with, but I did not work in a factory and I knew nothing. Honestly, I could surprise you with what I did not know. I used to think of marriage as a mere matter of companionship. It never occurred to me that children or the purpose of marriage had anything to do with sex.[12]

Aside from rare accounts such as these, we lack personal testimonies of family planning from men and women of fertile age in the early twentieth century in Ireland. Yet, oral history has the potential to offer a window into individuals' lived realities and can also provide insights into common perceptions surrounding the experiences of previous generations. In some of the oral history interviews conducted for this project, respondents reflected on their parents' experiences and how these differed or were similar to theirs. These reflections provide some insights into the experiences of older generations but also illustrate the persistence of silences, obstetric trauma, shame, and lack of reproductive choices, well into the twentieth century. Respondents also tended to characterise their parents as being devout in their adherence to Church teachings and passive in relation to issues of sexuality and family planning, which arguably hints at a type of collective or popular memory in relation to the experiences of older generations.[13] Yet,

---

[10] Alexander J Humphreys, *New Dubliners: Urbanization and the Irish Family* (London: Routledge and Kegan Paul Ltd, 1966), p. 120.
[11] *Ibid.*   [12] *Ibid.*, pp. 138–40.
[13] For more on collective and popular memory, see Abrams, *Oral History Theory*, pp. 95–9.

continuities were also acknowledged. While many interviewees recognised differences in standards of living, schooling and opportunities compared to their parents' generation, it is evident that their contraceptive choices, or lack of, were similar to their parents.

Mothers' experiences were often referred to by female respondents and offered a way for them to situate their own life experiences. Martina (b.1955) stated:

But then I look back at my mother's life and that was worse than what mine was. She was with the same man all her life and that was just as bad or worse because ... I don't know, there were no opportunities for her, do you know what I mean? Compared to how it was, I mean, I feel, my life.

In Martina's view, women of her mother's generation 'were restrained mentally and spiritually. And physically a lot of the time. So, they didn't have ... They had no choices at all.' Likewise, Clare (b.1936) from the rural west felt that in contrast to her mother, 'I suppose I had a career, I had a job. My mother didn't.' Noreen (b.1954) felt that women's work in the home was undervalued. She stated: 'they were very crucial in society but very little value left on them, you know?' Similarly, Sally (b.1956) told me: 'I can see that my mother was trapped with children. Had four of us. And the eldest being four going on five and the youngest a couple of months'.

Lily (b.1946) from the rural north felt that women's lives were dictated by a lack of choice around sexual and reproductive health matters. She explained: 'Yeah, I'd say our mothers just laid back and had sex and got pregnant, and laid back and had sex and got pregnant, you know, the size of the families? It obviously was that way, you know. And the men just went on regardless. They had no real input into it all, you know.' Carol (b.1954) felt that her mother, who had been born in 1916, 'certainly wouldn't have had any control over, over contraception or anything like that. Or wouldn't really have understood it, I think to be honest'. Mary Ellen (b.1944) from the rural west of Ireland stated:

I think they just had children. They didn't understand it at all, sexuality. Maybe I'm wrong but I feel they knew very little about it. And they had their children. My mother had four children but other families had lots more. Lots more. Maybe my mother's age with ... I don't know, I think she was in her 30s, well into her 30s when she married, maybe I'm wrong, but I just think it wasn't discussed. And those children kept appearing after 9 or 10 months. And the family kept ... it was the norm. But I think way back ... I think it was just sex to the female. More a male thing. I really don't know but ... they didn't ... it wasn't discussed. And it was just when two parties got together that was it. And oftentimes I don't think they understood how the female anatomy worked.

These testimonies suggest that many of the female respondents viewed their mothers as having little agency in the areas of family planning and sex. There was a sense among interviewees that women of previous generations had limited knowledge of sex and birth control and that they played a passive role in these matters. Yet, although respondents in general were unclear about whether their parents used family planning methods, some recalled their mothers discussing the use of the rhythm method or safe period. Maria (b.1957), for instance, explained that her mother:

used to say that the rhythm, 'cause she would've used rhythm, seven children, rhythm, she would say rhythm was a feast or a famine.

Similarly, Judith (b.1950) from Dublin found out through her aunt that her mother had used the safe period:

And I never asked, but I remember, again one of my aunts telling me. There was three of us with four years between us. That she was supposed to have practised the safe method. And where she heard about that, I don't know.

Although the rhythm method was not a reliable form of family planning, it is clear that some women, such as Maria and Judith's mothers, were actively trying to restrict their families. And, as this chapter will show later on, they were not exceptional.

Trauma and silences around reproductive health experiences were common for the earlier generations. Nellie (b.1944) for example, recalled her mother's traumatic experience of childbirth:

I suppose I was very precious, because my mother and father were 10 years married before they had any child. And she probably had surgery, but she never talked about it. Which, she got pregnant anyway, and she had a child. The child was born here at home, and she nearly died herself. The child died. The child was a forcep delivery. Terrible. Terrible, terrible. And painful. It wasn't talked about. And they were waiting so long to have to take the child and bury it, was a tragedy really.

Helena's (b.1945) mother had fifteen children. Helena recalled her mother 'She used to joke it was her holiday, going to the [name of local maternity] hospital every year was a holiday'. Helena's mother also had seven miscarriages, one of which Helena witnessed:

Yeah, I can remember her one time being taken downstairs, and I'm sitting on a chair, and it's soaking with blood. And I remember trying to wash the blood out of the towels the following morning, and I couldn't get it out, yeah.

Her mother's trauma had a significant impact on Helena too. Helena recalled each time her mother became pregnant that 'you didn't know whether she was gonna die or not, yeah'. She recalled on one occasion 'realising that she was pregnant again. (laughs) I went around to every church in the town. There were seven churches in the town, praying that she'd have a safe delivery. I- I can remember that fear.'

Similarly, Mairead (b.1953) who grew up in Dublin recalled her mother's experiences as an adoptee and the impact of silence in relation to information about her birth parents. She said:

She was actually adopted. And she thinks she was adopted by her aunt, but they would never actually tell her in those days, you know. [..] It's funny in those days people wouldn't, it was so a no-no to have a child out of wedlock, you know. I get emotional still, you know.

Mairead became tearful when recalling her mother's experiences, highlighting how such traumas can impact the next generation.

Many of the oral history respondents were also keen to stress the influence that the Catholic Church had on their parents' lives. Áine's (b.1949) mother, for example, had eight children. She reflected on how following the teachings of the Church on birth control had impacted on her parents' lives:

It was just, it was horrible and she was led and said by them whereas my dad wasn't. He wanted to use birth control, whatever, you know. Anyhow as we often said to him, 'You wouldn't give any of us back now would you Dad?', but anyhow. So, it wasn't the life that she would have wanted, and she really had a tough life you know, because she was a free spirit like myself, you know.

Lizzie (b.1946) from the rural west of Ireland recalled her mother's experience at losing a baby. She explained:

Now, as I said, for instance they were controlled by their religion and superstition really in a way because we had seven girls and a boy was born that died and that boy, my mother never saw him, you know that, she never, never saw him because at that time they never brought a dead baby back to the mother. And at that time they didn't, as well, they didn't bury them in the cemetery and they had no blessing, no nothing. Absolutely nothing.

As Lizzie explained, at that time, an unbaptised baby could not be buried in a Catholic Church graveyard. Children's burial grounds, or *cillíní*, were used as the resting places for unbaptised or stillborn children who the Church considered unsuitable for burial in consecrated ground.[14] Lizzie's father

---

[14] See: Eileen M. Murphy, 'Children's burial grounds in Ireland (Cillíní) and parental emotions toward infant death', *International Journal of Historical Archaeology*, 15:3 (September 2011), pp. 409–28.

went up, fair dues to him, in the night with another man and he buried it in the new graveyard. He buried his child in the graveyard and he told the canon at the time that he wouldn't touch it, that was his property.

Lizzie acknowledged that her father, a chemist, was 'educated and looked up to in the town so he could get away with it.' Nevertheless, this was a powerful act of resistance. The loss of this child had a significant impact on Lizzie's mother, one which she could never speak about. Lizzie's mother's silence around the death of her child illustrates the impact that this had on her, and in Lizzie's view, the Church's rules in relation to the burial of unbaptised children exacerbated the trauma.

Catholic Church teachings, in the view of oral history respondents, also helped to shape their parents' attitudes towards sex and birth control. Mark (b.1952) from a town in the south-east of the country, recalled his mother's attitudes after reading in the newspaper about a woman who died after complications from being on the pill. He recalled that 'she said "That's God's will, that shouldn't be what people are doing" and my mother is a wonderful person and very Christian but she bought all this bullshit, hook, line and sinker, you know.' Ellen (b.1949) felt that her mother

was very strict, very religious, yeah. And she said the only way you don't have children is don't have sex. That's it. And it did happen, because I know another woman, now she would have been a bit older than me all right. And I know that she got married, and she had two children, and then she moved into the spare room because she didn't want any more children. That was the end of that, that was her contraception. Which wasn't great, but, yeah it was like that.

Daithi (b.1950) felt that his 'family were clearly influenced by religion. I'd say my father and mother were almost anti-contraception. I would say they didn't have access to it at all. You know? And, and therefore, had 11 kids'. Rosie (b.1938) from the rural Midlands felt that for her parents, family planning 'just didn't exist and it wouldn't be discussed either. They'd be always against abortion, they'd always be against family planning because the Church said it wasn't right.' Yet, other interviewees recalled their parents having more progressive views. When Colette (b.1946) told her mother (b.1904) that she was expecting her third child, she could 'see her mouth tightening. She was saying "I thought nowadays…". You know, my mother was all in favour'. Colette recalled her mother on another occasion stating, "I can't understand what business it is of any priest or any bishop or having been … what goes on between a couple behind a closed bedroom door."

An analysis of individuals' accounts of their parents' experiences of and attitudes towards family planning suggests that many respondents viewed their parents as passive and lacking knowledge in this area. The general consensus was that men and women of fertile age in the early decades of the twentieth century simply adhered to Church teachings. However, it is clear from some of the accounts that some individuals were actively taking steps of resistance, such as through the use of the rhythm method in the case of Maria and Judith's mothers, or by rejection of societal norms in relation to the burial of unbaptised children, in the case of Lizzie's father. Mothers' trauma could, as Mairead and Helena's accounts show, have a distressing impact on their children. Moreover, there were evidently silences around issues such as family planning and sexuality which could suggest a reluctance from parents to discuss these issues with their children, but also perhaps illustrate that for survivors of trauma, 'the ability to speak is blocked completely'.[15]

1.2   'A Dangerous and Nefarious Trade'

Given the archival silences around family planning in the early twentieth century, newspaper accounts can provide evidence of how individuals may have obtained access to contraception. In the period prior to criminalisation, there is evidence to suggest that, as in other countries, there was a bustling trade in contraceptives in Ireland. In 1925, an article in radical Irish newspaper *Honesty* explained:

What are known as 'rubber goods' can also be had without difficulty, the only difference between Dublin and English cities in this respect is that here they are not publicly exposed for sale in attractive shop windows; but, nevertheless, the 'business' is proceeding and developing.[16]

According to Diarmaid Ferriter, further information emerged about the black market for contraceptives when there was debate about repealing the CLAA during the late 1960s and early 1970s.[17] For example, Keith Joseph Adams from Dublin wrote to the Taoiseach Jack Lynch in 1972 to provide information about his knowledge of the period from 1929 to the phasing out of contraceptives. Adams had worked as an assembler in the sundries department of a pharmaceutical wholesale company called May Roberts which dealt with medical goods.[18] Adams and his colleague

[15] Abrams, *Oral History Theory*, p. 184.
[16] 'Dublin's moral plague spots', *Honesty*, 28 February 1925, p. 9.
[17] Ferriter, *Occasions of Sin*, p. 194.
[18] Letter to Taoiseach Jack Lynch from Keith Joseph Adams, 29 August 1972. [NAI, 2003/ 16/453]. This case is also discussed in Mary E. Daly, 'Marriage, fertility and women's lives in twentieth-century Ireland (c. 1900–c. 1970)', *Women's History Review*, 15:4, (2006), pp. 571–85, on p. 574 and Ferriter, *Occasions of Sin*, p. 194.

T. Farquaharson had responsibility for the stock which consisted of items such as thermometers, finger stalls, trusses, sponges, and dressings. Revealingly, Adams wrote that he and Farquaharson had:

sole charge of a press with a yale lock, no body not even the Manager or Director had entry to this press. The reason: it was stocked with cigarettes, confections and razors and blades, also carried a stock consisting of 2 gross rubber preventives and we were responsible for the stock.

Adams explained that he and Farquahrson supplied 'about four or five chemists occasionally in the city', including Blakes on Fownes Street and Liffey Street, Rosenthal's chemist on Merrion Row, Hamilton Long on O'Connell Street and Price's chemist on Clare Street. In addition, every fortnight, a chemist called Blair in Cork city ordered a gross and on occasions a gross would be posted on an order to NAFFI or the Junior Army and Navy Stores to the fort on Spike Island and Fort Camden at Lough Swilly. Perhaps recognising the influence of religion on individuals' family planning practices, Adams provided a detailed breakdown of the religions of staff working in the company, stating that 'of that staff one third were Protestant and of that staff no one availed of contraceptives with the exception of one protestant occasionally. We would usually cover this up by putting through an order for a sponge'. Adams wrote that he 'never knew of anyone of the said staff to avail of preventitives [sic] in the case of R.C. [Roman Catholics] conscience makes cowards of us all and if one was involved in an accident it would be far better to have rosary beads in your pocket'.[19]

As Sandra McAvoy has shown, some members of the Committee on Evil Literature which met in 1926 alleged that books on contraception were readily available in Ireland; Fr. Devane asserted that Marie Stopes' booklet *A Letter to Working Mothers* could be obtained from Kearney's of Stephen Street in Dublin, while the Revd M. Quinlan claimed that both Eason's and Hanna's bookshops stocked publications on birth control.[20] Moreover, advertising materials submitted to the Committee on Evil Literature showed that individuals could obtain contraceptive devices by mail order, if not through local sources.[21] In 1924, for instance, an advertisement for 'surgical rubber goods and appliances' appeared in the *Kerry News* for Le Brasseur Surgical MFG Co. Ltd in Birmingham, with readers advised to call or write for a 76-page Illustrated Catalogue and

[19] Letter to Taoiseach Jack Lynch from Keith Joseph Adams, 29 August 1972 [NAI, 2003/16/453].
[20] McAvoy, 'Its effect on public morality', on p. 43.
[21] McAvoy, 'The regulation of sexuality', p. 255.

'Manual of Wisdom'.[22] Information on birth control was also accessible through advertisements in British newspapers and periodicals which could be bought in Ireland.[23] For example, in 1921 the *Freeman's Journal* carried an advertisement for George's Surgical Stores in London for 'rubber goods of every description for travelling, day and night use. Best quality only'. Readers could write for a catalogue sent under plain cover for free.[24] As well as this, Irish newspapers in the 1920s carried numerous advertisements for condoms, described as 'rubber goods'. Blake's Medical Stores in Middle Abbey Street, Dublin, for instance advertised 'surgical rubber goods, suspensory bandages, enemas, sprays, syringes, elastic stockings and all rubber appliances, Price list free' in the *Westmeath Independent* in 1919.[25] However, most Irish suppliers of condoms were not so blatant in advertising their wares.

Advertisements for Kearsley's 'Widow Welch's Female Pills', which were likely to have been abortifacients were carried by Irish newspapers in this period also.[26] In 1920, an advertisement for the pills from C & G Kearsley appeared in the *Sunday Independent* stating that they were 'prompt and reliable for ladies' and could be obtained from 'all Chemists, or Post free' from London.[27] The advertisement also appeared in the *Limerick Leader* in 1926, describing the product as 'a well-known remedy for female complaints'.[28] Following the introduction of the Censorship of Publications Act in 1929, however, such advertisements were banned in Irish newspapers, but Irish men and women would have been able to see such advertisements in British newspapers imported into the country.[29] Yet, as Mary E. Daly notes, a 1933 tax on imported newspapers and periodicals resulted in a drop of sales in newspapers, and 'threats to seize newspapers such as The Sunday Times in future if they carried advertisements for contraceptives or contraceptive advice soon resulted in their omission from the Irish edition'.[30]

In debates in the Seanad over the CLAA in 1935, some senators had warned that banning birth control would only serve to drive the

---

[22] 'Surgical rubber goods and appliances', *Kerry News*, 19 September 1924, p. 2. The advertisement was printed in a number of Irish newspapers during the 1920s, e.g., *Connacht Tribune*, 11 August 1923, p. 13.

[23] Pašeta, 'Censorship', p. 204.

[24] 'Surgical appliances', *Freeman's Journal*, 11 April 1921, p. 1.

[25] 'Medical', *Westmeath Independent*, 4 October 1919, p. 6.

[26] Greta Jones has highlighted an advertisement which appeared in the *Cork Free Press* in 1912. See Jones, 'Marie Stopes', p. 258.

[27] 'Female pills', *Sunday Independent*, 14 March 1920, p. 4.

[28] 'Hearsley's Original Widow Welch's Female Pills', *Limerick Leader*, 10 February 1926, p. 1.

[29] Jones, 'Marie Stopes', p. 258.

[30] Daly, 'Marriage, fertility and women's lives', p. 575.

contraceptive trade underground. Senator Kathleen Clarke stated that while she was in agreement with the Church and State in their condemnation of contraceptives she was 'totally opposed to the Government's method of trying to deal with this crying evil'. Based on her experiences of prohibition in the United States which drove individuals to engage in an illicit trade of alcohol, Clarke believed that:

> prohibition in connection with this will work out in much the same way. I believe you will drive the trading in and the use of these things into secret and illicit channels in which you will not be able to get after them. You will not alone bring the State and the laws of the State into contempt by inserting prohibition in this Bill, but you will bring the Church and religion into contempt.

In Clarke's view, the prohibition of contraception would drive individuals to rebel against the law – 'the fact that they are prohibited from doing it often creates a desire within them'. Clarke argued that the trade in contraceptives in the country was not so great as to warrant prohibition, instead, 'we want something else; we want something more human than laws'. Senator John Philip Bagwell agreed with Clarke, stating 'What you will do by this legislation is, you will drive underground what is now overground. Whether that is a good thing or not is a matter of opinion. Personally, I do not think it is.' Nevertheless, in spite of these objections, the bill was passed with Section 17 which related to contraception left intact.[31]

Indeed, Clarke and Bagwell's predictions were accurate. Following the introduction of the CLAA, there were a number of cases of prosecutions against individuals who were importing or selling contraceptives illegally, with significant penalties attached. In many of the cases, it is clear that the judge in question wanted to make an example of the convicted person and appeals to fines or prison sentences were rarely granted. Discussion of these cases reveals concerns about 'foreign' influences on the Irish State but also shed light on notions of respectability among the pharmacists who were keen to distance themselves from this trade. After the first three years of the Act, however, there appear to have been few cases brought to the courts, or at least, these were not reported in the press.

The first two cases under the CLAA which related to the import of contraceptives did not result in arrests or fines. Messrs. Henry Bell, a chemist firm based in Waterford, was the first to be accused of

---

[31] Criminal Law Amendment Bill, 1934, Report Stage. Seanad Éireann debate – Wednesday 6 February 1935, 19:15. https://www.oireachtas.ie/en/debates/debate/seanad/1935-02-06/4/

importation, or attempted importation of contraceptives under the CLAA. In August 1935, four containers of goods arrived in Waterford quays from British Drughouses Ltd and upon inspection by a Customs and Excise official, were found to contain 'one gross of contraceptives', namely quinine pessaries.[32] The Justice stated that there was not any suggestion that the chemists 'made trade of these things'.[33] During the case, Arthur Pitt, managing director and one of the owners of the firm, said that he had received prescriptions from doctors for the supply of the items mentioned and stated that the items were used as remedies for certain diseases and for cattle. He claimed that the item in question would be made up for doctors' prescriptions and not put in new boxes, and that over the last 17 years, he had never been asked for the item over the counter nor did his firm stock contraceptives.[34] The case was dismissed owing to extenuating circumstances under the Probation Act. In August 1936, Lep Transport Ltd. were fined £100 for the importation of contraceptives in October 1935.[35] In an appeal in November 1936, a representative for the company claimed that they did not know what the package contained and that they had nothing to gain by it except the 3s. 6d. importation fee. The goods were imported on behalf of Blake's Medical Stores, Fownes Street, Dublin. The Judge reversed the decision because he was not satisfied beyond all doubt that the company had known the contents of the package.[36] Interestingly, Blake's Medical Stores were not prosecuted for importing the contraceptives. Keith Joseph Adams' letter mentioned earlier suggests that this chemist had been involved in the contraceptive trade prior to the introduction of the CLAA.

In February 1936, a swoop by detectives and customs officers was made on chemist's shops in Dublin. A large number of chemists and depots were visited in a search for contraceptives, with the *Irish Press* reporting that 'a big haul was made in one instance'. An official from the Revenue Department stated that forbidden goods were usually seized at the port, but that recently, 'the goods were reaching this country in parcels, with declarations so vaguely or inaccurately worded, that they escaped detection'.[37] Pharmacists such as then vice-president of the Pharmaceutical Society of Ireland, James O'Rourke, were quick to distance themselves from the purveyors of such goods. O'Rourke had been

[32] *Birth Control News*, 14:8, April 1936, p. 87.   [33] *Ibid.*, p. 93.
[34] 'Prosecution against Waterford firm', *Munster Express*, 20 March 1936, p. 7.
[35] '£100 fine in prohibited goods case', *Irish Times*, 14 August 1936, p. 12.
[36] 'Decision reversed', *Irish Times*, 3 November 1936, p. 2.
[37] 'Police raid chemists', *Irish Press*, 26 February 1936, p. 1.

involved in debates around contraception since 1931, when, as Sandra McAvoy has shown, he dominated discussions over the 1931 Pharmacy Bill and 'pursued a ban on sales of contraceptives with an evangelizing zeal that suggested at least sympathy with the ideals of Catholic Action'.[38] Five years later, he was still heavily involved in these debates. In an interview with the *Irish Press*, he stated:

A number of establishments in Dublin use titles and signs which convey the impression that they are all chemists, and it is notorious that for many years these premises have been the main centres for the distribution of the prohibited wares. In addition, it is well known that a number of other centres, mainly under the control of persons of foreign extraction have been engaged in the traffic.[39]

O'Rourke's testimony here is significant as it highlights a trade in contraceptives that existed in Dublin but also points the blame firmly on 'foreign' persons. In addition, O'Rourke tried to affirm the respectability of Irish chemists in obeying the law, and explained that the journal of their society refused to publish 'advertisements of a certain character'. Similarly, F. E. Smith, secretary of the Chemists' Branch of the Irish Union of Distributive Workers and Clerks emphasised that his association 'has always looked with disfavour on the transaction of business of such a type, and we would like that there should be no misrepresentation, or misunderstanding in the minds of the public', suggesting that the practice was not widespread and was confined to a few isolated cases.[40] In March 1936, following the prosecution of Messrs Henry Bell Ltd. chemists in Waterford for the attempted importation of contraceptives, O'Rourke wrote to the *Irish Press* to condemn the statement by the counsel for the defence who said during the trial that the case 'was of great importance to pharmaceutical chemists in the Free State'. O'Rourke assured readers that the Pharmaceutical Society of Ireland 'which represents all creeds, has always taken up an attitude of the strongest opposition to this traffic'. O'Rourke emphasised that 'this traffic is of no concern whatever to Irish Pharmacy, with the exception of a few black sheep such as are to be found in every profession'.[41]

Examples continued to be made of individuals who were found to be dealing in the contraceptive trade. In July 1936, Charles Brocklebank, of the Medical Stores, Fownes Street, was accused of unlawfully keeping contraceptives for sale, harbouring prohibited goods and being involved in the importation of contraceptives.[42] In February 1936, following the interception of goods by Customs, Brocklebank's premises was searched

---

[38] McAvoy, 'Its effect on public morality', p. 48.
[39] 'Chemists and raids', *Irish Press*, 27 February 1936, p. 1.   [40] *Ibid.*
[41] 'Chemists and recent prosecution', *Irish Press*, 17 March 1936, p. 14.
[42] 'Jail sentence and fine', *Irish Times*, 4 July 1936, p. 4.

and a locker containing cartons which stored small tins of rubber sheaths, in addition to eight similar cartons containing the same type of contraceptives were found in the cellar of his premises.[43] Brocklebank argued that these goods had been at the premises for two years, that they were not for sale, and that the parcel intercepted by customs had been a plant by the director of another firm with whom he and his brother had worked before starting their own business.[44] Brocklebank was fined a total of £250 in addition to six months' imprisonment with hard labour, with additional fines to be allocated if he did not pay on time. In imposing the fines, Mr. Little 'said that he hoped that the putting into effect of that section of the Act would have a salutary effect and that they would not be troubled with such prosecutions in future'.[45] In an appeal in 1936, the fines were allowed to stand but the sentence of imprisonment was remitted because of the 'adverse effect' this would have on the defendant's future medical career.[46] Similarly, Christopher Grouse from Dublin, was prosecuted in May 1937 for illegally importing contraceptives. Grouse's residence was searched under warrant and two sealed envelopes containing fifteen contraceptives were found in a drawer in his living room. Grouse initially denied knowledge of these but then stated he had purchased them in Belfast and not declared them when passing through Dundalk on the train.[47] Grouse was fined £100.[48] In 1938, two men, Frank McCreech and Bernard Brennan, based at Bride Street, Dublin were fined £50 each for illegally possessing contraceptives for sale.[49]

Those engaging in the contraceptive trade tended to be denoted as outsiders. As Mosse has suggested in his work on sexuality, nationalism, and respectability in twentieth-century Europe, 'such outsiders were regarded as potential revolutionaries, as frightening as any who mounted the barricades'.[50] In the case of male abortionists in post-independence Ireland, particular attention was drawn to their non-Irish ethnicities and non-Christian religions in order to portray them as outsiders.[51] Jewish grocers and chemists appear to have been particularly targeted by the legislation on contraception. As Trisha Kessler's work has shown, in the early twentieth century, Jewish shopkeepers were viewed as 'unwanted competition amidst rising fears that large numbers of Jews were entering

---

[43] 'Criminal law charges', *Irish Times*, 3 July 1936, p. 13.
[44] 'Jail sentence and fine', p. 4.   [45] *Ibid.*
[46] 'Student's appeal', *Evening Echo*, 2 November 1936, p. 2.
[47] 'Dublin District Court', *Irish Times*, 25 May 1937, p. 2.
[48] '£100 fine for importing prohibited goods', *Irish Independent*, 1 June 1937, p. 10.
[49] 'Two men fined', *Irish Times*, 18 February 1938, p. 2.
[50] Mosse, *Nationalism and Sexuality*, p. 151.
[51] Delay and Liger, 'Bad mothers', pp. 297–300.

Ireland'. Rhetoric around Jewish migrants 'termed Irish economic practices as legitimate and those of Jews as illegitimate' and 'implicit in this narrative was the suggestion that Jewish economic ways were potentially harmful to the nation'.[52] The case of Ivor Kronn in 1936 exemplifies this rhetoric and shows how anti-Semitism could be invoked in court rulings. Kronn, a Jewish grocer was summoned in July 1936 on eight counts under the CLAA for unlawfully keeping contraceptives for sale, selling contraceptives and importing contraceptives.

The discovery of Kronn's involvement in the contraceptive trade had come about when a sixteen-year-old boy, Lewis Davies, was arrested in connection with another offence and was found to have two contraceptives in his possession. The police then visited Kronn's premises in Lower Clanbrassil Street and discovered a number of contraceptives there and at his private residence. In his evidence in the court case, Davies stated that at the end of January 1936, he had gone to Kronn's shop with his cousin David Woolfson. Woolfson had given Kronn one shilling and in return was given three contraceptives which were brought from a room behind the shop. Davies gave his cousin a shilling and obtained the contraceptives, giving his cousin one and retaining two, which the police found in his possession. Woolfson alleged that he did not want them for himself. Kronn explained during the case of the goods that 'married men used them to prevent children', to which Woolfson replied, 'I prefer the children'. Evidence was also produced to show that Kronn had ordered 14lb of contraceptives valued at £31 12s from the London Rubber Company which had arrived in Dublin in January that year. The closing statement of the Judge, Mr. Little, clearly highlighted Kronn's Jewish identity. In his conviction speech, Little stated that the defendant 'clearly belonged to a community among whom the Old Testament was revered'. Little further emphasised ideas of race suicide and the damaging impact of birth control on the nation, arguing 'the greatest danger in European civilisation to-day was the question of birth control'. Kronn received a significant sentence of £200 in fines (four fines of £50) as well as six months' imprisonment with hard labour. If the fines were not paid within 14 days, another 13 months would be added to his sentence.[53] An appeal by Kronn in October 1936 resulted in the fine being reduced to £100 but the prison sentence was to stand.[54] Kronn's case was not exceptional. Obstetrician and gynaecologist, Michael

---

[52] Trisha Oakley Kessler, 'In search of Jewish footprints in the West of Ireland', *Jewish Culture and History*, 19:2, pp. 191–208, on p. 195.
[53] 'Criminal law charge', *Irish Times*, 2 July 1936, p. 8.   [54] *Ibid.*, 23 October 1936, p. 14.

Solomons (1919–2007), recalled the prosecution of a Jewish chemist, Sam Rosenthal who ran The Modern Pharmacy, on Merrion Row:

As a young man I had listened to my father's indignant reaction when a local chemist, Rosenthal of Merrion Row, was visited by Gardaí, fined, and threatened with closure if he continued to sell condoms.[55]

Five summonses against Rosenthal in respect to goods prohibited under the CLAA were dismissed in July 1936.[56] And, in July 1936, a case was taken against David Glick, a chemist's assistant. A 1911 census record indicates that Glick was Jewish, his father Bernard Glick is listed in the census as a 'commercial merchant'.[57] Glick had been on holidays in August 1935 and had purchased three dozen contraceptives in London. Glick was found to have possession of two dozen of these in his home. He claimed that these were for his own private use and that he had not declared them at Customs as he did not think it was necessary. Glick was fined £100 for the importation of the contraceptives.[58] And, in 1938, Munshi Singh and Hazoor Singh, two men from Lahore, India, were sentenced to four months' imprisonment for the sale of contraceptives. Newspaper reports of the case evidently racialised the two men. An article in the *Connacht Tribune* began with the sentence 'Last week, two dusky visitors arrived in Castlebar, adorned with turbans and carrying suitcases which contained certain prohibited articles in violation of the Criminal Law Amendment Acts [sic]'.[59] Munsi Singh was described in one report in the *Irish Times* as 'a holy man in the Buddhist religion' while another report described the two men as 'two Hindoo gentlemen'.[60] According to the *Irish Independent*, the men had been in Castlebar for a period telling fortunes, selling silk fabrics and offering to buy old gold. Munshi Singh told the Justice that he had bought the contraceptives in a chemist shop in Dublin but had not sold any.[61] The Justice said that the men were 'engaged in a dangerous and nefarious trade forbidden by the law'.[62] In their appeal the following month, however, doubts were raised that the men had actually been selling the contraceptives as the articles were found in their pockets rather than in their pedlar's bag. Given that

[55] Michael Solomons, *Pro Life? The Irish Question* (Dublin: The Lilliput Press, 1992), p. 22.
[56] 'Criminal law charge', *Irish Times*, 2 July 1936, p. 8.
[57] Census record for Glick family, Wolseley Street, Dublin. http://www.census.nationalarchives.ie/pages/1911/Dublin/Merchant_s_Quay/Wolseley_St_/67552/
[58] 'Criminal law charges', *Irish Times*, 3 July 1936, p. 13.
[59] 'Two dusky visitors arrive', *Connacht Tribune*, 21 May 1938, p. 7.
[60] 'Irish news in brief', *Irish Times*, 13 May 1938, p. 3 and 'Circuit court, Tuesday', *Connacht Telegraph*, 18 June 1938, p. 4.
[61] 'Castlebar charge', *Irish Independent*, 13 May 1938, p. 5.
[62] 'Engaged in a nefarious trade', *Western People*, 21 May 1938, p. 4.

there was no evidence that the contraceptives were for sale, the convictions were reversed and the charges dismissed.[63]

Moving into the late 1930s and the 1940s, however, there appear to have been less prosecutions for the sale of contraceptives. There are three potential explanations for this: it is possible that the highly publicised prosecutions which took place in the 1930s had acted as an effective deterrent to individuals to avoid engagement with this trade. Alternatively, it may have been the case that the authorities were beginning to turn a blind eye to such crimes. A third potential explanation might be the impact that the Second World War had on black market networks.[64] As Claire Jones has noted, the war disrupted domestic contraceptive production in Britain as 'supplies of rubber, spring steel for use in rubber cervical caps and quinine for the manufacture of chemical pessaries were significantly reduced and grew worse as the war went on'.[65] Regardless, contraception continued to be viewed by opponents as a 'foreign', corrupting influence well into the twentieth century, as will be discussed in Chapter 8. As the next section will show through letters from Irish men and women to Marie Stopes, the legal restrictions on access to contraception as well as censorship on information relating to birth control had an important impact on individuals' reproductive choices.

1.3   Letters to Marie Stopes from Ireland

Marie Stopes (1880–1958) was a British palaeobotanist, birth control campaigner and eugenicist.[66] In 1918, following her disastrous first marriage, Stopes published her first book on sexual relationships, *Married Love,* which was followed up later that year by the book, *Wise Parenthood,* which contained advice on birth control.[67] She went on to establish birth control clinics in Britain and campaign for birth control through her publication *Birth Control News*. Stopes encouraged readers to write to her and a huge archive of thousands of letters from correspondents around the world as well as replies from Stopes is held at the Wellcome Collection. This includes letters from Irish correspondents.[68]

---

[63] 'Hindoos in Castlebar circuit court', *Connaught Telegraph,* 25 June 1938, p. 5.
[64] With thanks to Cara Delay for suggesting this possible explanation.
[65] Claire L. Jones, *The Business of Birth Control: Contraception and Commerce in Britain Before the Sexual Revolution* (Manchester University Press, 2020), p. 48.
[66] For a recent biography of Stopes see Clare Debenham, *Marie Stopes' Sexual Revolution and the Birth Control Movement* (Palgrave, 2018).
[67] Lesley Hall, *Sex, Gender and Social Change in Britain since 1880* (Palgrave, 2012), pp. 82–3.
[68] See: Lesley Hall, 'The archives of birth control in Britain', *Journal of the Society of Archivists,* 16:2, (1995), pp. 207–18.

A letter from a 24-year-old woman living in Sligo in 1918 is typical. The woman explained that she had been married for two years. She and her husband did not want to have a baby for six or eight months after they got married 'and we practised what you call coitus interruptus, and I was left stimulated and unsatisfied each time'. Their son was born 'by mutual wish' 16 months after their marriage. She explained to Stopes her frustration at the many books they had read from the 'Self and Sex series' by Vir Publishing, stating 'Some way it's the same thing in all of them, that no union should take place except for procreation only. Surely it strikes fear into a woman's heart every time coitus takes place that she will conceive when she doesn't want to.' The woman explained her rationale for trying to space her pregnancies using the withdrawal method and asked Stopes for advice about douching after intercourse:

Since the birth of our boy we have reasoned out the sexual act more than heretofore and my husband can usually contain himself to give me an orgasm before he reaches his climax on withdrawal – now he wishes me to ask you – whether its syringing with vinegar and water or just washing out immediately afterwards that will kill the sperm immediately – if he stayed in – we tried when we were married first quinine pessaries but they affected my head and I did not know how that was until I read your book. We don't want another baby too soon as we agree that when they come tripping one another they cannot be as healthy as if they were 2 or 3 years apart. Being married yourself you won't mind giving us your advice.[69]

This letter gives insights not only into this couple's family planning methods but suggests that the couple's rationale for spacing their pregnancies came from a belief that doing so would result in healthier children. Cormac Ó Gráda and Niall Duffy's study of letters sent by Irish and Scottish men and women to Marie Stopes has shown how 'the postal service provided a voice to some of those living far from the early family planning clinics, that it guaranteed confidentiality, and that it was inexpensive'.[70] Their analysis of the Irish letters suggests that men were more likely to write than women, and that women were more likely to write on birth control with men more likely to write on recurrent sexual problems. Irish letters were more likely to come from the northern counties which later became Northern Ireland and provide evidence of a demand for 'spacing' children.[71] In my analysis of the letters, I will

---

[69] [WC, PP/MCS/A/42]
[70] Cormac Ó Gráda and Niall Duffy, 'The fertility transition in Ireland and Scotland, c.1880–1930' in S.J. Connolly, R.A. Houston and R.J. Morris (eds.), *Conflict, Identity and Economic Development: Ireland and Scotland, 1600–1939* (Preston: Carnegie Publishing, 1995), pp. 89–102, on p. 98.
[71] *Ibid.*, p. 99.

focus on those which requested advice on birth control. Of course, as Ó Gráda and Duffy have pointed out, these letters were primarily coming from middle-class and literate men and women.[72] Nevertheless, for an era where there is such limited archival evidence of personal experiences of family planning, and without the opportunity to interview men and women who lived in this period, they are an important source for under-standing the problems faced by men and women living under legislative restrictions to access in the early twentieth century.

Evidence from the letters suggests that Irish men and women struggled to gain access to information on birth control and Stopes' publications even in the period prior to the introduction of the 1929 Censorship Act. An Irish man, writing to Stopes in 1918 stated:

As a young husband I have been intensely interested in your book 'Married Love'. At the same time I do not think you realise how difficult it is for the ordinary man to get any reliable information as to the safest means to control birth. If you can inform me, or put me in the way of obtaining information as to the approved anti-conceptional methods I shall be deeply grateful.[73]

Similarly, a woman from Dublin writing to Stopes in April 1922 explained that she had tried to obtain one of Stopes' books but had not succeeded. She wrote 'I am a married woman with four young children and I am very keenly interested in your subjects' and asked if Stopes could send her a copy or tell her where to obtain one. Stopes' secretary replied with details of her book *Wise Parenthood* 'which gives full details concerning Birth Control. If you have any difficulty in obtaining these locally (as you probably will) I should advise you to apply direct to the publishers'.[74]

It is likely that letters addressed to Stopes from Irish men and women may have been detected by customs officials. A man writing to her from Dublin in 1933 for instance addressed his letter to Stopes' married name 'as you are not popular in official circles here and letters might be opened for inspection'.[75] In reply to a man who wrote to her in 1935 to com-mend her work on contraception and ask about obtaining more of her publications, Stopes replied:

I am glad to have an interested reader in your country. You can get any of my books sent in plain envelopes from the Society which I founded and which is running in London. The two of which I enclose slips would probably interest you. The difficulty, however, may be that your Customs people may stop them. If you don't mind the trouble I should very much like to know how you managed to get hold of 'Contraception'. Is it permitted? Did you buy it from an ordinary

[72] *Ibid.*, p. 98.   [73] [WC, PP/MCS/A/86].   [74] [WC, PP/MCS/A/229].
[75] [WC, PP/MCS/A/13].

bookseller? Because as you know the Roman Catholics have been very active in interfering with the sale of my books.[76]

Information on Stopes' activities and publications appear to have been disseminated through the British press in Ireland in this period and evidence from the letters suggests that Stopes' ideas were gaining traction among a number of men and women. Writing in November 1918, a woman from Wexford explained that she had read an article by Stopes in the *Sunday Chronicle*, an English newspaper. The woman wrote that she had lost two children, one had been stillborn and the other had died as a result of spina-bifida. She wrote that because of this experience, she and her husband did not wish to have any more children and wanted advice on a remedy or where she could get more information, stating 'I have sought for some very persistently but without hope and should be ever obliged if you could throw some light on this matter'. The woman clearly felt embarrassed about writing to Stopes for advice, mentioning 'this is a subject one does not like approaching and as a consequence, I have kept putting the matter off ever since I read and re-read your article'.[77]

Similarly, a man living in Queen's County (later Laois), and also a reader of the *Sunday Chronicle*, wrote to Stopes in 1921 to ask advice on birth control. He and his wife had four children and wanted to avoid having any more. His wife was 'not at all strong owing to one of her kidneys having fallen after our last baby and our Dr said it would be better if she had no more children. But he did not tell us how to prevent them'. The man also explained that his salary as a lawyer's clerk was not sufficient enough to provide all they required in addition to further expenses from another child. He asked Stopes 'would you be so kind as to tell us how we may prevent a further increase in our family, or if it is possible (apart from abstinence from intercourse) without injury to my health, or further damage to my wife's. I am sure you can understand how easier it is for us to ask you, a stranger, these questions, than to approach our local Dr or any other friend in the matter'.[78] The man's comments about his doctor highlight the difficult dilemma that individuals were placed in without proper access to effective birth control as well as illustrating a broader reluctance from members of the medical profession to provide advice. In her reply, Stopes sent details of her publications which advised on different methods of birth control and suggested the man should write directly to the publisher to obtain them. She also wrote 'I know that Ireland is a difficult country, and you may not be able to obtain from your local chemist the things necessary. If this is so, write direct to Messrs.

---

[76] [WC, PP/MCS/A/68].   [77] [WC, PP/MSC/A/2].   [78] [WC, PP/MSC/A/210].

E. Lambert & Son, Manufacturing Chemists, 60, Queen's Road, Dalston, London.'[79] A woman from Cork writing to Stopes in 1923 explained that she had followed Stopes' case in the *Daily Mail* and that she was 'very much in favour of your views on the "Birth Control" & of the rise of contraceptives'. The woman had two sons, one aged 2 years and 2 months and one aged 1 year old. She asked Stopes to forward on one or two of her books stating that 'several of my friends, including of course myself, would very much like to possess your worthy books which are unfortunately unobtainable here'.[80] Information on Stopes' books continued to be disseminated through the British press in Ireland into the 1930s. A married man from Waterford wrote to her in 1937 stating he had seen her books advertised in the *Daily Mirror* and asked if she would send him a booklet describing the books available for sale.[81]

Stopes was well aware of the difficulties that Irish men and women had in accessing her texts and contraceptives more generally. In 1929, Miss A, a woman living in Cardiff, wrote to Stopes to say that she was planning to leave Cardiff to be married and that she and her husband would be living in Co. Wicklow. Miss A asked:

I am anxious to know if you could tell me whether birth control appliances are available anywhere in Dublin and if so, where. There are I know the very strongest prejudices against anything of this kind throughout Ireland, and also I believe a legislation relative thereto which differs from our own. At present I only know Ireland very slightly, but I gather that throughout the country neither ignorance nor prejudice in such matters are confined to the peasant classes.[82]

Stopes replied promptly, advising the woman to be fitted with a cap at her clinic, or to visit the nurses at the travelling clinic in Wales before her marriage. She further explained:

As regards your question about Ireland, I do not know whether contraceptives can be purchased there, I fancy they are criminal in Ireland. You should take a supply with you and get your further supplies by post, but whether they will reach you I cannot tell at all.[83]

In her responses to letters asking for information on contraception, Stopes tended to advise respondents to visit one of her English clinics, however, for many respondents, this would have been financially prohibitive. For instance, in reply to a woman from Dublin writing in 1922, Stopes suggested that she should come to London to be personally fitted

---

[79] [WL, PP/MSC/A/210].   [80] [WC, PP/MCS/A/58].   [81] [WC, PP/MCS/A/88].
[82] [WC, PP/MCS/A/10].   [83] [WC, PP/MCS/A/10].

with a cap as 'I know of no-one in Ireland who could help you with this, and it is very important that the cap should fit properly'.[84]

Some of the letters received by Stopes were very personal in nature and highlight the fear and anguish experienced by many women without lack of access to contraception or information about family planning.

A letter from a woman living in Cork writing in 1923 highlighted the impact of Catholic teachings against contraception:

> Dear Dr. Stopes, my case is like this: my husband is Catholic, he will not prevent and I am not strong enough to keep having a child. I married young 20 yrs, and I have just started on the road for my fifth child, my husband is what one would call eccentric, he is 12 yrs my senior, he is always studying, and must keep suffering and if I complain he says I am always grumbling, my means will not allow of my getting help, when I was courting he gave me the idea that I would be somebody quite comfortably off, I was only 17 yrs when he came over to Ireland and three years later I came across and married him, I am away from all my people and old friends and I cannot stand the strain of continuously being sick, no man is worth it I think I have as much as I can manage with four young children, the oldest is 7 years. Look at all the yrs before me and if I do not learn of something to prevent me from being all the time in bad health, I am afraid life would be a burden, I am splendid in health until I fall, then my misery starts.[85]

The woman explained that she was over two months pregnant and asked Stopes for advice on how to procure an abortion:

> there is I have heard a bottle called 'Black Mixture' I have no way of getting it because the nurse that would send it is travelling the world. I suddenly thought of you and I knew if anyone would help you would, I do not mind what your fee is, if only I was in London, that is my home, I could explain my life to you, it has been one big disappointment and only that I have all the children I wouldn't stay here.[86]

Cara Delay's work on illegal abortion has suggested that in Ireland, physical harm methods such as the consumption of herbs, purgatives, and pills was a more common means for women to procure an abortion.[87] The woman stated in her letter that she had already taken 'quantities of pills but I am so strong that it was no use, I feel sure the black mixture would put me right'. In her view 'when God laid down the laws of nature he never meant us to be human incubators, nature is there, and so is our intelligence to know what our strength can stand, one is just as wrong to abuse as the other, my husband is peculiar on that point that I am just like a machine for his use'. Moreover, she expressed her difficulties in obtaining abortifacients, stating 'Cork is such an old-fashioned goody-goody place

---

[84] [WC, PP/MCS/A/167].   [85] [WC, PP/MCS/A/163].   [86] [WC, PP/MCS/A/163].
[87] Delay, 'Pills, potions, and purgatives'.

that they would not sell you what you wanted if they thought it was for a wrong purpose. I do not want to be free for getting around or to be going with other men, all I want is to be and keep in good health to make my household happy and to be able to do my duties, which one cannot do if one is feeling ill'.[88]

No reply was included with the letter from Stopes, however, she was staunchly anti-abortion so it is possible that she simply did not reply to the request.

Recognising the demand for family planning services on the island of Ireland, in 1936, a year after the introduction of the CLAA, Marie Stopes opened her Mothers' Clinic at 103, The Mount, Belfast, which was in a working-class district of the city. An article in the *Birth Control News* in September 1936 announced the establishment of the clinic to 'provide gynaecological and birth-control help for poor Irish mothers' and requested contributors from supporters of the Society for Constructive Birth Control (CBC) 'for this most urgently needed help for Irish motherhood'.[89] While Stopes recognised that situating the clinic in Ulster meant that 'this source of help will not be so available to those in the Irish Free State as it should be', there was the expectation that the Belfast clinic would 'serve the whole geographic country of Ireland' and that women could travel by bus or train between Dublin and Ulster.[90] Writing to an Irish supporter from Donegal in 1937, Stopes explained that while the clinic was living on a 'very hand-to-mouth existence', she noted 'people are coming up from Dublin and elsewhere to the Belfast clinic now.'[91] The expectation was that the clinic would result in 'more healthy and happy Irish boys and girls, and fewer miserable and tormented lives'.[92] As Greta Jones has shown, the clinic advised married women on birth control as well as helping with infertility. Consultations were free but the patient had to pay for the cost of appliances.[93] Reflecting on a year of work in 1937, Stopes believed that the Belfast clinic had been 'of great help, I believe, to the country of Ireland as a whole, not only to that city'.[94] The clinic did not have political support and faced opposition from the Catholic Church in Belfast, while few medical men were prepared to come out in support of birth control.[95] As Jones has shown, 'many of the women already knew of or practised some form of fertility control prior to attending the Mothers'

---

[88] [WC, PP/MCS/A/163].
[89] 'In Ireland', *Birth Control News*, September 1936, 15:4, p. 37.
[90] 'Ireland', *Birth Control News*, November 1936, 15:6, p. 63.
[91] [WC, PP/MCS/A/A116]
[92] 'Ireland', *Birth Control News*, November 1936, 15:6, p. 63.
[93] Jones, 'Marie Stopes', p. 265.
[94] 'Behind the scenes in the year's work', *Birth Control News*, December 1937, 14:5, p. 53.
[95] Jones, 'Marie Stopes', p. 268.

Clinic' with practices including abortion, breastfeeding, abstinence, coitus interruptus, sponges and condoms.[96] Attendance at the clinic was usually motivated by the ineffectiveness of these methods.[97]

Testimony from a nurse at the Belfast Clinic published in *Birth Control News* in 1937 outlined the problems facing women in the Irish Free State:

A patient came up from Dublin to be fitted. She says it is dreadful in the Free State now, for it is impossible to get any kind of preventive. They had always, up to recently, been able to get X's pessaries from the chemists, but now it is a criminal offence for chemists to stock them. She thinks it is so unfair that the Roman Church can force its will on the Protestants also. Her neighbour, who is a Catholic, is to have her seventeenth child in March. This woman is full of T.B., half her children have died and those who are living are tubercular, and yet the Priest tells her it is right for her to go on bearing a child every year.[98]

The nurse's testimony highlights the problems faced by Protestant women who were subject to legal barriers of access to contraception but also the challenges faced by Catholic women who wanted to adhere to Church teachings. Her testimony also suggests the power of the local priest in encouraging women to have large families, a theme which persisted well into the twentieth century as Chapter 5 will show. Another report on the clinic described how an unmarried Catholic woman had come to the Belfast clinic asking for an abortion, telling the nurse 'that she had had three abortions in 1936 produced by a chemist in Dublin to whom she had paid in all £20.' The chemist apparently had to leave Dublin and the woman came to Belfast having heard there was a birth control clinic there. However, as the report stated 'she had a totally wrong idea of the work of the Clinic and went away much disappointed that birth control clinics disapprove of abortion'.[99] Reflecting on this particular case, Stopes wrote that she believed the significant opposition from the Catholic Church was because 'sound and wholesome control of conception places motherhood in a woman's own hands. But if she is kept ignorant and driven to abortion or producing unhealthy infants in her misery, then she is at the mercy of someone who has to be paid, be it priest or doctor'.[100]

Stopes' replies to women who wrote to her were often empathetic. Writing to Stopes in 1943, a woman from Kilkenny explained that she had read Stopes' letter in the *New Review* and wondered 'if you would ever be so terribly kind as to help me? You said in your letter that strangers sometimes write to you so please don't think it is awful cheek on my part'. The woman wrote that she had had four children 'and two

---

[96] *Ibid.*, p. 269.   [97] *Ibid.*, p. 269.
[98] 'From our Belfast clinic', *Birth Control News*, March 1937, 15:10, p. 111.
[99] 'No free state clinics', *Birth Control News*, May 1937, 15:12, p. 145.
[100] 'Behind the scenes in the year's work', *Birth Control News*, December 1937, 14:5, p. 53.

mishaps' in eight years and that the 'worry and fear' about subsequent pregnancies 'is absolutely ruining my whole life, I even have nightmares about it, day & night the dread of it haunts me. So will you please send me some instructions? I shall be forever grateful to you'. The woman stated that she had asked doctors, nurses and chemists for advice 'but no good, and of course in this country one can't buy things'.[101] In her reply, Stopes apologised that she could not send her correspondent printed instructions as 'anything we send is opened and destroyed' but advised the woman 'strongly to go personally over the border to 103, The Mount, Belfast, where my representative will give you such help as I would give myself, without any charge'.[102] The clinic closed in 1947 as Stopes' expenses increased as a result of the war, however, during its existence it saw 3,000–4,000 first-time patients.[103]

Letters to Stopes were sometimes published in *Birth Control News* in order to highlight the need and demand for birth control services in Ireland. A letter from a woman from Dublin published in 1937 requesting information on how to procure an abortion highlighted the impact of a lack of information on contraception. The woman explained that her doctor had referred her to contact Stopes and that she had '3 other children eldest aged 5 besides an infant 6 weeks old which I am nursing. I went under a serious operation last July and I took fits at the birth of the present infant which almost cost me my life. I was also in danger of fits in the previous children owing to a kidney trouble so that I dread a repetition'.[104] In an editor's note in the publication, it was stated that Dr. Stopes 'will not and cannot answer such letters. To do so in a manner approved by the writer would be a criminal offence. The letter itself is an incitement, and the writer of it is guilty of a criminal offence'.[105] Another letter published in the same issue from Mrs. C.C., also based in Dublin, explained that she had recently had a stillbirth at eight months. She stated 'This was my first baby and I was very much disappointed because I am very fond of children and long for one of my own, but as I am anaemic at present my husband and I do not want to start another baby till I am fully recovered. I wonder if you could help me with some safe form of birth control as I do not wish the same thing to occur again. Hoping you will understand and help me'.[106] What is interesting about some of these accounts is that these Irish women were framing their desire for effective birth control in terms of concerns about the impact that having subsequent children would have on their health.

---

[101] [WC, PP/MCS/A/88]   [102] [WC, PP/MCS/A/88]
[103] Jones, 'Marie Stopes', pp. 270–1.
[104] 'Correspondence', *Birth Control News*, June 1937, 16:1, p. 11.   [105] *Ibid.*
[106] *Ibid.*

It is evident that there was an appetite for birth control among some men and women in Ireland and support for Stopes' ideas. The owner of a bookshop and newsagent in Dublin contacted Stopes in 1926 to alert her to the sitting of the Committee on Evil Literature stating, 'all literature relating to Birth Control is being attacked and the Committee is being asked to exclude it and advertisements relating to it from the Free State'. Stopes and the man entered into correspondence, and she asked him to send her any information relating to the Committee such as reports or newspaper accounts of its sittings. In a subsequent letter to the man, she stated 'In view of the fact that I do not want your letter opened, would you mind addressing it not to me personally, but to Mr. Bagge at the above address, as I have a feeling that my name on the envelope will probably lead to it being opened'.[107]

There were also Irish individuals who agreed with Stopes' work in England and were evidently interested in introducing her ideas to Ireland. One woman, writing to Stopes in 1937 asked whether it would be possible for Stopes to meet her and her sister 'with reference to introducing to Ireland the rights you have conferred on poor women here.'[108] It is unclear whether Stopes and the woman met, although subsequent correspondence in 1940 suggests they did. In another letter from 1940, the woman wrote:

As I explained I do not entirely see eye to eye with you as regards method. However, our general purpose of giving more health and happiness to women and children is the same. This probably sounds impatient coming from an unknown individual like myself. However, your propaganda had much to do with my becoming a nationalist and starting four years ago to fit myself to eventually set up a 'Preparation for Marriage' centre in Dublin. For this I gave up my private experimental school for small children which was the apple of my eye.[109]

Writing again the same year, she thanked Stopes for meeting her and that it would 'probably be three or four years before I get my ideas going'.[110] It is unclear if the woman did go on to formalise her plans but her correspondence, and that of other members of the public in Ireland who wrote to Stopes, suggests there was support for her ideas and that her publications were reaching some men and women.

Irish doctors were also limited in access to contraceptive devices and advice. The Marie Stopes archive contains a number of letters from Irish doctors who wrote to Stopes for information. Writing in 1926, a Monaghan doctor explained that 'Being a constant reader of John Bull I notice you strongly advise the use of contraceptives in suitable cases.

---

[107] [WC, PP/MCS/A/76].   [108] [WC, PP/MCS/A/71].   [109] [WC, PP/MCS/A/71].
[110] [WC, PP/MCS/A/71].

I have a patient who really needs something in that way.'[111] Similarly, a female doctor writing from Cork in 1923 asked Stopes where a patient might obtain 'the cap which you recommend for Birth Control'.[112] A Dublin specialist in gynaecology and obstetrics wrote to Stopes in 1936 to ask if it might be possible to obtain the 'composition of the greasy solubles which you recommend for use with the caps and dia- phragms'. He remarked that several of his patients used these but were finding that 'owing to the increased vigilance of the Customs authorities in this country they are being held up in transit. If I could give them the necessary prescription they could be made up at the local chemists as an ordinary preparation'.[113] Stopes replied stating that the matter had been placed before their committee and that they regretted that they could not provide the formula because 'when such requests in former days have been acceded to, such unfortunate results have accrued' with commer- cial firms advertising 'our President's name in a manner most detrimen- tal to her and to our Society'. However, they advised that there would soon be a clinic opening in Belfast where pessaries and other contracep- tives could be obtained with more ease.[114]

Moving into the 1950s, some individuals received birth control advice and contraceptives by post from the Family Planning Association in London. As Greta Jones notes, in the 1950s the FPA received requests for information from Ireland and 'succeeded in sending information to the Republic' by posting parcels out in plain packing and addressing them by hand.[115] In April 1953, for example, Dublin-based doctor Marie Hadden wrote to the FPA to ask if they had 'any publications suitable to give to a young man and woman contemplating early marriage who are anxious to plan their family to suit their programme of careers for both?' Recognising that a reply from the FPA could be intercepted, Hadden asked them to reply 'under plain cover because – as you are no doubt aware – your society's work is not very well received in this country at present'.[116] Indeed, publications sent by the FPA to individuals were intercepted by Customs and Excise. A surviving 1954 letter from the Office of the Revenue Commissioners at Dublin Castle to the FPA, indicates that they were returning a copy of the prohibited book *Any Wife or Any Husband* which the FPA had addressed to a man based in Cork.[117] The FPA secretary replied to this letter expressing 'our extreme

---

[111] [WC, PP/MCS/A/271].   [112] *Ibid.*   [113] [WC, PP/MCS/A/261].
[114] [WC, PP/MCS/A/261].   [115] Jones, 'Marie Stopes', p. 270.
[116] Letter from Dr. Marie A. Hadden to the FPA, 28 April 1953. [WC, A21/7].
[117] Letter from Office of the Revenue Commissioners to the FPA, 12 November 1954. [WC, A21/7].

surprise that such a book should be prohibited, as it is published for the purpose of helping those couples who are experiencing difficulties in the marriage relationship.'[118]

Other individuals obtained contraceptives directly from England. Máirin Johnston (b.1931) a member of the Irish Women's Liberation Movement, recalled in an oral history interview that she and her then husband obtained condoms by post from England:

I don't know what they were called then, but we used to call them French letters. We didn't call them anything else.

Johnston remembered seeing an advertisement that said:

'Rubber goods, sent under plain cover.' It didn't say what they were, just 'rubber goods sent under plain cover' and there was a box number, and you sent your cheque or whatever, in an envelope and you sent it off to this box, and back came the rubber goods. They were like tubes of a bicycle, they were so thick.

Similarly, Dermot Hourihane (1933–2020), a founder member of the Fertility Guidance Company, also explained in an oral history interview that he obtained condoms by mail order from the FPA in England. However, for the majority of individuals, without the knowledge of these organisations, options for family planning were limited to natural methods.

1.4   Conclusion

As this chapter has shown, in early twentieth-century Ireland, contraception was framed as a British or European negative influence. Pharmacists distanced themselves from the illegal sale of contraceptives owing to a lack of respectability with this association. Moreover, those who were engaged in the contraceptive trade were, like abortionists, othered as a result of their race or religion, in an attempt to suggest that birth control was not an Irish or indeed Catholic practice in the newly established Irish Free State. While the personal family planning experiences of individuals born in the early twentieth century are difficult to uncover, oral history interviews with individuals about their parents' experiences illustrate the impact of Church and State regulation on 'ordinary' people's lives. They also reveal interesting things about common perceptions of the experiences of older Irish generations and how younger generations situate their own experiences in contrast to these. Moreover, it is clear that silences reveal both a reluctance on behalf of parents to discuss these

---

[118] Letter from FPA to the Revenue Commissioners, Dublin Castle, 26 November 1954. [WC, A21/7].

issues with their children but could also point to the impact of trauma. Letters to Marie Stopes and the experiences of individuals detailed in her publication *Birth Control News* suggests that there was an appetite in Ireland for information on effective methods of family planning. This, combined with evidence of the black market in Ireland suggests that some individuals were at least attempting to resist Church and State authority, even if they were ultimately unsuccessful.

2   Sexual Knowledge and Morality from
       the 1940s to the 1970s

In April, 1971, the following letter appeared in Angela Macnamara's problem page in *Woman's Way* magazine:

We are two girls of fourteen. Two boys treated us very badly at a party and we and they lost control of ourselves. We didn't know what they were doing as our mothers never told us anything about life. Could they have done anything dangerous? Would it be wise for us to talk to a priest about what happened?[1]

Letters such as this one, which were not uncommon, are indicative of the confusion and ignorance among many about sexual health. They suggest that there were problems with modes of communication and that many young Irish men and women were not being taught anything by their parents about reproduction. Moreover, the fact that the two girls asked Macnamara if they should go and talk to a priest about the issue highlights the place of the priest as a regulator of morals within the community. This account is not unusual either; one oral history respondent, Ellen (b.1949) recalled a friend going to her priest for confession after she experienced a sexual assault, and her period was late:

She didn't tell me exactly what he did, but her period was late, and she thought that she was pregnant. So, she went to confession, and she told the priest, and the priest told her she couldn't be pregnant with what happened. But she hadn't told me, but she had, whatever, she had told him. She was about 24 at the time and she didn't even realise whether she could be pregnant or not, by whatever he had done, you know?

Knowledge of reproduction and contraception was limited for many Irish men and women growing up for much of the twentieth century, and the Irish State systematically failed to provide any formal sex education despite calls for it from the early twentieth century. The Carrigan Committee, which met between 1930 and 1931, effectively ignored the recommendations of a number of female witnesses, such as Dr. Dorothy

---

[1] 'Angela Macnamara's help page', *Woman's Way*, 9 April 1971, p. 52.

Stopford Price and Dr. Delia Moclair Horne who suggested that there was a strong need to provide young women and girls with sex education, and particularly for young women affected by poverty or institutional-isation.[2] As James M. Smith has shown, the Carrigan Report evaded this testimony, effectively suppressing calls for formal sex education, with echoes of this concealment to be found 'in the Catholic hierarchy's resistance to pre- and postnatal care in debates surrounding the "Mother and Child" scheme (1951) and, more recently, in attempts to thwart the "Stay Safe" program (1993)'.[3] Mandatory sex education was not introduced into Irish schools until 1997 with the establishment of the Relationships and Sexuality Programme.[4]

The attitudes and legislative initiatives of the Irish government in the 1920s and 1930s cast a long shadow over the rest of the twentieth century. Lack of access to contraception combined with the power of Catholic teaching meant that there was considerable fear around pre-marital sex, which also influenced how sex education was disseminated in the period with a focus on morality rather than physiology. As Tom Inglis has shown, the Church helped to create and maintain understand-ings of what constituted 'good moral behaviour'.[5] Pregnancy outside of marriage was seen as inherently shameful. Many of the respondents did not engage in sex before marriage because the fear of pregnancy and ensuing shame that would be brought on their families was too great. In the absence of formal sex education, young men and women were provided with moral codes regarding sexual activity, which were in turn policed by families and communities. Ultimately, this chapter shows how attitudes to sex in the period were shrouded in a culture of fear which was perpetuated by Catholic Church teachings. Yet, at the same time, women's magazines and television programmes such as The Late Late Show attempted to push against these boundaries through more open discussion of matters relating to sex and family planning.

2.1   Lack of Sexual Knowledge

The majority of oral history interviewees emphasised a lack of sex educa-tion, either from their schools or from their parents. Imelda (b.1935)

---

[2] James M. Smith, *Ireland's Magdalen Laundries and the Nation's Architecture of Containment* (University of Notre Dame Press, 2007), p. 15.
[3] *Ibid.*
[4] Ann Nolan, 'The transformation of school-based sex education policy in the context of AIDS in Ireland', *Irish Educational Studies*, 37:3, (2018), pp. 295–309.
[5] Tom Inglis, *Moral Monopoly: The Catholic Church in Modern Irish Society* (Dublin: Gill and Macmillan, 1987), p. 216.

who grew up in Dublin, explained, 'To be honest with you, we didn't know where a baby or anything came from. We had to find out for ourselves and everything. We were taught from one another and all like that'. Sarah (b.1947) from the north of the country, told me, 'Nobody talked about it at school, or at home. You had to learn the hard way'. Con (b.1940) also explained that 'everything was left up to yourself to figure out or find out you know'. In her study of female sexuality in childhood in 1930s and 1940s Dublin, Hazel Lyder reported similar findings and has suggested that in relation to sex education, 'parents, lacking sufficient knowledge and language and labouring under the obligation of the sexual taboo, adhered to a code of silence'.[6] Sex education at secondary schools was non-existent for the majority of participants. Eibhlin (b.1943) recalled that the nuns in her school 'certainly didn't say as much, only, "Stay away from boys"'. Máire Leane's study, which entailed oral history interviews with 21 Irish women born between 1914 and 1955, also found that a lack of concrete knowledge about the facts of life was reported by 19 of her 21 interviewees.[7] Lack of sexual knowledge was not a uniquely Irish feature of this period. In her oral history study of family planning practices in Switzerland (1955–1970), Caroline Rusterholz reported that the majority of her participants stated that contraception and sexuality were taboo topics within their families and that they lacked knowledge of these issues during their childhood and adolescence.[8] Oral history testimony is supported by contemporary sources. Michael Solomons, wrote in 1983 about his work as a gynaecologist at Mercer's Hospital in the 1960s, stating 'Both women and men were suffering due to a lack of basic knowledge about sex. It became clear to me that more people were interested in sex than knew anything about it'.[9] Similarly, in her report for the Social Work Department of the Rotunda Hospital, Dublin in 1966, Eleanor Holmes wrote that 'proper sex education, too, has been almost entirely lacking in all strata of society'.[10]

As Carole Holohan has shown, during the 1960s, sexual themes and issues such as contraception and divorce became an increasingly visible part of popular culture as a result of imported television programmes and popular music.[11] In 1962 *Hibernia* magazine discussed the issue of sex education and the need for an educational programme which reflected the needs of the time as well as moral principles. Meanwhile, some

---

[6] Lyder, 'Silence and secrecy', p. 81.   [7] Leane, 'Embodied sexualities', p. 32.
[8] Rusterholz, 'Reproductive behavior', p. 54.   [9] Solomons, *Pro-Life?* p. 18.
[10] *Clinical Report of the Routnda Hospital, 1st January 1966 to 31st December 1966*, p. 68.
[11] Carole Holohan, *Reframing Irish Youth in the Sixties*, (Liverpool University Press, 2018), p. 129.

journalists accused the Catholic Church of pastoral neglect of young people.[12] Eleven years earlier, J. McCarthy, writing in the *Irish Theological Quarterly* in April 1951, suggested that responsibility for the sexual instruction of young people should lie with their parents, and that a 'due and properly ordered physiological education, which is integrated into and animated by the Catholic concept of marriage, is possible and commendable'.[13] Writing in the October issue, James A. Cleary discussed the changes in Irish society which meant that sex education was more needed than before. Cleary drew on his experience preaching Missions and Retreats in Ireland and other countries over thirty years. He highlighted the issue of women entering the workplace or university after leaving school and encountering men in these settings.[14] Cleary also believed that young women's curiosity was being roused at university 'where the very literature they must read contains numerous allusions to ordinary sex-matters'.[15] Moreover, he drew attention to the problem of films depicting scenes of a sexual nature in cinemas as well as the importation of 'sex-books and sexual magazines from England and America', dance-halls and company-keeping.[16] By the 1950s, dancehalls and cinema provided young people with the opportunity to participate in teenage culture and interact with peers.[17] Dances were the most common meeting place for young couples coming of age in the 1950s and 1960s. Dances were traditionally not held on Saturday nights so that young men and women would still be able to go to Mass on Sundays, and ballrooms were closed for the forty days of Lent, a practice which survived in rural areas well into the 1960s.[18]

James Cleary believed that sex instruction was particularly important for Irish girls, drawing attention to the fact that Irish women had to wait longer for marriage, with the average age of marriage being twenty-nine. The late age of marriage at this time, particularly in rural Ireland, has been explained by scholars such as Mary E. Daly and others as being a result of 'large families, the absence of any regulation governing succession, and the lack of alternative occupations' which ultimately 'gave parents considerable control over land inheritance and consequently over marriage'. In addition, for men and women who had the responsibility of

---

[12] Holohan, *Reframing Irish Youth*, pp. 129–30.

[13] J. McCarthy, 'Preparation for marriage', *Irish Theological Quarterly*, 18:2, (1 April 1951), pp. 189–91 on pp. 190–91.

[14] James A. Cleary, 'Is sex instruction needed in Ireland?', *Irish Theological Quarterly*, (1 October 1951), p. 373.

[15] *Ibid.*, pp. 373–4.   [16] *Ibid.*, p. 378.

[17] Eleanor O'Toole, *Youth and Popular Culture in 1950s Ireland* (Bloomsbury, 2018), p. 186.

[18] Holohan, *Reframing Irish Youth*, p. 118.

looking after their parents or siblings, marriage might never occur, or others postponed marriage until these responsibilities no longer existed.[19] Cleary stated that 'it is not rare in Ireland to meet Catholic girls of twenty or twenty five, even teachers, who are *completely* ignorant of sex-matters'.[20] While Cleary believed that mothers should provide their daughters with information, he felt that many were unwilling, embarrassed or incompetent to do this.[21] However, as Elizabeth Kiely has shown, there was a general perception in Irish society up until the 1980s that young Irish people had little or no right to sexual expression or consumption, and this was reflected in 'the perception that a formal sex education would destroy their innocence and possibly arouse sexualities that were best left latent.'[22]

Some Catholic sex education initiatives were prompted by concerns around emigration, which was perceived to be a significant threat to young people's morals.[23] Jennifer Redmond posits that young Irish women who emigrated lacked knowledge of sex due to censorship and lack of open discussion around the issue but were 'symbolically marked as sources of sexual knowledge and desires that would get them 'into trouble' upon leaving the country'.[24] Some Irish secondary schools did, therefore, begin to provide some sex education from the mid-1960s, however, this was usually very basic or focused on issues of morality rather than the physiology of reproduction. Gráinne (b. 1937) remembered some discussion of sexual activity in her Leaving Cert year; however, this advice was ambiguous:

The last couple of weeks before we left, the nun that was head over our group, Sister Cornelia, she was over the senior school Leaving Cert class and I think she kind of gave a little bit of a discussion about sexual activity and things like that, but it was so vague and you'd hardly know what she was talking about. But that's the only person who ever discussed anything like that.

By the late 1960s, not much had changed. Hugh (b.1951) recalled the following of the sex education he received at his secondary school in a small town in the west of Ireland:

We had one or two lectures in secondary school about sex, but I mean they weren't very frank as regards the mechanics about it or anything else. Contraception wasn't

[19] Daly, *The Slow Failure*, pp. 115–18.   [20] Cleary, 'Is sex instruction needed', p. 379.
[21] *Ibid.*
[22] Elizabeth Kiely, 'Lessons in sexual citizenship: the politics of Irish school based sexuality education' in Máire Leane and Elizabeth Kiely (eds.), *Sexualities and Irish Society* (Dublin: Orpen Press), pp. 297–320, on p. 292.
[23] *Ibid.*, p. 292.   [24] Redmond, 'The politics of emigrant bodies', p. 83.

mentioned at all, you know. Except you daren't … well first you daren't have sex and secondly you daren't get a girl pregnant.

Barbara (b.1950) from a town in the south-west recalled a nun in her school trying to give her class an explanation of periods:

I remember one time a nun tried to tell us … It was mostly about periods and things and she was so embarrassed that she actually went out of the room herself. She was a reasonably young nun. I mean maybe the older nuns now would be able to toughen it out, but she didn't. She actually ran out, the face was burning off her as she ran out of the room and that was the end of her lesson.

While responsibility for sex education thus often lay with parents, many respondents felt that it was a challenge for them to openly discuss such matters. Rosie (b.1938) from the rural Midlands recalled her mother talking to her and her sister about periods. She said:

And she was ironing in the kitchen, and we were sitting down. She said, 'I want to talk to you.' And, she told us about our periods, and she told, she told us why we got periods and things like that. It took five minutes, or 10 minutes, and she, she went on ironing then, and I saw she thought, 'Well thank God, I've done me duty.'

Other mothers gave more rudimentary information. Carmel (b.1952) remembered 'She just said that you'd bleed once a month, the sanitary towels were in the bottom drawer. She told us to put it on, to put it into a bag, and she'd get rid of it, but that was it.' However, Carmel's mother did not explain why women got periods: 'Nobody said why it's happening. We were just told that's what you do to keep from ruining your clothes.' Ann (b.1945) from a town in the south-west told me that when she got her period aged 14, her mother 'just said to me, "You'll be getting those now every month." And that was it.' For girls who were not expecting to get their period, however, it could be a terrifying experience. Siobhan (b.1942) remembered her first period in the following way:

We had the old fashioned little switches, you know the one with the square. And I walked … I got up, I used to sleep walk, and I got up and I walked into that at 2 or 3 in the morning. And I screamed that morning when I woke up. I said, 'I'm covered in blood'.

Similarly, Úna (b.1942) remembered 'I was never told anything. I got my periods and I thought I was going to die'. Aoife (b.1947) also told me 'my first period arrived when I was about ten and a half, and I was frantic, because blood is dangerous, I knew I was going to die.' Deirdre (b.1936) also recalled:

I was 12 years old and my mother, she never even told me what it was, or anything you know. And, oh, they don't, back in them days, they don't talk about things like that. Oh, I didn't know what it was, and I didn't know what it was. And how I found out what it was, I had it twice before I ... there was a girl I used to know her, she had a lot of older sisters and I was telling her one day. She said, 'That's a period.' 'How do you know?' 'I have older sisters.'

The experiences of these participants were not distinctive to Irish women. A number of participants in Lara Freidenfelds' study of menstruation in the United States reported similar incidents, however, American women born in the 1940s and 1950s, unlike their Irish counterparts, were more likely to receive information from their mothers, pamphlets or school education.[25] Closer to home, as Caroline Rusterholz found for Switzerland from the 1950s to 1970s, the taboo around sex education meant that several of her female respondents recalled feelings of distress when they began menstruating.[26]

Some interviewees reported a sense of secrecy and shame around menstruation. Nora (b.1940) said 'Well I knew what was happening all right but my mother just kind of said, "Here, put them on you." And that's that and don't tell anyone. Be secretive about it, if you like. Jeepers, I think about now, when you see all the things advertised on the television and everything.' Similarly, Paula (b.1955) said 'I was horrified actually. I was horrified at the secrecy of it. And you leave them in a bag under your bed when you're finished. And then in the night time when the men are in bed, they're burnt in the fire. That seemed to be standard.' The shame was also compounded by the size of sanitary towels. Paula explained 'they weren't like nice and discreet ones like you have now. They were ones with big loops you attach. They were horrible actually.' Similarly, Cathy (b.1949) recalled that when she got her period, her mother 'got me the old fashioned Southall sanitary towels and they had a loop ... There was a belt and there was a thing on it and you looped them in the belt. That was what we had to wear. That thick. I hated them. Absolutely hated them'. The pads made Cathy feel self-conscious. She told me 'You couldn't really wear a pair of pants with them, because they were huge.' Similarly, in Lucinda McCray Beier's study, there was a strong code of secrecy and shame around menstruation which meant that many mothers in Lancashire in both the pre- and post-war period did not tell their daughters about periods.[27]

[25] Lara Freidenfelds, *The Modern Period: Menstruation in Twentieth-century America* (Baltimore: Johns Hopkins Press, 2009), pp. 38–73.
[26] Rustherolz, 'Reproductive behavior', p. 54
[27] Lucinda McCray Beier, '"We were as green as grass": learning about sex and reproduction in three working-class Lancashire communities, 1900–1970', *Social History of Medicine*, 16:3, (2003), pp. 461–80, on p. 467.

Some respondents recalled that this lack of knowledge persisted until marriage. Tessie (b.1938) told me 'Hadn't a clue. We were thick as planks, I swear to God, getting married. We truly hadn't a clue'. Likewise, Aoife (b.1947) told me 'once we were married, we had no idea how to do intercourse – no idea'. Ann (b.1945) similarly expressed the view 'Now that was the sex side of it. And it was ... oh I don't know ... it was like leading a lamb to slaughter'. Kate Fisher has suggested in her study of birth control practices in early twentieth-century Britain, that 'Women were not only more sheltered from the subcultures in which sexual information was spread but they also censored themselves, preferring to play an ignorant role'.[28] In the case of my study, however, men also commonly professed to a lack of knowledge around sex and family planning in their younger years. Ronan (b.1933) told me 'No, I hardly knew anything about the woman's period until I got married. [...] And my mother sent me up to the priest to get instructions.'

Lack of knowledge could extend to pregnancy and childbirth. Clodagh (b.1940) told me 'You weren't sure what way you were having this baby though.' Martina (b.1955) speaking to me about her first pregnancy and childbirth experience, told me 'I mean, it sounds crazy now when I say that but in actual fact, no idea. And even when I went in to have that baby, I still had no idea of what the procedure was.' Likewise, Elaine (b.1950) said that she knew 'Very little. Very little. It was ridiculous. What they know now, I think I had a second child before I knew it. You know? The first one was such a shock. I didn't know what was happening to me.' Sarah (b.1947) also recalled a friend's experience: 'Her waters broke, she didn't have a clue what ... she never knew about the waters breaking, and this kind of thing.'

Contemporary publications also referred to this lack of knowledge. In 1965, 'Marriage counsellor' in *Woman's Way* magazine stated that 'many young girls and boys actually reach the altar without any sound knowledge of sex' and stressed that it was the responsibility of parents to impart knowledge to their children.[29] The article provided clear guidance on how to provide sex education to children and advised parents who felt shy around the issue not to neglect their duty in this regard.[30] Parents were, however, often reticent to talk to their children about the facts of life. Instead, some parents would explain the birth of a new child by saying they were found under a cabbage plant, or other

---

[28] Fisher, *Birth Control*, p. 75.
[29] 'Marriage counsellor: telling them the facts of life', *Womans' Way*, 3 September 1965, 21.
[30] *Ibid.*

analogies. Diane's (b.1949) parents owned a fish shop in a small town in the north of the country and they explained to her that her younger sister 'came in with the salmon – we used to get salmon in boxes, and we found Mary in the salmon, that's where Mary came from.' Diane felt that although her mother 'was a very modern, go-ahead woman, she would have been very reticent about sex and contraception and the rest of it, it was all hush-hush, and it was because of the Catholic Church, of course'. Mary Anne (b.1955) similarly recalled, 'I think I was told I was gotten through a cabbage plant'. Instead of clear guidance, parents tended to make opaque statements. I asked Emer (b.1939) if her mother told her anything about how people got pregnant and she said, 'My mother said not a word, she said, "You'll learn soon enough".' Similarly, Teresa (b.1946) from a small village in the south-west said 'Oh no sexual education, not at all, it was "soon enough" and no. "Soon enough", even with your periods, my mother didn't even talk about it, do, you know, what she said, "You'd be better off not to know", like that kind of'. Similarly, Angela Davis has suggested that for women growing up in the 1920s and 1930s in England, topics such as sex and childbirth were 'taboo' subjects which were not discussed within most families and that this reticence around discussion of sexual topics 'cast a long shadow into the 1960s'.[31]

Participants in Máire Leane's study, which involved interviews with 21 Irish women born between 1914 and 1955, also referred to vague warnings issued by parents which only served to cause confusion.[32] The majority of individuals in my study also recalled parents' embarrassment in addressing issues around sex, and terms such as 'be careful' and 'mind yourself' were often used in place of explaining what behaviour their teenage or young adult children should be avoiding. These statements could be read as an assumption that their children knew what they were referring to with these warning. However, many of the interviewees did not know at the time what these warnings actually meant. Richard (b.1954) remembered 'Just my father said to be careful and just a few words but really very little'. Hannah (b.1950) told me 'My mother never spoke to me, only, "Be careful".' Similarly, Dennis (b.1937) recalled coming back from a tour of Killarney with his girlfriend and his mother saying to him 'She said "I hope", she says, "you were good"', which he did not understand. Virginia (b.1948) likewise remembered: 'You were told to be careful, but you didn't know what be careful meant. (laughing)

---

[31] Angela Davis, '"Oh no, nothing, we didn't learn anything": sex education and the preparation of girls for motherhood, c.1930–1970', *History of Education*, 37:5, (2008), pp. 661–77, on pp. 667–8.
[32] Leane, 'Embodied sexualities', p. 33.

You know? You didn't know what they were telling you'. Mairead (b.1953) remembered 'We wouldn't have had much sex education. My mother used to say "Keep your knees together". Things like this'. Mary Anne (b.1955) also recalled being given the same advice by her mother but not understanding it:

'Oh, mind yourself'. Me being green as grass, 'What you mean mind yourself? Mind yourself walking down the street, what? Mind yourself, what?' And so a hundred years afterward I knew what she meant, 'Mind yourself'. Mind yourself, don't get pregnant.

Some respondents who grew up on farms explained that they learnt from observing animals. Christopher (b.1946) from the rural south-east, for instance, told me 'I think the advantage of coming from let's say a farm background is that you have seen the – in let's say the dairying or the animal and you have seen let's say the reproductive process'. Likewise, Katherine (b.1948) who also grew up on a farm explained 'As a kid, you're out, you're holding poor horses for this, and that, and the other thing. And you're ... There's a stallion around, and you're ... You know. You're very ... I suppose you're, you're open, like I mean, very open to it'. Similarly, Bernadette (b.1947) explained:

I don't know how I knew, but I did know. But I grew up on a farm, and you knew. I mean you saw the bull servicing the cow. This is very crude now. You saw the boar being brought to service the sow. You saw all this going on. The vet came, and the vet helped if there was a calf being born, and we'd be told to go in when the vet ... but of course, we wouldn't go in. We would go, we'd go into some shed and we'd peep around the corner, and we'd see the calf coming out, and we'd see all that. As we got older, then we were probably there anyway, you know?

Interestingly in Bernadette's testimony, she was told by her parents to go back into the house when the vet arrived so that she would not see the calf being born, suggesting that her parents wanted to shield her from this aspect of the reproductive process.

Shame and secrecy also surrounded the pregnant body. As Máire Leane has shown, 'the construction of the pregnant body as offensive to the public gaze impacted on pregnant women in very concrete ways'.[33] In fact, as Jennifer Redmond and Judith Hartford have argued 'revulsion towards the female, fertile, sexualised body in the classroom appears to have contributed to the rationale' for the 1932 marriage ban.[34] Women

---

[33] Leane, 'Embodied sexualities', p. 46.
[34] Judith Hartford and Jennifer Redmond, '"I am amazed at how easily we accepted it": the marriage ban, teaching and ideologies of womanhood in post-Independence Ireland', *Gender and Education*, (2019), pp. 194–5.

in Leane's study recalled that during pregnancy they consciously excluded themselves from public spaces and wore loose-fitting coats when they went out.[35] Similarly, in my study, some respondents recalled how the condition of pregnancy was often hidden. Elaine (b.1950) recalled how when she was pregnant and she was going into town, her mother would tell her '"Put on a looser coat, will you? Put a looser coat on you". You know, it was totally hidden'. Similarly, Myra (b.1947) remembered 'If you saw someone who was pregnant, "what's wrong with them?" "Mind your own business". They didn't say oh, they're having a baby. We were very innocent'.

Given the lack of formal sex education in most Irish secondary schools and the fact that a lot of parents tended to be hesitant to talk to their children about the facts of life, the main way of finding out information was through peers, the media or in the case of young women, through magazines. Eamonn (b.1933) from the rural south-west said, 'Never mentioned by the parents. You learnt that in bits and pieces around the fields or maybe at football matches or wherever. You picked it up and sometimes you never learned'. Dennis (b.1937) found out the facts of life from a cousin. He explained, 'No, I didn't find out till I was about 14. It was my cousin who told me one day. I said, "Ah, you're joking." (laughs). I didn't believe him'. Similarly, Nora (b.1940) told me 'No, you did not. Not very much anyway, girl. Only what you read or what your friends told you. It's the same as your periods, nobody even told you about them really'. Brigid (b.1945) from a small town in the south-west received some information from her older cousins: 'They were filling me in, so I was never ignorant of the facts, I'd say. Quite early on I was well aware of what was going on. Talk in school, that was how I learned'. Bernadette (b.1947) who grew up in the rural west of Ireland also recalled finding out from a neighbour. She said 'Well, my first information about where babies come from was from a girl who lived next door. She was one of the wild ones that ended up going to England. But she told me, she said, "They come out of there", pointing to her navel. I always remembered that, but of course, she was wee. Someone must have told her that'. Jean (b.1953) who grew up in a small town in the north of the country explained 'In my case, it was my older sisters, Anne's just a year older than me. And she had a friend. We just lived in council houses, we were all very friendly. But there was a load of children at that stage. And it was her older sister told us. Told her, and told us'.

[35] Leane, 'Embodied sexualities', p. 46.

However, peer-learning meant that urban myths and misinformation could be spread. Mary Ellen (b.1944) from the rural west of Ireland felt that because young men and women were getting their information from 'reading books or conversing between each other and that', that individuals 'often times they got the wrong slant about it'. Úna (b.1944) recalled an incident with her first boyfriend when she was aged 17: 'I was after getting a tooth out and I wouldn't let him kiss me, in case I became pregnant'. Paula (b.1955) from a town in the west of Ireland recalled an encounter with a boy where he 'Really liked me so dragged me down a lane and started kissing me and started moving his body against me and stuff'. Following the encounter:

Oh, I was in convulsions. I remember telling my friends at school. I said, 'Oh, I'm afraid I might be pregnant'. And I was age 14 definitely, if not 15. So I wouldn't have … That's how naïve I was. I didn't know that you actually had to engage in sexual intercourse to be pregnant. That's just one memory I have of back then.

Paula also recalled anxiety about kissing and the idea that certain types of kisses could lead to pregnancy:

'Cause if you French kissed, you could get pregnant. You know? You had this ridiculous idea. You were quite anxious about all these things. And kept it at a certain level. You know? And yeah. So, that was me anyway. Wasn't everyone? But it was me.

2.2   Sex Education Booklets for Adolescents

A small number of sex education booklets were published in the 1950s and 1960s with guidance for young men and women about questions of sex. The earliest of these appear to have been two publications from the 1950s written by Rev. Thomas Anthony Finnegan. Finnegan (1925–2011) was ordained as a priest in 1951 and served as a chaplain of St. Angela's College, Sligo, before going on to become Junior Dean of St Patrick's College, Maynooth, and later bishop of Killala, Co. Mayo from 1987–2002. His first publication, *The Boy's Own: A Practical Booklet for Teenage Boys* (1954) first appeared as a series in the Marist Fathers' monthly publication *Our Lady's Family* before being collated for publication together. *The Boy's Own* dealt primarily with issues of sexual morality such as purity, bad thoughts and bad language, and framed these themes in the context of sin. A section on Bad Actions explored 'sexual powers' and 'sexual pleasure'. Finnegan emphasised that 'this pleasure is permitted only in marriage, because it is only in marriage that children may be brought into the world. That is God's law, and deliberately to go against it is very seriously sinful, even if only in thought'.[36] The book went on to say 'the devil will try to get you into the habit of sin, because he knows that bad habits are often hard to overcome. In this matter you must be very manly', and suggested that if the reader had difficulties or questions, they should ask their father or priest.[37] Readers were advised to avoid temptation against purity through prayer and other activities, avoidance of bad companions and frequent attendance at Mass and Holy Communion, every morning if possible. Again, the trope of manliness was reiterated with the author stating 'Jesus will make a man of you, strong with His own strength'.[38] Girls were to be treated with utmost respect and it was the young man's responsibility to protect their virtue.[39] The book contained no information on the physiology of sexual intercourse and reproduction but focused its attention on the moral aspects of sex.

The *Boy's Own* was followed up with a 1966 publication by Finnegan called *The Girl's Own: Questions Young Women Ask*. In contrast with his earlier publication, *The Girl's Own* contained much more frank discussion of issues around love and romance, dating and 'troublesome thoughts'. The book was written in an accessible question and answer format. This book, like its predecessor, followed Catholic codes of sexual morality and emphasised that sexual activity should only take place within marriage. In the section on kissing, for instance, readers were advised that 'passionate kissing and embracing – which are designed by God to prepare for this act – can properly take place only in marriage. That is the reason why such kissing and embracing are mortally sinful for the unmarried'.[40] Chastity and modesty were encouraged, and girls were warned to avoid boys with 'low moral standards' and immature young boys.[41] Such ideas were not unusual in Irish society at the time and some interviewees felt that women had the responsibility to maintain chastity in a relationship. Nicholas (b.1953) felt that 'the onus was wholly on the woman not to engage in sexual acts. That's the way I see it. Of course, it sounds a bit rough. But men pursued and the women managed the situation'. Similarly, Sandra (b.1951) recalled her father telling her 'Women are the keepers of male morals'. In Sandra's view 'This is what he used to say. And in those days, women kind of took on that role.'

Aidan Mackey's 1965 publication *What Is Love?* was a guide aimed to be given by parents to their adolescent children. The foreword explained that the book dealt with questions such as 'Why do people get married?'

[36] T.A. Finnegan, *The Boy's Own: A Practical Booklet for Teenage Boys* (1954), p. 15.
[37] *Ibid.*, pp. 15–16.   [38] *Ibid.*, p. 16.   [39] *Ibid.*, p. 17.
[40] T.A. Finnegan, *The Girl's Own: Questions Young Women Ask* (1966), p. 12.
[41] *Ibid.*, p. 8.

and 'What exactly is "falling in love"?'. While the book did not claim to give information about 'sex…or about how sex works…It will help you to avoid wrong ideas and actions which could do a great deal of harm to you – harm which could last all your life.'[42] Adolescence was described as a time 'of excitement and adventure and discovery. It is also a time of some danger'.[43] Young people were warned not to act on their impulses. In particular, this advice was aimed the young girl who allowed boys to 'take liberties' or 'paw her'. Mackey wrote that 'Girls who cheapen themselves in this way are not admired or respected by boys. You can judge that from the names which boys give to such girls', these included 'second-hand', 'shop-soiled' and 'fly-blown'.[44] Readers were encouraged to avoid 'impurity' and to only use the 'gifts' God had given them 'for the right reasons and at the right time, and do not waste and spoil them by meddling before you are old enough and knowledgeable enough to understand and enjoy them as God meant them to be enjoyed'.[45]

By the late 1960s, a sex education booklet called *My Dear Daughter* published by the Sisters of Notre Dame in Liverpool was being used in some girls' schools and was often recommended by agony aunt Angela Macnamara to girls who wrote in to her columns requesting information on the facts of life. The book, like others, tended to focus on issues of morality. Paula (b.1955) from a town in the west of Ireland recalled the book being taught at her school:

We had a thing called *My Dear Daughter*, that the nun would do with us. And it would be common. You know? And somebody would come around to give a lecture. And I absolutely hated it. And every girl in my class hated it because it was all cloaked. A big issue was made out of it before it happened. Oh, so and so is coming. So you started to get stressed about buzz words been mentioned that were taboo words that weren't mentioned and yet were mentioned and you thought well, what detail is going to be gone into? It was all spoken around in a way, you know? But you never got a clear, concise informative picture of things.

As several historians have shown, Irish agony aunt, Angela Macnamara became an important voice on the issue of sex education in the 1960s.[46] Macnamara provided talks to girls at convent schools in Dublin on issues such as 'company-keeping', dating and courtship.[47] Paul Ryan's engaging study of Macnamara's agony aunt column in the *Evening Press* from 1963–1980 shows how her column 'was one of the few sources of

---

[42] Aidan Mackey, *What Is Love? A Guide to Right Attitudes to Love and Sex for Children and Younger Adolescents*, (1965) p. 4.

[43] *What is Love?* p. 11.   [44] *Ibid.*, p. 13.   [45] *Ibid.*, p. 14.

[46] See: Holohan, *Reframing Irish Youth*, pp. 130–2; Catriona Clear, Paul Ryan.

[47] *Ibid.*, p. 130.

sexual information in Ireland especially during the 1960s'.[48] For Ryan, 'Macnamara's power lay in the monopoly of information about sex that she held over a section of the population, particularly in 1960s Ireland'.[49] Caitriona Clear's study of women's magazines in 1950s and 1960s Ireland shows how Macnamara provided vital information for girls and women of all ages on a variety of issues.[50] Macnamara's book *Living and Loving* was published in 1969 with the aim, in her own words, of helping readers 'reason out for yourself the good and responsible attitude Christians should adopt towards dating and courtship'.[51] Sexual activity was defined as something that should only occur within marriage, with Macnamara suggesting that uncontrolled 'desire to express love in physical terms' would result in chaos, warning of the danger of pregnancy and that 'babies would be born whom nobody wanted, and for whom there would be no secure home'.[52] Young men and women were advised to exercise the utmost self-control and to avoid 'petting' which was 'objectively wrong because it is a loveless act when it can lead easily to remorse, guilt and frustration'.[53] Unlike other earlier guides, a clear explanation of how conception occurs (between a husband and wife) was provided.[54] The dangers of pregnancy outside marriage were also dwelled on by Macnamara as a warning. She wrote:

A girl who is aware that her behaviour with her boyfriend is too passionate should test her reactions by supposing that she actually had the misfortune to become pregnant by him. Think exactly what the results would be. She is now responsible for the life of another human being. Could she tell her parents, and what way would they react? What of relations, teachers, neighbours? It is no good her blaming anyone else. She knew the possible consequence of the risks she was taking.[55]

Menstruation, seminal emission and masturbation were also explained in depth. Young women were advised of the importance of modesty.[56] The key methods of contraception were listed (surgical sterilisation, drugs, interrupted intercourse, use of the diaphragm, use of the condom, use of the coil, the infertile period) but it was noted that all contraception was forbidden by the Catholic Church although 'responsible family planning is encouraged'.[57] Only the infertile period was described in depth.

---

[48] Paul Ryan, *Asking Angela Macnamara: An Intimate History of Irish Lives* (Dublin: Irish Academic Press, 2012), pp. 204–5.
[49] *Ibid.*, p. 197.   [50] Clear, pp. 81–93.
[51] Angela Macnamara, *Living and Loving*, (Veritas Publications, 1969), p. 3.
[52] *Ibid.*, p. 9.   [53] *Ibid.*, p. 13.   [54] *Ibid.*, p. 12.   [55] *Ibid.*, p. 27.   [56] *Ibid.*, p. 34.
[57] Macnamara, *Living and Loving*, p. 37.

In some cases, and particularly for the younger members of the cohort, parents provided their children with booklets such as the above. Pól (b.1948) explained to me that he was taught nothing in school but recalled his father's embarrassment as he 'threw a book at me, you know, "What every boy should know", sure I can figure it out'. Judith (b.1955) who grew up in Dublin, recalled being given a booklet on the facts of life by her mother 'But no conversation. Just said, "Here. Read that"'. Judith told me of the booklet:

But of course all I saw on the top was 'for girls'. So immediately I wanted to know what was 'for boys'. So I went rooting in her room. And found the booklet she had. And it was, I suppose, for the parent to talk with – and then there was a section for boys and a section for girls. Of course, I got out the section for boys and read it.

Jacinta (b.1954) who also grew up in Dublin had a similar experience. Aged nine, she found a booklet in her mother's bedside locker with

A girl's side and a boy's side and I read the whole lot. It didn't mean much to me because I didn't really understand. When I was ten, she gave me the girl's side with the boy's side ripped out. I'd already read both. I thought it was funny. What to expect. It doesn't mean a lot to you at the time, its pre- it happening.

2.3   Women's Magazines and the Media

Carole Holohan has argued that while the Catholic Church continued to 'exert significant moral influence over the lives of the majority Catholic population', the 1960s marked 'something of a turning point' as the print media began to openly discuss the topic of sex.[58] Women's magazines were an important source of information for many young women on the basic facts of life, but also on contraception. Writing in the magazine *Woman's Way* in 1964, editor Sean O'Sullivan lamented that 'even to-day, untold hundreds of thousands of people get married and except for what HE has picked up from the gutter or learned the hard way in Confession, they don't know any more about the facts of life, marriage or sex than Mammy or Daddy did'.[59] Articles on family planning, which were frequently published in the magazine, highlight significant ignorance among young women. In 1978, for example, Clare, aged 22 (described as a secretary and single with a six-year-old daughter) explained, 'I regret not having known more about family planning when I was younger. I was just

[58] Holohan, *Reframing Irish Youth*, p. 128.
[59] 'By the way', *Woman's Way*, 14 June 1964, p. 10.

sixteen and doing my Leaving Certificate when I was five months pregnant'.[60] Similarly, Cora, a 19-year-old student explained 'I've been studying in Dublin for over a year now and find attitudes very different from what they are at home. I went to a convent school and sex was only briefly mentioned in the biology class, but we were told nothing about family planning'.[61]

Indeed, the regularity with which letters relating to the basic facts of life were published suggests that many remained truly ignorant about basic physiology. Caitriona Clear has argued that the problems in Angela Macnamara's columns were genuine and suggests that the fact that Macnamara usually had at 'least one obliquely worded "answer only" problem' in her page suggests the page's authenticity.[62] Moreover, in the 1960s and 1970s, due to the growing popularity of problem pages, Macnamara and other Irish agony aunts struggled to keep up with their correspondence.[63] Clear's analysis of the problem pages of *Woman's Way* magazine between 1963 and 1969 has shown that out of 1,186 letters to the magazine, 31.5% concerned sex education/information, 30.9% concerned courtship (not sex), 13.8% dealt with 'miscellaneous', 10.8% with extended family/parent-child, 6.7% were questions about work/education and 6.3% were concerned with marital conflict.[64] As Clear has shown, Angela Macnamara was 'unequivocally opposed to artificial methods of birth control for married, and it need hardly be added, for single people', holding this view throughout the 1960s and modifying it slightly in later life.[65] Yet, she was also wary about recommending natural methods of family planning.[66] The young people's magazine *New Spotlight* dealt with issues relating to sexuality in its problem pages in the 1960s and 1970s, with responses to more sensitive issues being published in the 'P.S.' section without the original letter. Many letters revealed considerable ignorance regarding sexual matters.[67] As in Clear's study of women's magazines, many of the letters from young people writing for advice from *New Spotlight* were 'coded or direct requests for moral/religious judgement'.[68]

Magazines were clearly an important source of knowledge for young women. Sarah (b.1947) explained that in the absence of information from her mother, she 'kind of more less read magazines, or books, those kinds of thing'. Judith (b.1950) felt that she gleaned a lot of her sex

---

[60] 'The pill generation', *Woman's Way*, 22 September 1978, p. 11.
[61] *Ibid.*, 22 September 1978, p. 12.   [62] Clear, *Women's Voices*, pp. 27–8.
[63] *Ibid.*, p. 28.   [64] *Ibid.*, p. 82.   [65] *Ibid.*, p. 89.   [66] *Ibid.*
[67] Holohan, *Reframing Irish Youth*, pp. 133–4.
[68] Clear, *Women's Voices*, p. 115 cited in: Holohan, p. 136.

education from magazines, stating, 'You know they had magazines. Generally I think that's where you get lots of your information from. The problem page. Or articles. Probably mainly English magazines like *Woman* and *Woman's Own*'. Noreen, (b.1954) also recalled:

And probably what I do remember, maybe more my sexual … sex education from, I remember getting a hold of these magazines called *True Love* magazines in that time. Sure they were all just raunchy stuff, you know? It was probably innocent raunchy stuff by what's exposed nowadays, but it was new to me. So you would pick it up from magazines.

Letters to Angela Macnamara's agony aunt column highlight the lack of knowledge among young people. In 1964, a woman wrote to Macnamara stating that she had become pregnant outside marriage. She explained, 'I was never told anything about how babies are conceived and though I sensed that our love-making was too intense, I did not dream that we could so easily go too far'.[69] Similarly, 'Westside Story' writing in 1966, stated:

I am 17 and don't know the first thing about the facts of life. I think it's a disgrace. I know you give talks in girls' schools, but our school is in the back of beyond, and they haven't got round to seeing the wisdom in having a straight-speaking married woman in to talk to us. Of course I know odds and ends, but I'd feel so insecure going on a date that I'd be terrified to accept one. Naturally our class are interested in boys, but you'd die if you heard the garbled versions we have of love and life. Can you help us by suggesting books?

Macnamara suggested the book *My Dear Daughter*, as well as *Dating for Young Catholics* by Monsignor Kelly and *Modern Youth and Chastity* by Father Gerald Kelly, but emphasised that giving children books was not adequate, and that girls and boys required 'discussions with understanding, frank adults'.[70] Some letters to magazines from young people show that not all Irish girls and women were willing to accept traditional Catholic and moral teachings. 'Teenage Girl' writing in 1965 asked, 'Isn't it unfair that Catholics are expected to have as many children as possible? Why is this so?' In her reply, Macnamara stated 'It is *not* so', and argued that parents had a duty not only to bring children into the world but to ensure that they were properly educated and provided for. Macnamara stated that the number of children could be regulated through abstinence from sexual intercourse.[71]

---

[69] 'Angela Macnamara's letters page', *Woman's Way*, 30 June 1964, p. 49.
[70] 'Can you help me?', *Woman's Way*, 23 September 1966, p. 34.
[71] *Ibid.*, first fortnight February 1966, p. 49.

Television had an important impact in disseminating information about contraception. By 1963, there were 150,000 television licence holders in the Republic of Ireland. Imported programmes from Britain were more likely to normalise sexual themes and address issues such as contraception and unmarried motherhood, and even before the advent of Telefís Éireann, some parts of the country received transmissions from BBC and ITV.[72] The advent of The Late Late Show, hosted by Gay Byrne from 1962, also meant that more 'controversial' issues began to be discussed on Irish national television.[73] In March 1971, Byrne dedicated an entire episode to the theme of 'Women's Liberation', with a panel consisting of Irish Women's Liberation Movement members Mary Kenny, Máirín Johnston and Nell McCafferty as well as Senator Mary Robinson, Maynooth lecturer Mary Cullen and television producer Leila Doolan. Following the Contraceptive Train in May 1971, Mary Kenny appeared again on The Late Late Show with Colette O'Neill. Kenny 'held up the condoms for the TV camera (discreetly wrapped in their packets, and not inflated)'.[74]

Many respondents pointed to The Late Late Show as being crucial in opening up discussion of more controversial issues such as contraception. Diane (b.1949) remembered 'The time that Gay Byrne interviewed people about contraception, The Late Late Show was very ... it was our great means of communication and getting information'. Mary Ellen (b.1944) felt:

It was really with The Late Late Show on television that things opened up because Gay Byrne used to have lots of interviewees like that. He'd discuss ... they would discuss issues that were unheard of being discussed on TV and people were watching the Late Late, very much so at that time. So it encouraged people to talk more openly about those issues. Before that it was a taboo.

Mairead (b.1953) felt that Gay Byrne 'brought it [sex] out in the open, people would never talk about anything'. Carol (b.1954) also felt that The Late Late Show had significant influence, because 'it had a wide appeal to people and a wide audience and it did bring the topics that people just didn't discuss, that were taboo with them'. A number of respondents also recalled the 1987 episode of The Late Late Show when Gay Byrne showed a condom on television. Nicholas (b.1953) from a city in the west of Ireland stated, 'Gay Byrne was the first to introduce a condom onto the television on The Late Late Show. So, whether, whether that was a good

---

[72] Holohan, *Reframing Irish Youth*, p. 131.
[73] For detailed discussion of The Late Late Show see: Finola Doyle-O'Neill, *The Gaybo Revolution: How Gay Byrne Challenged Irish Society* (Dublin: Orpen Press, 2015).
[74] Mary Kenny, *Something of Myself and Others* (Dublin: Liberties Press, 2013), p. 155.

or a bad thing the one thing that was definite about it was that it was controversial'. For Aoife (b.1947) who also watched the episode, 'that was the first time I ever saw a condom or heard what it was called'.

2.4   The Impact of Religion on Attitudes to Sex

Religion was a significant part of the lives of respondents growing up. Clodagh (b.1940) for example, explained:

Well, we were brought up you see as they say that was our life you see you were brought to church, of course it was Catholic school, got First Communion, Confirmation, you never questioned anything, that was life and you believed everything you were told.

Catholicism inevitably had an impact on attitudes to sex. Several participants recalled how they felt that physical intimacy was a sinful activity. Áine (b.1949) explained 'you always got the vibe that, you know, sex was dirty, filthy'. Such ideas stemmed from Church teachings growing up. Marian (b.1935) explained to me, 'If a fella put his hand on your knee it was nearly a sin. That kind of thing. Kissing was about the nearest you got to ... but of course when I met my husband I knew he was the one. There was a lot of pressure. I think that's why we probably got married ... everybody got married young and you had all this in your head. No you don't do this, you don't do that, kind of thing. It was a sin...'. The perceived sinfulness of physical activity meant that many individuals were afraid to engage in physical intimacy as adolescents. Eugene (b.1939) explained 'you'd be afraid to put your hand on a girl's... at that time. You'd be shy about it. You'd be very slow'. When I asked him why this was, Eugene explained, 'Ah sure the priest. They were all – the clergy you know'. He then went on to recall a dance in his area where 'a neighbour of mine was dancing real tight and he came over to him and tapped him on the shoulder.' Indeed, many interviewees recalled similar incidents where sexual activity was policed by priests. Pól (b.1948) who grew up in a small town in the west of Ireland felt that:

it was all sinful, you know what I mean? It was sin, it was sin and French kissing was a mortal sin. Kissing with closed lips was a venial sin. Because you didn't know where ... what did the priest say once to me? If a girl opened her mouth and you kissed her God knows where it would lead to.

As Louise Fuller has shown, in the 1950s, there was a range of devotional Catholic activities. These included the Holy Hour, Benediction, the Forty Hours, confraternities, sodalities, novenas, processions, missions, the cult of indulgences, Lenten fast and abstinence and exercises of mortification, First Friday devotions, confession and the rosary.[75] By the 1970s, some of these activities had become less popular or were de-emphasised by the Church. For the majority of the participants in my study, however, most of whom were coming of age from the 1950s to the late 1960s, these activities had an important impact on their psyche. Hazel Lyder found that many of the women in her study of female sexuality during childhood in 1930s and 1940s Dublin recalled 'strong, if oblique, messages being given about sexual morality on these occasions'.[76] Retreats led by redemptorist priests were recalled by a number of oral history participants. Dennis (b.1937) from the south-west of the country described the annual retreat in his village in the 1950s as follows:

In our village, we'd have an annual retreat. You know what those things are? The missioners would come in and the missioners were Redemptorists mostly. There'd be hell ... and the women were one week, the men were another. They weren't even in the church together and there'd be hell. The whole moral situation, of bad company keeping, sex and all that was pounded. There were other things. Don't get me wrong, stealing and lying and cheating. All those things were also part of the regime. But the sex thing was the one that ... There would be a night devoted to company keeping and that would be the ... That was the 50s.

Bob (b.1931) also recalled the missions as follows:

I remember from the Redemptorists and hellfire on the... we all were terrified about this. Young girl and look at you rotting in the grave now or something, she's damned to hell and this kind of fire and brimstone kind of sermons at that time. Terrified people.

Declan (b.1944) who was younger than Bob and Dennis, also recalled the missions in his parish in the 1950s and early 1960s. He remembered an annual lecture 'it was always a Tuesday night, that was the sex, the lectures on sex then'. Declan recalled, 'it was all about sex and company and all that'. Lizzie (b.1946) also recalled the missioners who would come to their parish, 'and they'd be up there. I mean, everything was adultery, and everything was a mortal sin. And I mean if you only have looked at your neighbour's husband, it nearly was adultery'. Úna (b.1944) also recalled the fear that she felt attending missions, reflecting on the power of the priests at the time, 'I mean you were afraid of your life with the priests'. For Úna this fear persisted even after marriage. She recalled the fear she felt around having sex for the first time on her honeymoon:

---

[75] Louise Fuller, *Irish Catholicism Since 1950: The Undoing of a Culture* (Dublin: Gill & Macmillan, 2002), p. 224.
[76] Lyder, 'Silence and secrecy', p. 79.

And I was giving him plenty of time, so that he'd be in bed and then I came out, I sat on the side of the bed. He knew I was nervous, but … Oh yes, because I was always kind of made afraid and then there used to be missioners, missionary priests and they'd be banging the pulpit and you were going to go to hell. I mean, at that time. We were brainwashed.

Even though Úna was doing nothing wrong in terms of Catholic teachings around sex, it is clear from the above quote that the Church's stance around sexual morality exacerbated her feelings of apprehension about having sex for the first time. Her use of the term 'brainwashed' was not unusual from my respondents either; many of whom reflected candidly on their adherence to Catholic teachings as young people in contrast to their changed views in older age.

Several interviewees recalled priests giving talks to them at school about the dangers of sexual activity. Maud (b.1947) remembered her class at school having a talk from a priest at the age of 15 or 16. She explained: 'They'd come into the convent and you couldn't speak. But they, in their own way tried to talk to you about sex'. Her main memory of the talk was being told, 'I remember that French kissing. Never, never kiss. Never let a boy kiss you. French kissing was a real sin'. Although certain activities were deemed to be wrong or sinful, respondents expressed their confusion at the time and lack of understanding of what they were being told. Martin (b.1952) from a town in the south-east of Ireland recalled:

One of the chief dangers to chastity was company keeping. Now they didn't tell us what chastity was, we just supposed it was a very bad thing. But also, they didn't tell us what company keeping meant. So, all I knew was that my father worked for a company. The whole family was doomed, kind of. Everything was skirted around. I just knew that if you went there you were in serious trouble.

Sexuality and company keeping were policed in other ways. Alice (b.1944) from the rural west of Ireland recalled, 'The priests used to go to the carnivals, and you had to keep a safe distance'. In a 1988 account, Evelyn Owens (1931–2010), the Labour Party politician and trade union activist, described how at the age when she and her peers were 'interested in boys or boys were interested in us', they would meet at the crossroads of Vernon Avenue and Belgrove Road in Dublin on the way home from school. She said: 'We had a local curate who was very anti the idea of boys and girls talking. So the big trick was not to get caught by Fr O'Keeffe on his bicycle coming home in the evening. If you did you jumped over a garden wall and hid. That was our introduction to company keeping'.[77]

---

[77] Mairin Johnston, *Dublin Belles: Conversations with Dublin Women* (Dublin: Attic Press, 1988), p. 113.

Confession helped to induce fear in young men and women.[78] The practice was also used by priests to help to reinforce the idea that sexual activity was sinful. Carol (b.1954) recalled a priest in her area in Dublin when she was growing up 'who would have frightened the life out of you. You'd hear him roaring out of the confessional box'. Hugh (b.1951) felt 'you assumed most people weren't having sex. We were brought up in such a repressive attitude that it was a mortal sin to have any sort of sexual encounters, if you had any sort of thing that you did do at all, you were forced to confess it'. Lizzie (b.1946) recalled going to confession aged 17 after her first kiss, telling the priest that she had committed a mortal sin. Dennis (b.1937) remembered the following experience in confession which clearly had a significant impact on him:

But I remember there was a cracked priest, anyway, but he was fairly strong on a mission, whatever, but going to confession and I went to confession to him, you see. I said, 'I committed bad actions'. 'What did you do?' 'I put my hand up a girl's leg'. He nearly went ape. Because I was leading her to hell and I was leading myself to hell and ... I didn't put my hand on a girl's knee for a long time after that.

Guilt around physical intimacy could extend into other areas of sexual pleasure. Julie (b.1947) from the rural west of Ireland candidly told me, 'But I remember, I suppose teenage years, you're, I remember actually lying in bed in the night and just wanting to experience, to arouse myself and then feeling so guilty'. And, as other testimonies in Chapter 5 will show, such guilt in relation to sex often persisted into adulthood.

2.5   The Stigma and Shame of Unmarried Motherhood

For much of the twentieth century, sex outside of marriage was strongly condemned and there was significant stigma towards this as well as unmarried motherhood and marriage breakdown in Ireland. In Clara Fischer's words, shame 'was mobilized in the pursuit of a postcolonial national identity, which centrally hinged on the moral purity of women, on the one hand, but was promoted and maintained alongside constructions of women and women's potential sexual transgressions as continuous threats to that identity, on the other'.[79] Sara Ahmed defines shame as 'an intense and painful sensation that is bound up with how the self feels

---

[78] Cara Delay, *Irish Women and the Creation of Modern Catholicism, 1850–1950*, pp. 84–6.

[79] Clara Fischer, 'Gender, nation, and the politics of shame: Magdalen laundries and the institutionalization of feminine transgression in modern Ireland', *Signs: Journal of Women in Culture and Society*, 41:4, (2016), pp. 821–43, on p. 824.

about itself, a self-feeling that is felt by and on the body'.[80] Furthermore 'to have one's shame witnessed is even more shaming. The bind of shame is that it is intensified by being seen by others *as* shame'.[81] The 1937 constitution defined women's role in Irish society as subsidiary to the institution of the family. For a woman who found herself pregnant outside of marriage, there were limited options – marriage to the father, emigration to Britain to have the baby in secret and give it up for adoption, or, in the majority of cases, seek assistance from a mother and baby home.[82] As Lindsey Earner-Byrne has argued, the shotgun wedding 'was a strategy of survival for many women facing single motherhood in Ireland'.[83] From the state's perspective, this was a cost-effective approach to the problem of unmarried motherhood as 'upon marriage the illegitimate child became the responsibility of the father rather than the state' but as well as this 'society was more forgiving of mothers who sought to legitimise their mistake by marriage, even if that marriage took place shortly before or after the birth'.[84] In 1988, journalist Nuala O'Faolain articulated the lack of options facing women who became pregnant outside marriage in the early 1960s, writing, 'There was no contraception or nobody knew about contraception. It was just your tough luck if you got pregnant. If you got pregnant you had to marry the bloke. You just *had* to. If the woman's boyfriend did not want to marry her, the only other option was to have the baby adopted'.[85] As well as shotgun weddings or adoption, some unmarried mothers had their children adopted by a relative. We know in other instances that shame and stigma was so strong that some women resorted to illegal abortion or infanticide.[86] Only one of my participants, Alice (b.1944) from a rural part of Ireland, mentioned an attempt to bring on an abortion on one occasion when, as a single woman, her period was late, and she believed she was pregnant. One common way women used to bring on an abortion was by drinking gin and having a hot bath. She recalled:

I've never told this either to anybody. Somebody told me that if you had gin to have an abortion, I bought a bottle of gin and put it into the bath, to the bath. I didn't know you had to drink it. [...] Thank god I wasn't pregnant anyway.

Alice's account here highlights how knowledge about how to procure an abortion could be misinterpreted, but also her relief at not being pregnant.

---

[80] Sara Ahmed, *The Cultural Politics of Emotion* (Edinburgh University Press, 2014), p. 103
[81] *Ibid.*   [82] Earner-Byrne, *Mother and Child*, pp. 179–80.   [83] *Ibid.*, p. 180.
[84] *Ibid..*   [85] Johnston, *Dublin Belles*, p. 61.
[86] On illegal abortion, see Delay, 'Pills, potions, and purgatives' and 'Kitchens and kettles'. On infanticide see: Rattigan, *What Else Could I Do?* and Farrell, *A Most Diabolical Deed*.

From 1968 onwards, with the introduction of the 1967 Abortion Act in Britain (with the exception of Northern Ireland), Irish women began to travel to have abortions there. We know that in 1968, 64 Irish residents travelled to have legal abortions in England and Wales, with this figure doubling each year up until 1972.[87] As Lindsey Earner-Byrne has shown, at a 1974 conference organised by Cherish, it was stated that 43 per cent of pregnancies of unmarried Irish women between the ages of 25 and 29 were terminated in England, compared to 29 per cent of their English counterparts, suggesting that for many young Irish women, 1970s Ireland was not a viable place to be a single mother.[88] Arguably, due to the significant stigma and lack of adequate state support, single motherhood was not a feasible option for the majority until at least the 1990s.[89]

In Britain, levels of stigma and shame directed towards unmarried mothers depended on the character of local communities and cultures, but Melanie Tebbutt suggests that it was 'less pronounced among the generation born after 1945' even as teenage pregnancy became a new focus of moral concern.[90] Pat Thane suggests that in England, the myth of the permissive society in the 1960s overestimates the extent of change that took place in Britain in this period, and while there was more openness towards the discussion of unmarried mothers, this change was 'slow, uneven, and contested'.[91] In Ireland, however, the stigma of unmarried motherhood persisted until late into the twentieth century and fear of pregnancy outside of marriage had a significant impact on respondents' attitudes towards pre-marital sex. Lindsey Earner-Byrne and Diane Urquhart have recently argued that in both the Republic of

---

[87] 122 in 1969, 261 in 1970, 577 in 1971, 974 in 1972, 1193 in 1973, 1421 in 1974 and 1573 in 1975. Figures from: Dermot Walsh, 'Pregnancies of Irish residents terminated in England and Wales in 1975', *Journal of the Irish Medical Association*, November 18, 1977, 70:17, p. 498.

[88] *Cherish: Proceedings of the Conference on the Unmarried Parent and Child in Irish Society 1974*, (Kilkenny, 1975), p.32, cited in Lindsey Earner-Byrne, 'The Boat to England: an analysis of the official reactions to the emigration of single expectant Irishwomen to Britain, 1922–1972', *Irish Economic and Social History*, 30 (2003), pp. 52–70, on p. 70.

[89] The unmarried mothers' allowance was introduced in Ireland in 1973, following significant lobbying by Cherish, the first support group for unmarried mothers. According to Lorraine Grimes, 'Those who were relying on the allowance struggled and only women with well-paid jobs could keep their children even after the allowance was introduced'. Lorraine Grimes, *Migration and Assistance: Irish unmarried mothers in Britain, 1926–1973*, (unpublished PhD thesis, NUI Galway, 2020), p. 136.

[90] Melanie Tebbutt, *Making Youth: A History of Youth in Modern Britain* (Palgrave, 2016), p. 127.

[91] Pat Thane and Tanya Evans, *Sinners? Scroungers? Saints? Unmarried Motherhood in Twentieth-Century England* (Oxford University Press, 2012), p. 139.

Ireland and Northern Ireland 'shame and secrecy formed fundamental bulwarks of societies which placed a high premium on sexual "purity"'.[92]

Many interviewees reflected on their fear of bringing shame on their family if they became pregnant outside of marriage and that this fear was enough to deter them from having pre-marital sex. Ann (b.1945) who grew up in a town in the south-east of Ireland, explained:

Now I was never brazen or … How can I say? … adventurous. I was always a good girl. My grandma used to tell me, 'You're a great girl'. But I was and whereas I'm not saying nobody ever had sex before marriage, of course they did. But it wouldn't enter my head. You know? It just didn't. And I think it was the best contraception ever. Or contraceptive. Because, oh my god, the thought of having to go home if I got pregnant. I couldn't. I'd kill myself, I'd say, before that would happen.

Christine (b.1947) from Dublin similarly reflected on this issue, stating:

I often wonder what kept me on the straight and narrow, if you like, before we got married was a fear of my mother, a fear of God. But a more fear of my mother that I could not go home and tell my parents that I was pregnant.

Shame can also act as a deterrent whereby 'subjects must enter the "contract" of the social bond, by seeking to approximate a social ideal'.[93] Lily (b.1946) from the north of the country, who was brought up Presbyterian, felt similarly around the issue of sex before marriage. She told me, 'I wasn't having sex. There was no way I would have. And if a person got pregnant anyway I'd have to leave home, you know'. She went on to say, 'you just would be told, like, that "if you get pregnant don't come home". That was the contraception that we used'. Likewise, Bridget (b.1945) explained, 'you never slept with anyone outside of marriage. So even my husband now like we never did until we got married, do you know? And so that kind of didn't enter into it, do you know? [..] Because that was the way it was done'. Bridget felt that if she had become pregnant it would have been the 'worst thing that could happen to you. Oh my mother would have lost her reason, do you know?' Hannah (b.1950) similarly recalled hearing about a girl becoming pregnant outside of marriage:

I heard about a girl, 'Where is she now?' 'Oh, she's gone. She's going to have a baby'. Like that was the worst possible thing you could probably have brought upon your family. I suppose that was very compelling. You were so afraid.

---

[92] Earner-Byrne and Urquhart, *The Irish Abortion Journey*, p. 11.
[93] Ahmed, *The Cultural Politics of Emotion*, p. 107.

Mothers may also have instilled this sense of shame around the issue of unmarried motherhood in their daughters. Ellen (b.1949) from the rural south-east, for instance, told me of her mother:

She was good in one way, but she was a very cross woman in another way. And her big fear always, I think was that I would get pregnant or I wouldn't be married, and it was a thing... I even had it in my head that if it ever happened to me I would never again go home. I had this in my head that if I got pregnant I would probably go away somehow and have the baby adopted. I would never go home. But this was just what you had in your head sort of. So with the result I suppose that when I had boyfriends I was... I'd let them kiss me and whatever, but we never let it go any further than that.

Ellen's overriding fear of disappointing her mother meant that she did not engage in any physical activity with boyfriends beyond kissing. She told me, 'There would be no question about it...[engaging in sex outside of marriage] none of us did. Absolutely out of the question. You'd be so afraid of the church and your parents and everything. You would be a finger point, if people knew it. It was such a shameful thing'. Kate (b.1944) also expressed a similar sentiment, stating, 'Having sex before [marriage], we never did, because it was against the law, so you just did what the church told you and you never did'. Similarly, Brigid (b.1945) who grew up in a small town in the south-west of the country, told me that her mother threatened to throw herself in the local deep water quay 'if anything will ever happen to any one of ye, in other words, if any one of ye got pregnant...we weren't even allowed to say the word "pregnant"'. Audrey (b.1934) who grew up in Dublin, received a similar message from her mother:

Oh, my mother did tell me, she was good to talking to me. She was very good about it. But then it was always, laced with, you have to do what you're told, and you don't, you do have a say and you don't. You don't have sex before you're married. In fact I used to say 'if I ever did give into a fella, they'd have to fish me out of the canal, I wouldn't even wait to see if I was pregnant'. That kind of thing, you know. We grew up with this fear of ...

Strict family attitudes in relation to the issue of pregnancy outside marriage reveal much about notions of respectability in twentieth-century Ireland. As Beverley Skeggs has argued, 'respectability is one of the most ubiquitous signifiers of class', but respectability also embodies moral authority.[94] Sexual knowledge and behaviour were closely related to respectability. For much of the twentieth century in Ireland the

[94] Beverley Skeggs, *Formations of Class & Gender: Becoming Respectable* (London: SAGE Publications, 1997), pp. 9–10.

unmarried mother and her child were viewed as outcasts in 'respectable' Irish society.[95] For parents whose daughter became pregnant outside of marriage, there was tremendous shame and stigma which could be damning within a small community. Lizzie (b.1946) for instance felt 'It'd be drummed into you to respect your family. That you were to respect your family and not let your family down. It was, don't let your family down and that was instilled in you so much, that you just didn't do it'. Chastity was viewed as a marker of respectability. A doctor interviewed by *Woman's Way* magazine in 1983 stated, 'Single people didn't have intercourse when I was a student over twenty years ago. That wasn't due to a fear of pregnancy. Nice girls didn't do it and if they did, men would find out and wouldn't marry them'.[96] Dennis (b.1937) reflected on this issue in the following way:

Put it this way, is that any girl who got into trouble as such, by trouble it meant you got pregnant. That they were actually quite ostracised and everybody ... 'She's no good' or 'she's not respectable' or as they would say, 'She came from a respectable family'. That was the ultimate. If her family had a record of previous debauchery, then it was, 'Ah yeah, sure what would you expect'. But if she was in a respectable family it was...

In McCray Beier's study of three working-class communities in Lancashire from 1900-70, 'parents' attitudes towards potential or actual pregnancy demonstrated their own respectability'.[97] Mark (b.1952) recalled his father saying of unmarried mothers, 'Ah, sure what would you expect coming from that stable'.

For those who did engage in some type of sexual activity, in Cathy's (b.1949) words, they 'really had to be careful'. Without access to contraception, engaging in sex before marriage was incredibly risky. While sex education was limited, participants were aware that full intercourse would potentially lead to pregnancy. Dennis (b.1937) felt that he and his peers had been instilled with a sense that pregnancy could happen easily. This helped to imbue a sense of fear around sexual intercourse:

We felt it could happen rather easily. If you had sex with a girl, you had a 50/50 chance of becoming a dad and all the responsibility. The whole thing was ... It was enough to frighten you off anyway.

---

[95] Maria Luddy, 'Unmarried mothers in Ireland, 1880–1973', *Women's History Review*, 20:1, (2011), pp. 109–26, on p. 123.

[96] 'The sex angle', *Woman's Way*, 8 April 1983, p. 12.

[97] McCray Beier, 'We were as green as grass', p. 470.

Even engaging in other sexual activities, however, could result in fear. Lizzie (b.1946) said 'Though you'd be tempted to do it, but you went three quarters of the way there and took the chance, and then you'd be petrified'. Several respondents reported 'only going so far' or 'not going the whole way', which could mean either avoiding penetrative sex or sometimes implied use of the withdrawal method. Carmel (b.1952) for instance said, 'I suppose you just knew that if you did something, a certain thing, you would become pregnant. And you just avoided that'. Carol (b.1954) said, 'You could kind-of footer around, but you couldn't, you know, go the whole way. So that was, you know, not unless you wanted to end up in trouble'. Lizzie (b.1946) also told me, 'You see, you still did things that you shouldn't do, because human nature being human nature, you still did it though you knew it wasn't wrong and you knew the consequences of it'. When I asked her how people avoided getting pregnant in these situations she said, 'They wouldn't go the whole way. They wouldn't go the whole way, but there again, you were never guaranteed, it was a chance to take'. Pól (b.1948) from a small town in the west of Ireland explained it as follows:

Because well the guilt of it and I suppose the whole thing of oh if they become pregnant and stuff. So like I would think most girls would let a fella go as far as, if they were in a long term relationship they would let them go as far as they could go but they wouldn't actually do any of the thing until they got married, which left people frustrated and stuff back then. But I'd imagine, but a lot of times people wouldn't even go that far, you know?

Pól's testimony highlights the guilt attached to engaging in intercourse before marriage but also the fear of pregnancy that was instilled in young people. Colm (b.1940) when asked whether couples in his age group waited until marriage before having sex laughed and said, 'I tell you, you done a lot of fumbling around. Let's put it that way'. Hannah (b.1950) who grew up in a small town in the north-west of the country explained, 'You got involved in heavy petting and all the rest of it. That was it. You didn't sleep with them'. Similarly, Teresa (b.1946) when asked how couples avoided pregnancy before marriage said they would 'just avoid sex if you can but I mean there was a lot of passion, there was a lot of passion'. Carol (b.1954) felt that this was a reason why people got married sooner, explaining, 'You didn't hang around, partly because you didn't want to get pregnant because it wasn't a good idea to be going home pregnant. And I was, I suppose, technically a virgin when I got married, because you know, you just didn't'.

Getting pregnant outside of marriage was thus commonly described by respondents through the use of terms such as 'fear', 'terrified', 'scared'.

Sara Ahmed suggests that while fear is an unpleasant experience in the present, 'the unpleasantness of fear also relates to the future' because it 'involves an *anticipation* of hurt or injury.'[98] Cathy (b.1949) for example, stated, 'I was terrified that anything would happen to me'. Clodagh (b.1940) from the rural Midlands explained, 'And we were terrified to get pregnant before we got married and you would be terrified of doing anything nearly in case you might get pregnant and I wouldn't go home and tell my mother or my father'.

Respondents were not always aware of what happened to women who became pregnant outside of marriage but their disappearance or the sense of not knowing helped to contribute to a fear around getting pregnant. Noreen (b.1954) for instance, told me: 'You would've known that something had happened and those girls disappeared. They were sent away. So you know that there was something, but you didn't know what. Again, it was all cloak and dagger kind of stuff'. Similarly, Lizzie (b.1946) recalled, 'you always had this big fear and you would have feared that if you did become pregnant, something would happen to you but you didn't know what it was'. As Maria Luddy has argued in the context of the condemnation of unmarried motherhood, 'moral judgement had social power in Ireland'.[99] The majority of the interviewees in my study discussed friends, neighbours or family members who had been sent to a mother and baby home; this may have been because of the fact that my interviews were conducted in 2018–19, a period when the issue was regularly discussed in the media. Cathy (b.1949) for instance, recalled a woman she knew growing up who became pregnant outside of marriage:

But her mother kept her at home and once she became... Once she got a bump, she wasn't allowed outside the door. So, she stayed at home and I remember going down to visit her one evening with my friends and she was in the bedroom. Not necessarily in bed, but she hadn't been out for a few weeks and she wasn't going to be out until after she had the baby. And then I think before the baby was born, obviously, I don't know if she just went straight to hospital from the house or whether she went into a home for a week or something to have the baby. Had the baby and it was adopted, that was it.

Indeed, fear of pregnancy and the potential of ensuing shame and negative parental responses appears to have persisted for young people coming of age in the 1970s. For Jean (b.1953):

[98] Ahmed, *The Cultural Politics of Emotion*, p. 65.
[99] Maria Luddy, 'Sex and the single girl in 1920s and 1930s Ireland', *The Irish Review*, 35, (Summer, 2007), pp. 79–91, on p. 89.

That was the worry really when you think of it. That was the bottom line, you just didn't want to get pregnant because it was frowned about really at the time, when you think. Now if it had happened, if it had happened that would have been okay, but that was it, you just didn't want to get pregnant really. That was it.

For those who did engage in pre-marital sex which resulted in a pregnancy, the shotgun wedding was a common outcome. Colm (b.1940) from the rural Midlands, for example, recalled, 'There was lads done it once and they were caught. And they had to go off and get married. Which was wrong too. There was more people married in this country, because the girl was pregnant'. Maria (b.1957) became pregnant aged nineteen. She married her boyfriend within a short period and had her first child aged twenty. In Maria's case, her parents were supportive and did not pressure her to marry. However, she felt 'But there was still the pressure to think, well how are we going to normalise this? So we did marry. You know what I mean? So society rather than ... I suppose you're in an awful fuzz really ... mentally about what you'll do...'.

Mary Anne (b.1953) from the rural south-west became pregnant aged 23, and 'because I was pregnant, I had to get married'. In Mary Anne's view 'it was the only option then'. Mary Anne and her husband later moved to England. She came home to Ireland for holidays, but felt that her parents treated her daughter with antipathy. She felt 'because I had to get married, there was that resentment towards her'. Sally (b.1956) from the rural east of the country became pregnant aged 17. She stated:

I was 17 going on 18, and at this stage I think I'd earned my place in the house as being very determined. Because I was still running the financial side of the family. So I just said to my mother, I'm getting married, and that's it. She didn't approve and I went ahead anyway and got married, and she never liked my husband. And she never quite forgave me, except for when my son was born.

Martina (b.1955) who also found herself pregnant aged 17 reflected on the lack of assistance available to her in 1973. Martina felt that her getting pregnant was largely down to her lack of sex education and naivety: 'I got pregnant, I was only 17 and no wonder I hadn't an idea about sex education or anything'. Martina had been working in a bar in her local town but was told to 'pack her bags' by her employer. She returned home to her parents and 'I told my mother and I was told, "You've made your bed now, you lay in it." So, in other words, get on with it now. You've made a mistake and ... So, my mother and my sister organised my wedding'. Martina had considered going to a mother and baby home in Dublin:

I didn't want it at all. And in fact, a friend of mine had taken me up to Dublin to see this priest in Dublin. [...] And he involved with one of these mother and baby homes. And I went up to Dublin and met him. And I mean, he'd have taken me in, but somehow or another I didn't want to go to Dublin either.

She decided to go ahead with the wedding. At her reception, she remembered 'looking out the window and I said, "Oh my God, my life's over"'. In Martina's view, getting married rather than going to a mother and baby home 'was the best of a bad lot'.

Catholic doctrine backed up the general belief that, in the words of Lindsey Earner-Byrne, 'the name of Irish motherhood was besmirched by the few who became pregnant outside the legal and religious boundaries of the family'.[100] Disapproval could also come from the clergy. Martina (b.1955) recalled, 'I think all the priest wanted was get you married. The most important thing is that when you have that child that you're married. So, there was no ... There was no options, there was no anything. I knew he was disapproving, I can assure you. And at that time there was a very strict canon in my home place. And I know he was disapproving, so you were up against disproval everywhere you went'. Likewise, several respondents recalled shotgun weddings taking place in the early morning or on the side altar. Brigid (b.1945) from a small town in the south-west recalled:

I knew one girl in [small town] who was like that. ... became pregnant, and she got married at six o'clock in the morning, down in a church down there in [small town] down the road here, because she'd have to get married outside of hours and out of the way, in the dark, and everything like that.

Martina (b.1955) also felt that there was an enduring stigma even though she was married: 'And as well as that, having a baby at that time, 1973, it was a different Ireland. You were frowned upon. And even though you were married, sort of everybody knew you were married because you got pregnant'. Indeed, although marriage was seen as a more respectable option, as Nuala O'Faolain commented in her memoir, *Are you somebody*, following a shotgun wedding:

Then you had to think of some way to explain things, when the baby arrived, seven months into the marriage. Couples suddenly emigrated to England and Australia. Women moved across the country and gave birth and hid the babies and put pillows under their skirts, when their mothers came to see them. Hundreds of babies were firmly said to be 'premature'. No matter how progressive the circle you moved in, you lose everything if you became pregnant outside marriage.[101]

---

[100] Earner-Byrne, *Mother and Child*, p. 179.
[101] Nuala O'Faolain, *Are You Somebody? The Life and Times of Nuala O'Faolain* (London: Hodder and Stoughton, 1997 edition) p. 86.

Myra (b.1947) recalled one such incident of a 'premature' baby:

I had a best friend and we were at the wedding. We were at the wedding but I didn't know she was pregnant getting married at all, and about four months after she was married, I heard she was having a premature baby at four months. I said to John – I was very innocent you know. I said to John, gosh I said... 'Myra', he said, 'Would you cop on to yourself', he said, 'You couldn't have a full baby at only four months'.

Chastity was also policed by the community and by individuals' mothers. Mary Muldowney has suggested that 'judgemental attitudes were implicit in the closing of ranks against perceived non-conformists to women's role in the family'.[102] Helena (b.1945) told me, 'We got engaged very quickly, and married within about three months. And there was some nosy old woman up the road. I only heard this later, and she said, "Oh, oh, she's pregnant." So, lucky enough, it was 10 months before my first child was born (laughs)'. Helena added, 'It's dreadful the way you were watched years ago'. Ellen (b.1949) similarly recalled, 'there was one woman and when everyone would get married she'd write the date they got married on the back of the door, and then she'd be counting to see how soon they were having the baby'. Mary Margaret (b.1945) explained to me that she got pregnant on her honeymoon but that her doctor told her she would give birth in April. She told the doctor, 'No I can't, I can't have a baby in April ... I was only married on the 1ˢᵗ of August, it has to be May'. Because people might think she had had sex before marriage, she was 'in the horrors' and expressed to me her relief when she had the baby in May, which was 9 months and 2 days after her wedding date. She said that this meant 'her reputation was saved'. This was by no means unusual and sometimes respondents' mothers were responsible for the significant stress placed on their newlywed daughters. Ellen (b.1949) had her first baby nine months after her wedding. She said, 'My mother gave me a hard time over that as well. Yeah, she reckoned that if you have a baby straight away after you're married it was a sign you tried before. And no matter how many times I told her "No I didn't." She wouldn't believe me'. Similarly, Aoife (b.1947) explained that her first child was born nine months and six days after her marriage. She said, 'And right towards the end of the pregnancy, Mother was shocked. She used to say, "Now, just make sure that child doesn't arrive too early – the world doesn't want to know about your enthusiasm". She was horrified, horrified that I'd had sex'.

---

[102] Mary Muldowney, 'We were conscious of the sort of people we mixed with: The state, social attitudes and the family in mid twentieth century Ireland', *The History of the Family*, 13:4, (2008), pp. 402–15, on p. 410.

2.6   Conclusion

Looking back on her experiences as a young woman, Virginia (b.1948) stated:

It was more a God of fear than a God of love that we knew when we grew up. And honestly, so you wouldn't think about those kind of things. It was just going so wrong, and it was that guilt that it carried, wrongly. But that's how it was, yeah.

As this chapter has shown, men and women's experiences in relation to sexual knowledge as adolescents and young adults were shadowed by stigma and the emotions of fear and shame. As Joanne Bourke has argued in relation to fear, 'historians always need to ask: what is fear *doing*? The history of the emotions cannot ignore power relations'.[103] Evidently, by propagating a culture of fear and shame around sexuality and denying individuals access to basic sex education, the Church and State attempted to uphold rigid ideas about how men and women should behave. This culture had long-lasting effects. Fear could lead to unhealthy attitudes to sex later on in life and a lack of adequate sex education combined with the stigma of unmarried motherhood meant that for many individuals, sex was something to be feared, and unrealistic parameters were created around appropriate moral and sexual behaviour. Moreover, as Chapter 5 will show, for many respondents the idea that sex was wrong persisted into adulthood and the use of contraception made them feel significant guilt. The confession box continued to be an important sphere for reinforcing these ideas.

The majority of interviewees received no sex education. Information on sex was picked up in haphazard ways and the vacuum of knowledge was often filled with misinformation and confusion. Engaging in sex outside marriage with lack of access to contraception could result in pregnancy outside marriage which was laden with shame. The fear of potential shame could often act as a deterrent from sex but also contributed to a climate of anxiety around sexuality. While some booklets on sex education emerged in the 1950s and 1960s, these helped to reinforce ideas about what constituted 'good' moral behaviour. Parents were also generally reticent to discuss sex education with their children, instead, attempting to transmit moral codes through oblique messages or simply avoiding discussions altogether. Women, and particularly mothers, were also tasked with the responsibility of policing other's moral behaviour in their families and communities. Women's magazines and television programmes such as The Late Late Show instead reflect a tension between older ideas around

---

[103] Joanna Bourke, 'Fear and anxiety: Writing about emotion in modern history', *History Workshop Journal*, 55:1, (Spring, 2003), pp. 111–33, on p. 123.

sexual morality and newer, progressive ideas around sexual health: they were an important source of knowledge and discussion about sexuality and family planning, and attempted to push against these moral restrictions. However, ultimately, women continued to be tasked with the burden of upholding an unrealistic ideal of womanhood which had been propagated by the Church and State.

3   Birth Control Practices and Attitudes to Contraception in the 1960s and 1970s

Reflecting on the experiences of couples today and the impact that a lack of access to reliable contraception had for her, Siobhan (b.1942) explained:

I mean, the contraception thing … it's a pity now, I envy … I sort of, I would have loved to have known what it was like to have got married and have no children for five years. I would have loved that, and that's the one thing … I shouldn't be having regrets, but that – I would have loved that. I envy the couples getting married now that can start … I mean I would have loved that.

As outlined in the introduction, contraception was not legalised in Ireland until 1979, and even then, it could only be obtained for *bona fide* family planning purposes, or through a family planning clinic in an urban area. Some legal restrictions lasted into the 1980s and 1990s. For example, condoms could only be obtained on prescription until 1985 when the change in the law meant that they could be obtained over the counter in licensed premises such as chemists by individuals over the age of 18. Moreover, clear guidance and information on family planning was limited.

As the previous chapter has shown, lack of adequate sex education and a climate of shame around sex which was reinforced by Church teachings, meant that contraception was not just legally inaccessible during the 1960s and 1970s, but was fundamentally stigmatised. This chapter highlights how, in the absence of legal access to artificial methods, natural methods of family planning, in particular calendar-based methods remained popular, particularly for couples who were born in the 1930s and 1940s. In addition, for many couples, having children was an accepted part of marriage; contraceptive methods only tended to be used after participants had already had children in order to 'space' subsequent pregnancies, or in order to 'stop' pregnancies following the completion of the family.[1] In contrast to Ireland, visions of England as a 'permissive' society persisted well into the twentieth century. The chapter also seeks

[1] For a detailed overview of the 'stopping' vs 'spacing' debate, see Simon Szreter, *Fertility, Class and Gender in Britain, 1860–1940* (Cambridge University Press, 1996), pp. 367–440.

to explore the dynamics of decision-making around family planning in the period, illustrating how women began to exhibit more agency around these choices, and that contraception was generally seen as a female responsibility. It will also illuminate the impact that lack of access to artificial contraception had on individuals.[2]

3.1   Information on Family Planning

During the 1960s and 1970s, information on contraception and family planning was disseminated through a number of sources. Magazines were an important source of information for participants such as Helena (b.1945) who explained that 'Magazines were the only place you could get that sort-of thing'. Sandra (b.1951) similarly remembered *Woman's Way* being significant. She recalled, 'People were discussing spacing your family. [...] And people would write in saying, "I don't want to have any more children, I have ten. How do I tell my husband?" and stuff like this. And she'd ... she'd probably write back and say ... That was the way we gleaned some of our information do you know what I mean?' Brigid (b.1945) recalled finding out about the Billings Method through *Parent's Magazine*, telling me, 'I suppose that's really where I got the most information from'.

Natural methods of family planning in line with Catholic teachings were popularised in women's magazines by agony aunts such as Angela Macnamara from the early 1960s.[3] In a two part series in *Woman's Way* in 1963, Macnamara discussed recent debates around birth control, ultimately arguing that artificial contraception went against Catholic teachings and that it would lead to sexual promiscuity and 'moral degradation'.[4] Instead, she promoted abstention as a form of birth control.[5] In 1965, the magazine also ran an article entitled 'Regulation of Family' by the magazine's marriage counsellor, described as 'a woman doctor', which promoted the idea of responsible parenthood through the use of the rhythm method.[6] Angela Macnamara also received regular letters to her agony aunt column asking about contraception; she tended to advocate calendar methods such as the safe period, temperature method, and

---

[2] In discussing the methods of contraception utilised, this chapter will focus primarily on natural methods and the use of condoms. The pill is discussed in more depth in Chapter 4, while permanent forms of contraception such as tubal ligation and vasectomy, which became more increasingly available from the 1980s, are discussed in Chapter 9.

[3] For a detailed account of Angela Macnamara's life and work, see Ryan, *Asking Angela Macnamara*.

[4] Angela Macnamara, 'On Control', *Woman's Way*, 14 November 1963, p. 14.

[5] Angela Macnamara, 'Science and control', *Woman's Way*, 30 November 1963, p. 55.

[6] 'Regulation of family', *Woman's Way*, 1 March 1965, p. 21.

later Billings method.[7] Information on natural methods of family planning were also provided in the magazine. In 1970, in the 'Young Motherhood Bureau' section written by Sister Eileen, an explanation of the temperature method was provided. Women were encouraged to avail of a special thermometer 'incorporating the new international Centigrade scale and with an enlarged distance between two grades' so that they could properly detect the slight rise in temperature that occurred with ovulation.[8]

Articles providing information on artificial forms of contraception were also common in *Woman's Way* magazine from 1966 onwards, particularly through articles written by Monica McEnroy. The magazine included a series of articles on the pill in 1966 and in 1968 the contraception issue was regularly discussed in its letters pages.[9] Similarly, in 1973, *Nikki*, a short-lived magazine aimed at young Irish women, published a 'Guide to Sexual Knowledge: Contraception' which provided information on the main forms of contraception, including caps, condoms, spermicides, the pill, *coitus interruptus*, and the rhythm method. Acknowledging that 'it's against the official teaching of the Roman Catholic Church', the magazine stated that in publishing the piece, they were 'accepting reality – the reality of abortion, or illegitimate children, of spoiled young lives. It doesn't help to preach a sermon to a pregnant teenager – nor to think "it'll never happen to *my* daughter". It does. That's why we printed this article'.[10]

The Billings Method was also popularised in Ireland from the 1970s by a huge network of lay women. Mavis Keniry, a mother of two, founded an educational service on the Billings Method from her home in Dublin in the early 1970s. She later expanded this to the Dublin Ovulation Method Advisory Service, which later became the National Association of the Ovulation Method in Ireland (NAOMI). By 1978, there were eleven ovulation method advisory service centres operating in Dublin and over eighty centres throughout Ireland. Women could also receive information through a postal advisory service. Keniry was also appointed to the ten-member International Committee of WOOMB (World Organisation for the Ovulation Method-Billings), attending their annual nine-day conference in Los Angeles in 1978.[11] Under the Family Planning Act of 1979, a provision was made that a comprehensive

---

[7] See, for example: 'Angela Macnamara gives a helping hand', *Woman's Way*, 10 November 1967, p. 59 and 'Help page: Angela Macnamara', *Woman's Way*, 6 December 1974, p. 68.

[8] 'Young Motherhood Bureau', *Woman's Way*, 16 October 1970, p. 48.

[9] For discussions of the pill in *Woman's Way* see: Laura Kelly, 'Debates on family planning and the contraceptive pill in Irish magazine *Woman's Way*, *1963 –1973*', (*Women's History Review*, online 2021).

[10] 'Sexual knowledge: contraception', *Nikki*, July 1973, p. 54.

[11] 'Natural family planning', *Connacht Tribune*, 3 February 1978, p. 31.

natural family planning service would be introduced to provide information, instruction and advice on natural forms of family planning, and that a grant would be provided to assist with research into natural family planning.[12] This meant that from 1980, NAOMI was provided with a grant to assist with its work. By then, there were 19 centres in Dublin with 100 women involved in teaching. Keniry estimated that by 1980 20,000 women in Dublin were using the Billings method and 50,000 throughout the country.[13]

Pre-marriage courses were also important in providing information on family planning to couples. Courses run by priests which were aimed at educating engaged couples appear to have started up around the mid-1950s. From 1955, pre-marriage classes were established in Dublin by the Jesuit Fathers and the Catholic Social Welfare Bureau.[14] An article in the *Irish Examiner* in 1955 explained that the aim of these classes was to give engaged couples 'a grounding in Catholic principles as well as in the various material aspects of marriage'.[15] However, speaking at the Christus Rex Congress in the same year, Rev. Daniel F. Murphy, stated that 'these took in only the minority, and in rural parts little or nothing was done by way of pre-marriage instruction'.[16]

Dennis (b.1937) and his wife used the safe period after they were married in 1965 to space the births of their three children. They found out about the method through the pre-marriage courses they attended separately as they were living in two different cities before marriage. He recalled that his course in a city in the west of Ireland 'was one of the first that was set up and there was a lot of gynaecologists'. He was living in digs at the time with a married couple with three young children. Dennis explained:

I came home anyway one night after my pre-marriage course with all this data on the safe period. I went in and Paul the husband says, 'Well, how did you get on tonight?' 'I'll be telling you now, later on', you see? They'd been married before pre-marriage days, before. He would have been about seven or eight years older than me, you see? I got out my pen and paper and I went through all how to with him. Then shortly after that, I got the house here and I moved up here. I met Paul about nine months later and he says 'Do you see that lad in the pram, that's yours!'

---

[12] Health (Family Planning) Act, 1979. Accessed: www.irishstatutebook.ie/eli/1979/act/20/enacted/en/print

[13] *Evening Herald*, 17 September 1980, p. 3.

[14] *Clinical Report of the Rotunda Hospital, 1st January 1966 to 31st December 1966*, p. 68.

[15] 'Dublin letter', *Irish Examiner*, 27 September 1955, p. 4.

[16] 'Rev. lecturer deplores marginal Catholicism', *Evening Echo*, 13 April 1955, p. 2.

While this is an amusing anecdote and was told by Dennis with humour, it nevertheless illustrates how knowledge was passed between individuals and the potential for information to be miscommunicated or misunderstood.

From 1969, formal pre-marriage courses were run under the auspices of the Catholic Marriage Advisory Council (later CMAC) which was established in Ireland in 1962, later renamed Accord. By 1976, there were 22 pre-marriage centres in the Dublin diocese and 33 centres elsewhere in the country.[17] Father Paddy Gleeson, who had worked as an emigrant chaplain in Northampton, England, was asked by the new archbishop, Dermot Ryan, to get involved in coordinating the pre-marriage courses in Dublin in the 1970s. Gleeson was inspired by his previous experiences working in Dublin in the mid-1960s, where he 'was conscious I suppose that a lot of couples were getting married maybe in a hurry for the wrong reasons'. The CMAC marriage guidance courses therefore provided an opportunity for couples to discuss key issues in advance of marriage and ensure that they were more prepared for what was to come. Moreover, the CMAC also established natural family planning centres for couples to obtain more information on those techniques if they wished.

Father Gleeson also produced a guide for priests conducting pre-marriage courses in 1978. For a three session course, he advised that the first session should be concerned with how much the couple knew about each other, how they came to fall in love, plans for their life together, and issues such as money and household chores. The second session should cover love, infertility, methods of family planning (this element usually being delivered by a doctor), sex and parenthood. The third session should deal primarily with issues of faith, the marriage ceremony and family and community.[18] Father Gleeson explained to me that at the courses he was involved in, the talk given by the doctor on family planning 'described all the methods. I mean the methods at that time would be you know, condoms, intrauterine devices I suppose you know and the pill I suppose, they'd be basically. And of course, the possibility of sterilisation as well'.

Individuals' experiences of pre-marriage courses varied and there were regional differences. Mary Ellen (b.1944) from a rural part of the west of Ireland got married in 1974. She recalled that her pre-marriage course touched on intimacy in brief and with regard to contraception:

[17] 'Apprenticeship for marriage', *Irish Press*, 30 December 1976, p. 9.
[18] Fr Paddy Gleeson, *Helping Engaged Couples: A Guide for Priests* (Veritas Publications, 1978).

They talked about the different forms of family planning and contraception and that. But it would be brief. The doctor would be very brief. It was very conservative information at that particular time. Because it was an unspoken language, sex, in society.

Christine (b.1947) and Stephen (b.1943) who got married in Dublin in 1969 recalled the pre-marriage course they undertook which was run by the Jesuits. Stephen recalled that during the course 'I don't think the word sex was ever used', while Christine explained, 'Family planning wasn't mentioned, nothing like that'. Noel (b.1952) from a small town in the west of Ireland, got married in 1975. He said the information he and his wife received about family planning in their course was 'very, very cursory'. Similarly, Pierce (b.1948) who got married in 1971 explained that the information provided on the pre-marriage course 'was very general sort of stuff', stating that it was not 'too invasive' or 'too personal' but 'it gave us a general outline of, eh, well enough to be going along with it, you know?'

Catherine (b.1953) who undertook her pre-marriage course in London found that the priest who ran the course had more progressive attitudes towards contraception:

He said 'Well, this is the Church's official attitude.' 'But', he'd say, 'but to be honest', he said, 'it's up to your conscience. If you think that it's okay to do that, who am I to tell you that you can't?'. So even back in 1974, you know.

Yet, even by the 1980s, natural methods were still being encouraged at Irish pre-marriage courses. Denise (b.1961) who was married in 1983 in a rural part of a northern county said that she 'was as wise when I went in as I came out. I hadn't a clue. People, you would be afraid to ask a question'. She recalled there being an emphasis on three key methods of 'natural' family planning:

I think it was something about temperatures and it was a rhythm and temperatures and something else. There was three things. And abstinence was a big thing. You know, just between do this and do that, you just don't do it. That's it, you don't do it. And you certainly don't use condoms and you certainly don't go on the pill. You know, these were the methods you were to use. And I said, 'There is no way I am starting to take my temperature, every bloody day'.

Some men and women may have gleaned information from booklets. In 1966, a number of the London-based CMAC booklets were reportedly available to purchase from Gill's bookshop in Dublin. These included titles such as *Beginning Your Marriage* (1963) as well as publications by Professor John Marshall, including *Family Planning* (1963), *A Catholic*

View of Sex and Marriage (1965), and *The Infertile Period* (1963).[19] Books on family planning and reproductive health that had been published in England were also read by some participants. For example, Clare (b.1936) from the rural west of Ireland, explained that she found out about the temperature method through her 'sister, a nurse in England, and I think she sent me books on it'. Maria (b.1957) from a city in the west of Ireland also recalled reading the British book *Everywoman: a gynaecological guide for life* (originally published in 1971) by Derek Llewellyn-Jones, which she also gave to her female work colleagues to read.

The first Irish book dealing with sex education for adults, was Michael Solomons' *Life Cycle: Facts for Adults*, published in 1963. Solomons had been inspired to publish the book as a result of his experiences in medical practice and his bewilderment 'of the ignorance that I had encountered among my patients', particularly in relation to problems individuals had conceiving which he felt were not down to 'infertility but poor technique'.[20] The book provided detailed information on topics such as marriage, sexual intercourse, conception, labour, adolescence, menopause and old age, and included diagrams showing the male and female reproductive systems and a glossary outlining key terms relating to reproductive health.[21] According to Solomons, the book was 'well received. There was little adverse reaction and it went into paperback'.[22] The book did not, however, provide detailed information on family planning or contraception, perhaps owing to the social climate at the time, and in order to escape censorship. The safe period was briefly referred to in the section that dealt with conception, but only to make the point that it was unreliable.[23]

The first detailed Irish guide to family planning, *Family Planning: a guide for parents and prospective parents*, was published eight years later by the Fertility Guidance Company in 1971. In the introduction to the booklet, family planning was framed in terms of responsible parenthood.[24] The booklet sold 800 copies in its first month and new editions

---

[19] 'Patients' postbox', *Woman's Way*, 18 November 1966, p. 37. Marshall was a counsellor and chairman of the CMAC (1952–1996) who had, in his early career, published the first guide to the basal temperature method of natural family planning. He had been brought onto the 1962 papal commission by Pope John XXIII, as a medical representative and defender of the Church's stance on artificial contraception. Geiringer, *The Pope and the Pill*, pp. 37–8.

[20] Solomons, *Pro-Life*, p. 18.

[21] Michael Solomons, *Life Cycle: Facts for Adults* (Dublin: Allen Figgis, 1963).

[22] Solomons, *Pro-Life*, p. 18.   [23] Solomons, *Life Cycle*, p. 46.

[24] *Family Planning: A Guide for Parents and Prospective Parents* (Dublin: Fertility Guidance Co., 1971), p. 4.

were reprinted in coming years.[25] The book comprised of two main sections, the first on 'effective family planning methods' explored the pill, the intra-uterine device, the diaphragm and sterilisation while the second section 'less effective family planning methods' examined the rhythm method, condoms, foams and jellies, withdrawal, and complete abstinence. Each of these methods was described concisely and clearly with the advantages and disadvantages of each explained. The guide also dealt with myths and misunderstandings about family planning. After sterilisation, the pill was proposed as the most effective form of family planning. The IUD was outlined as the next most effective because 'like the pill, its application is not directly related to love-making, and it requires no adjustment after insertion'.[26] The temperature/rhythm method was deemed to be less effective and 'seldom advisable when there is a real medical or social necessity for the couple to avoid pregnancy'. Nevertheless, the guide explained that 'when conditions are right, however, the temperature method can be useful for reducing a couple's fertility and spacing their children'.[27] The initial version of the booklet escaped censorship but featured in a 1973 Dublin District Court case which will be further discussed in Chapter 8. Reprints of the guide in later years were similar in terms of the content provided, but also included detailed colour diagrams, which meant that it was picked up by the Censorship Board. The 1976 edition of the book was banned by the Censorship Board on the grounds that it was 'indecent and obscene'. The IFPA took a High Court case against the Censorship Board which they won. The Attorney General appealed but the ruling stood.[28] The 1978 third edition, also contained illustrations, however, it was noted in the IFPA's 1978 annual report that 'some of the artwork has been changed'.[29] Information was also provided on infertility and pregnancy tests.[30] Interestingly, there was also a slight shift in language, perhaps reflecting changes in social attitudes. In the original guide, the couple were usually referred to as 'the husband' and 'the wife', however, in the third edition, they were simply referred to as 'the man' or 'the woman'.

Students were also active in disseminating information. For example, a contraception guide was produced by the welfare officer of TCD, Kathy

---

[25] Solomons, *Pro-Life*, p. 37.   [26] *Family Planning*, p. 13.   [27] *Ibid.*, p. 14.
[28] Solomons, *Pro-Life*, p. 42.   [29] *IFPA Annual Report for 1978*, p. 5.
[30] *Family Planning: A Simple Guide to Contraception and Fertility* (Dublin: Irish Family Planning Association, 1978).

Gilfillan in 1971. In order to avoid prosecution, the author of the guide was listed as the collective student body and it was only distributed within the university grounds.[31]

Women also discussed and circulated information on family planning among themselves. Christine (b.1947) for example, stated, 'but you know when you're women and you have children and you're sort of chatting among yourselves. That's how we came to learn things, from one another. And some of course were a bit more knowledgeable than others, but that's how we learned about it'. Similarly, Diane (b.1949) explained how she found out about family planning through reading and from friends coming back from being abroad:

Well, when you have friends you investigate and you read and some goes to America, maybe on holidays or they go to abroad and they come back with … some people travelled and even in the 60s and 70s we travelled and come back with information from other places.

Men may also have shared information on the topic. Jeremiah (b.1942) explained that he learnt about family planning 'from the media or whatever, you know? And from the boys'. Yet, as the following sections will show, family planning was often viewed as the responsibility of women.

3.2   Attitudes to Family Planning

Con (b.1940) who grew up in the rural south-west explained:

There was no such thing as family planning in those days or anything else, you know and it wasn't even a matter for discussion at that stage in life, you know, it would have been many years later before people even discussed these things or spoke about them, you know and there wasn't much advice now, it was learned by experience and that was it really, you know. That was that.

Several respondents, like Con, and particularly those from the older cohort of participants, when first asked about family planning and contraception, stressed that 'there was no such thing' or expressed fatalistic attitudes towards having children. A couple, interviewed together, Tony and Emer (both b.1939) who spent their childbearing years in a city in the west of Ireland, were also united in this view:

[31] Steve Conlon, *The Irish student movement as an agent of social change: a case study analysis of the role students played in the liberalisation of sex and sexuality in public policy* (unpublished PhD thesis, Dublin City University, 2016), p. 166.

TONY: There was no such thing as contraceptives when we were younger.

EMER: Oh God no.

TONY: Nobody knew anything about them.

EMER: No.

TONY: No.

Given that the period when these respondents were getting married and starting to have children (1960s and 1970s) witnessed increased discussion of contraception in the media, these responses may seem surprising. However, they are revealing on three levels. First of all, the participants were keen to emphasise a difference in the experiences of their generation compared to mine, using phrases such as 'when we were younger' or 'in those days'. Indeed, as the discussion went on, participants often drew attention to the differences between their experiences and those of people of fertile age today. Secondly, as Chapter 2 demonstrated, there was a resounding lack of knowledge in relation to sex and reproduction, and indeed, for the older members of the cohort, particularly those living in rural areas, this may have been more pronounced. Respondents in Kate Fisher's study of family planning practices in England and Wales in the early twentieth century also emphasised a lack of knowledge and asserted their innocence of matters relating to contraception.[32] Indeed, in the Irish context, this may also have been the case. For instance, Úna (b.1944) who grew up in a city, explained:

Family planning? Not at all. And there was no such thing. There was nowhere to go at the time, do you know? It was something you didn't do. There was no family planning. That didn't come into it at all.

Many interviewees born in the 1940s also expressed an acceptance that having children was a normal part of married life. When asked about what she knew about family planning when she got married, Nellie (b.1944) from a rural part of the west of Ireland told me:

No. Absolutely nothing. You just knew that you wanted to have children and that would be it.

Maud (b.1947) who grew up in a rural part of the north of Ireland, explained that she 'didn't know any planning at all'. Her first child was born within a year of marriage and her second sixteen months later. She asked her doctor to prescribe her the pill but was refused. Her third child was born four years later but this gap was not planned, and she ascribed this space to illness. She had surgery after the birth of her third child and

---

[32] Fisher, *Birth Control*, pp. 26–75.

had no subsequent pregnancies as a result. Her sister, on the other hand, had six children, and Maud believed 'Now if I didn't have that surgery, I probably would have carried on'. In Maud's words:

She didn't do any planning or anything, because she was led to believe that was just how it was really. You went on and you had your babies. Didn't you?

Some female respondents such as Kate (b.1944) from a town in the south-east of Ireland, had a stoic attitude towards having children:

Oh yeah, it just... you got your baby, you got your baby, so you didn't...and you were pregnant again, so that was it. There was no big deal, oh my God.

Similarly, Irene (b.1942) who lived in the rural south-west contrasted her attitudes towards having children with those of women of childbearing age today:

I never minded becoming pregnant. And honestly... Didn't. And no, I didn't. I suppose it's just a way of life. It is a way of life. And that's so different. It's so different today isn't it?

For these respondents, it appears that in addition to there being an inability to access effective family planning methods, there was also a resistance towards family planning too. This may have been in part due to Catholic Church teachings at the time, as will be discussed further in Chapter 5, which placed emphasis on the idea that child-bearing was an integral part of marriage. It may also have been due to the social prestige of having a large family, as Kevin C. Kearns has suggested in his study of Dublin tenement life, stating that 'in working-class culture, there was a natural pride in having produced a small tribe of sons or daughters'.[33] Tom Inglis suggests that large families could be ascribed not only to individuals following Church teachings, but peer pressure from mothers and other women.[34] Having large families meant, however, that low employment rates persisted for Irish women as childcare was difficult to arrange and would not have been economically viable.[35]

Many respondents referred to 'pot luck' with regard to children and taking what came. Christina (b.1935) from a small town in the Midlands, stated:

And we, kind of you just take pot luck with... that's the way we did at that time. There was no such thing as contraception.

---

[33] Kevin C. Kearns, *Working Class Heroines: The Extraordinary Women of Dublin's Tenements* (Dublin: Gill Books, 2018), p. 132.

[34] Inglis, *Moral Monopoly*, p. 185.

[35] Lindsey Earner-Byrne and Diane Urquhart, 'Gender roles in Ireland since 1740' in Eugenio F. Biagini and Mary E. Daly (eds.), *The Cambridge Social History of Modern Ireland* (Cambridge University Press, 2017), pp. 312–26, on p. 317.

Emer and Tony had a similar attitude, stating that in contrast with younger generations, they did not plan the number of children they would have:

TONY: It was pot luck.
EMER: That's it.
TONY: Whereas now they plan their family, don't they? At that time you didn't.
EMER: If they come they come and that's it.
TONY: If you had another one that was it.

Similarly, Stephen (b.1943) and Christine (b.1947) explained to me that they didn't ask their doctor for advice about family planning after the birth of their first child:

STEPHEN: No, because we felt possibly that... We probably didn't... Did we really think about whether we'd need it? No?
CHRISTINE: We didn't think about it or talk about it, even. No, we just went on with life.
STEPHEN: Went on with life and things were probably a little bit easier with families in those days, there wasn't as much going on. You know? We were just husband and wife, we were in this house. I was working and you weren't because I was bringing in a reasonably good wage and we were happy in what we had. And we did what married people do and... what happened then? A second child came along but there was no planning, there was no thought that... 'We're going to have two'.

For Stephen and Christine, family planning was not a topic of discussion in the early years of their marriage as they both wanted to have children, and this decision was informed by a sense that having children was 'what married people do'. Moreover, as Stephen explained, with Christine working in the home, they felt that there was less of a need for them to consider spacing the pregnancies. Other interviewees expressed similar views, such as when Anthony (b.1934) was asked if he and his wife had considered how many children they wanted to have, he replied, 'No, we kind-of just took it as it came'. These fatalistic attitudes to having children perhaps reflect a few things: fundamentally, a lack of information on and access to contraception. But they are also revealing of the persistence of the traditional family structure in Ireland during the 1960s and 1970s which designated the husband as the breadwinner and confined his wife to the role of homemaker and mother. Several respondents reflected on these gender roles. Ann (b.1945) felt that while her husband was a 'a good man. A great father and great worker kind of thing. But I ran the show, if you know what I mean'. In Ellen's (b.1949) view:

the men were no good back then, I can tell you that now. Men didn't change nappies, men didn't dress children, men didn't do anything, feed them, do anything until they were well able to get up and run around and dress themselves sort of, you know? The men didn't do anything. [...] Men expected you to give up your job and stay at home and look after the house, and bring up their children. That was just I think the normal kind of a thing.

Annie (b.1939) who had eleven children, explained how organised she needed to be with housework:

Oh, you had to have everything ready the night before. Them times, they didn't have three or four pair of shoes, they had the one pair of shoes, and you polished them every night when they were gone to bed like. And leave out their socks and pants and you know, what they had for the next day. Oh you had. I remember I used to iron when they were all gone to bed and everything. And I could be ironing up to twelve o'clock like. Then the minute I'd sit down, sure I was falling asleep.

Changes in equality legislation including the removal of the marriage bar in 1973, as well as shifting values in relation to gender equality which were associated with the women's movement, meant that for the younger couples in the cohort, contraception and family planning were more important considerations.[36]

Some respondents also drew a distinction between their experiences and attitudes towards the possibility of planning one's family and those of their children, or my own generation. Paula (b.1955) from an urban part of the west of Ireland, explained that she had discussed the issue with her daughter who had asked about whether she and her sibling were planned and that her daughter found it hard to understand that there had been no planning involved or thought given to the number of children that her mother wanted. Paula explained:

No. I feel foolish acknowledging it because of your generation, people seem to be taken aback. Did I sit down and plan? No. We didn't plan. No. It was just I was pregnant and it was happy news and I was delighted.

A number of interviewees thus had their first child soon after getting married. Jim (b.1933) from Dublin, explained to me that he and his wife's first child, 'was conceived the day we got married. It had that feel about it'. Many respondents also reflected on a sense of lack of control over the number of children they would have. Bridget (b.1945) had her first child a year after her marriage, and went on to have four more children within the following six years. She explained:

But I suppose families at that time weren't so restricted numbers-wise, I think. It just kinda happened, you know? I think that's the way it was with most people at the time.

[36] Kennedy, *Cottage to Creche*, pp. 94–5.

Similarly, Sally (b.1956) who grew up in the rural east, recounted the feeling she had that there was no option but to have children, particularly because of a lack of contraception. In her view, pregnancy 'was there waiting for you. And it was like a train crash, you were born straight on the line, because there's no way of your being able to prevent it'.

Such attitudes appear to have persisted into the 1970s and 1980s. Nicholas (b.1953) from a city in the west of Ireland, explained that after marriage, 'I would have said that our thoughts would have been to have children as soon as it was quickly possible, practically possible'. Financial stability was not a major consideration, in Nicholas' view 'The biggest factor would be just having children'. Likewise, Pól (b.1948) from a small town in the west of Ireland, and his wife, married in their thirties and as a result 'contraception never came into it. Or family planning didn't come into it. We wanted children straight away and so, we were aware of it. But it wasn't even come up for discussion because we wanted ...' Clodagh (b.1940) from the rural Midlands expressed that she felt the purpose of getting married was to have a family and as a result, she did not have concerns about spacing her children:

I'll tell you really what you thought about was, you got married to have a family, that's what everybody done, you know you didn't think, 'Oh my God there's a whole load of them going to come together'.

Clodagh's testimony also highlights the social pressure she felt around having children:

You see you'd be terrified you weren't going to have kids, that would be the thing you'd be thinking about that way when you were getting married, that was what marriage was about, having children like and everyone just loved to have children that's the sort of thing you know.

When she didn't become pregnant after four months of marriage, Clodagh was worried she was not able to have children. This concern may have emanated from the pressure she felt to have children but the issue of infertility was also beginning to be more widely discussed in the press, such as in women's magazines.[37] However, Clodagh soon became pregnant with her first child and by the age of 28 she had a total of six children (including a set of twins) under the age of four and ten months. Four years later she had another child, and her eighth child was born when she was 46. Clodagh explained:

[37] See for example: Elizabeth M. Hayes, 'When a baby never comes', *Woman's Way*, 30 August 1968, pp. 14–15 and *Woman's Way*, 6 September 1968, pp. 34–5.

I mustn't have known much about birth control anyway, did I? No, but the first few you wouldn't be thinking about it. You wouldn't even dream about – it was only then when I had the six, it was, when I had – then I just said to myself, but the birth control there was no artificial birth control, you had to control yourself or ourselves, shall we say you know.

In Clodagh's case, as with many other respondents, family planning practices were not used until the couple had already had a number of children and wanted to space subsequent ones, while many other respondents only began to use contraceptive practices for 'stopping' when they had completed their family size. And in some cases, because the woman in the couple had reached menopause, family planning was no longer an issue. Several respondents did not engage in any attempt at family planning, again, perhaps due to an acceptance that having children was a part of marriage, but also potentially due to a lack of knowledge. Bridget (b.1945) for example, told me:

We were as green as could be, you know? We didn't really … you just kind of … I don't know. We didn't really, and you know if you asked, the honest truth was I suppose none of them were planned, do you know, that kind of way? It just happened. Do you know?

3.3   The Prevalence of Natural Methods

With a lack of access to artificial contraception, the only option for most couples who wanted to limit their families was to abstain from sex or utilise calendar-based methods such as the safe period, temperature method or Billings method. As Table 3.2 in the Appendix shows, the 21 oral history respondents who were born in the 1930s all tended to use natural forms of family planning such as the safe period, temperature method or Billings method, with the exception of four individuals and one couple who said they used no form of family planning, and two respondents who used the safe period, the pill and condoms during their fertile years. These findings correlate with Betty Hilliard's study of 105 women in Cork city which suggested that the women in her sample relied on 'combinations of luck, natural methods and their partner's co-operation to curtail their number of pregnancies'.[38]

Nuala (b.1935) who grew up in a small town in the Midlands and married in 1964, when asked what people would do to space their children stated: 'Go to different beds I suppose. I'd say that was the solution'. With regard to information on family planning, Nuala said,

[38] Hilliard, 'The Catholic Church and married women's sexuality', p. 36.

'I would say we didn't know anything about it any way.' Similarly, after the birth of their two children, Christine (b.1947) and her husband used abstinence. She explained to me, 'After the second, we were careful but that would've been abstinence, it wasn't anything else. No pill or any-thing else. We didn't know anything about them, at that stage'. Eibhlin (b.1943) also practised abstinence after the birth of her fifth child:

I was forty when I had him, so I sure did, yeah I was just being very careful because I didn't... I knew I was at an age when it wasn't good... well, it could be quite dangerous you know? And I said, definitely five was enough you know.

For the majority of interviewees who did engage in family planning, calendar-based methods were commonly used in the absence of other forms of reliable contraception. Of the 99 total respondents who had been married, 47 reported using a calendar method such as the safe period, temperature method or Billings. The Knaus-Ogino method of family planning or 'rhythm method' was developed from the findings of Japanese gynaecologist Ogino Kyusaku and Austrian gynaecologist Hermann Knaus who separately calculated the time of ovulation in 1924 and 1929 respectively.[39] Based on his findings, Knaus worked out that in normal circumstances, ovulation usually took place 14 days before the next period began.[40] In 1951, Pope Pius XII declared that the Knaus-Ogino method was acceptable to the Catholic Church, thus bringing it to worldwide attention.[41] However, the method was very unreliable as there could be many reasons for fluctuations in a woman's cycle.[42] Writing to the *Sunday Independent* in 1968, H. L. from Dublin commented that for the vast majority of people the rhythm method was 'a real game of guesswork, with no real guarantee of success'. In her view:

It is very hard on young married couples to have to limit their lovemaking to a few days every month, and believe me, it boils down to a few days each month if one wants to be absolutely sure of non-conception. For myself, I have no so-called safe period after a period as my cycle is 25–31 days. Under these circumstances it is very hard for me to have a satisfactory relationship with my husband as often times he is working late, and I am asleep when he gets in, or I am babysitting and he is asleep when I get in. The result is that I often have no intercourse for 3–4 months at a time. Needless to say, this is very frustrating and as a result both myself and my husband suffer from tension and nerves.[43]

---

[39] Donna Drucker, *Contraception: A Concise History* (MIT Press, 2020), p. 33.
[40] Robert Jutte, *Contraception: A History* (Wiley, 2008), p. 204.
[41] Jutte, *Contraception*, p. 205.   [42] *Ibid.*, p. 204.
[43] 'Rhythm: a real game of guesswork', *Sunday Independent*, 25 August 1968, p. 8.

Tessie (b.1938) and her husband used the safe period which she described as: 'You'd be trying to gauge in between and hope for the best, you know what I mean?' She and her husband used the method in combination with the withdrawal method. Ellen (b.1949) went to her doctor after having three children in two and a half years:

So, when I said it to the doctor then I said, 'What will I do?" And he said, "Well I don't agree with giving the pill but I'll kind of tell you about the safe period'. As they called it. So he just said, for five days after your period you're okay, but then for about two weeks you shouldn't do anything and then the week before the period again. You know, if you're fairly regular you could kind of work that out.

The safe period was often described by male respondents as being something that their wife was responsible for, or they alluded to the fact that women were more knowledgeable about this method of family planning. Colm (b.1940) explained that the 'safe period wasn't something that lads discussed. You know what I mean? It was a woman's problem'. Ronan (b.1933) and his wife started using the safe period method after having six children. They had not used any method prior to this. He explained, 'But we did, we did at that stage then, we started em, family planning you know and watching the safe time to have intercourse. But up to that no, nothing. So that was the beginning of it but that was after having six children'. From Ronan's testimony, it appears that his wife took responsibility for the method; he explained that:

the women would know more about these things than we would. And she would read books. She was a very good reader and she would you know. And to be sure, she'd be talking to her friends and other women and she'd learn that way. So between what she read and meeting other young married women in the same position.

For Ronan, however, 'It was all new to me. Ovums and all the rest of it'. Such statements contrast with Kate Fisher's findings for 1930s and 1940s Britain which showed that contraception was a male responsibility and that 'birth control was seen as an essential element of a husband's duty.[44] In the Irish context, for participants born in the 1930s, 1940s and 1950s, responsibility for contraception appears to have lied predominantly with the female partner.

The safe period method was less reliable and many of the respondents who used it found that it did not work for them. Gráinne (b.1937) who had eight children, told me 'It was talked sometimes about the safe

[44] Fisher, *Birth Control*, pp. 189–237.

period and everything, and my husband considered that was hogwash. And I think it was because it didn't work for us anyway'. Similarly, Winnie (b.1938) who had seven children, explained that she 'would vaguely have, you know, without, in my last couple of children probably, I would have tried to mind the different time of the month to... It never really worked. Didn't pay a lot of heed now to be honest'. Mary Margaret (b.1945) who successfully used the safe period in combination with breastfeeding to space her four children, admitted that there were 'a lot of mistakes made too, that was human nature'.

The safe period method relied on having a regular cycle and women with any variation on this struggled to use it reliably. Siobhan (b.1942) from the rural Midlands, had five pregnancies in total. She tried to use the safe period method after the birth of her first baby but found that she became pregnant with her second child. She explained 'I know for a fact that I was caught on the 24th day', which, under the rules of the safe period should have been an infertile day. Similarly, she later conceived on another occasion 'maybe three days after the period. Like, I worked that out. I knew myself. So I couldn't have worked a safe period system'. She explained that for her 'There was no safe period' and 'So, I was just terrified' as she believed that any time she had sex it could result in a pregnancy. Similarly, Lily (b.1946) who grew up in the rural north of the country, and had three children, used the safe period as a method of family planning when she got married after experiencing negative side effects on the contraceptive pill. She found that the safe period mostly worked for her, but with her first pregnancy 'I was caught – I was caught you know, I was caught when I'm like ... you know when they say your cycle is 28 days, mine used to be 32. And I was caught on the 28th day'. Siobhan and Lily's use of the term 'caught' highlights the unreliable nature of the safe period and the sense that pregnancy was out of their control.

Calendar based methods may also have been difficult for women with a number of children who may not have had the time to chart their cycles. Evelyn (b.1940) used the safe period for a while to space her pregnancies, but believed that:

Obviously, it's very difficult. I'm sure if people were clinically good at this sort of stuff and took the time, it's like anything, you'd probably be able to work things out right? For somebody with a lot of kids and who's busy, that would be difficult.

Similarly, Colette (b.1946) who lived in a small city, used the safe period primarily for religious reasons, switching to condoms later. She recalled the anxiety during her use of calendar methods when she was coming up to the time of her period:

Oh, you … coming up to the time when … I think it was when a period was due. You would be uptight, absolutely, and I mean I would suffer a bit with premenstrual tension. Not very badly or anything, but that combined with this. As I say, the most wonderful cramp you could have. Sore boobs. You know, oh God. […] Oh, I could never understand people in later years, 'Oh, she suffers terrible with her pains', would you go away, it was the best pain I ever had.

She contrasted this with her experience using condoms as 'No, I remember thinking that it's a shame I didn't start doing it years ago. You know? Because I mean it took all the worry and all the counting and all the rest of it and …'

The temperature method of family planning was developed by a Catholic priest, Wilhelm Hildebrand, who linked the measurement of basal temperature to birth control, finding that at the time of ovulation, a woman's body temperature rises by about 0.4 to 0.6 degrees Centigrade and that the temperature remained raised until around the start of the woman's next period.[45] This method, however, required the woman to keep a careful record of rises in body temperature.[46] The Billings method, developed by Australian married couple, Dr. John and Dr. Evelyn Billings, was a more reliable form of natural family planning. It involved observation of changes in the cervical mucus and charting in order to detect periods of fertility and infertility. As mentioned earlier, the method was popularised in Ireland from the 1970s by NAOMI.

The temperature method could also be constraining and respondents who used it perceived it to be unreliable. Clare (b.1936) described the method as 'taking temperatures and keeping records and all that', which she found 'boring'. She found that 'it kind-of worked, but you couldn't be 100% relying on it'. Similarly, Pierce (b.1948) and his wife used the temperature method after their first two children, which he described as 'You had to take your temperature. It was supposed to go up a bit or go down a bit', however, although his wife did it for a period of time, they still conceived a third child. 'So it wasn't working very well. (laughs)'. Likewise, Julia (b.1946) went to the doctor for family planning advice and was told about the temperature method, but 'I did that for a while but it didn't seem to … (laughs) I don't know if I was taking it right or not, but it didn't seem to work for me when you had four of them in three years'. Similarly, Ellie (b.1944) found out about the temperature method from an aunt who was a nun. However, she 'lost the thermometer one morning, and couldn't find it (laughs) […]"Oh, that's that."' A 1971 *Woman's Way* article reflected on the challenges individuals faced in using the method. While the article acknowledged that the method was

---

[45] Jutte, *Contraception*, p. 205.   [46] *Ibid.*

useful for women with regular periods and for women who wished to abide by Church teachings against artificial contraception, it had a failure rate of 7 out of every 100 women who used the method, with a higher failure rate for those who used the method in a 'half-hearted' way.[47] Myra (b.1947) tried using the temperature method but explained her confusion about it:

But sure I was doing it all wrong. I used to be sitting up in bed feeding the child and take this temperature. You weren't supposed to do anything like that, it'll tell you how stupid we were. You know, yeah, yeah, you were supposed to — when you woke up in the morning, you were supposed to take that lying down before you did anything else. So if you had a baby boy alongside you, like you couldn't do that but we were doing that.

While Myra seemed to blame herself for her inefficient use of the method, it is evident that little effective guidance was being provided at the time, which meant that women often picked up information in a haphazard way.

Calendar-based methods did, however, rely on having what Mary Ellen (b.1944) from the rural west of Ireland described as a 'considerate' husband. She felt that 'Not all men would be considerate. A lot of them would be very demanding men sexually'. A letter to *Woman's Way* in 1971 emphasised this point, stating, 'Women with husbands who refuse to work the safe period are in a sad position. If the husband is selfish about this aspect of marriage it often follows that he is mean and inconsiderate in other aspects too'.[48] Similarly, Christina (b.1935) who used the safe period, described her husband as 'very considerate'. Margaret (b.1954) who used the Billings Method also described her husband as 'extremely understanding' and 'very considerate'.

Abstention during fertile times could be difficult for some couples in terms of reducing the spontaneity of sex and potentially reducing sexual pleasure because of the fact that sex took place in at the point in the cycle when the woman was not fertile.[49] Colm (b.1940) felt that safe period 'I always looked on, it was sex by appointment. Not sex on instincts. Which I think that's, that ... I think that's wrong too'. Colm felt that sex on impulse was preferable to being told, in his words, 'Oh Jaysus, I can't go

---

[47] Kate Kennelly, 'Dilemma: report on family planning', *Woman's Way*, 22 January 1971, p. 24.

[48] 'Over to you...', *Woman's Way*, 23 April 1971, p. 6.

[49] In her study of birth control practices in England and Wales, Kate Fisher similarly found that some of her respondents reported that appliance methods were less favoured because they removed the spontaneity necessary for sexual pleasure. Fisher, *Birth Control*, p. 170.

to till next, what, Sunday'. Julie (b.1947) from the rural west of Ireland explained:

I would have known the theory of it all, but the theory is one thing, and the Billings method was the … we were supposed to be using, but that's fine, except that the time that you really want to be close to somebody is actually your fertile period. So it's actually doubly hard. My husband used to say he only had to look at me for me to get pregnant. He only need to look at me he used to say. That's not quite true.

Ellen (b.1949) also remarked on the problems of abstaining during the fertile time of the cycle, which for her, was about two weeks of the month under the guidelines of the safe period. She stated, 'But you know, human nature being what it is, you want sex at the time that you're supposed to have it'. Teresa (b.1946) from a small town in the southwest had a similar experience using the Billings Method. She found, 'it was awkward enough because – our friends and we'd be talking about it like that's a very controlled thing and being sexually active it isn't that you want to be sexually active when you're safe, you know'. Margaret (b.1954) who used the Billings method to plan her pregnancies, worked out that there were 12 days in her 31–32 day cycle which was a 'no go area and then the rest was possible if the mood was up to it.' She did not find the method completely satisfactory in that:

You were having it [sex] at your dry time of the month when you neither had the inclination nor the physical body symptoms that would make it easy for you to have sex. So it wasn't a good thing at all. I, I did not find it a good thing.

The scientific nature of the Billings Method was also off-putting to some women and cycle-charting could be onerous. Carol (b.1954) who found out about the Billings method on her pre-marriage course, described it as 'undignified and ridiculous … and it didn't work apart from anything else'. Eibhlin (b.1943) was told about the Billings Method by her friend who was a nurse. Eibhlin described the method as 'it was to do with mucus and stuff and that was kind of complicated for me'. She explained:

I had a friend […] and she was advising me because I had them pretty near together. I had one a year after the other like, you know. The first two, the first two there was only a year between them. And then the next one, there was two years so, it was like that. She was telling me about this Billings method and everything but I never really did it. I didn't really have much patience for that kind of … kind of stuff and there was very little contraception there. So it was kind of just to hope for the best, you know?

Bridget (b.1945) used the safe period to work out when she and her husband should abstain from sex. She had heard about the Billings method but, 'it seemed to me to be very complicated. So, I mean, I didn't even enter into the discussion'. She added that 'it was just too formal or something, or do you know?'

Others found that calendar-based methods worked for them. Nellie (b.1944) began using the safe period as she got older as a result of concerns about the increased likelihood of having a baby with Down's Syndrome. She explained, 'You just had a thing about ... you'd know when you'd be menstruating so you could have a fair idea'. Similarly, Sarah (b.1947) who grew up on a farm in the north of the country, found out about the Billings method at the pre-marriage course she attended with her fiancé in the early 1980s. She recalled, 'You kept a kind of chart of the monthly cycle, and the changes, and you knew then you were ovulating. That was kind of it, it worked all right'. Frances (b.1952) from the north of the country, used the Billings method and found 'Family planning for me was very simple, because I really and always had very regular menses, so I never had any problem with that'. Of course, calendar methods were also useful for couples who were trying to conceive a child. Bernadette (b.1947) from the rural west of Ireland, went to her doctor to seek advice on family planning as she was hoping to conceive. She began to use the temperature method to try 'to make out when you were ovulating in the month'.

Natural methods were also preferable for some respondents because they were in line with Church teachings. Eamonn (b.1933) from the rural south-west of the country, married his wife in 1961 and after having three children, they used the Billings method. He described this as:

So you weren't altogether starved of sex. There were certain days you refrained, and you paid close attention to the body heat and so on that it all entails. And it does work. If used properly, it does work. So if you want to go according to the Church, that's the way you go.

For Eamonn, this was the only method of family planning that was acceptable to him because it was in line with the Church's teachings on the use of contraception. Christina (b.1935) and her husband used the safe period after having six children, for economic reasons, because they felt that they would not have been able to 'afford many more' but also because it was in line with Church teaching and 'being a Catholic, I don't think if there was [artificial contraception] I would've used it'. Others used the Billings method as a result of an unsatisfactory experience with other forms of contraception. Maria (b.1957) used the contraceptive pill but found the method unsatisfactory because of the side effects she experienced. She and her husband later used condoms, as well as the Billings method to try and minimise the use of condoms, which they did not find completely satisfactory, and spermicides 'when you were being extra cautious'.

The withdrawal method was referred to by a number of respondents, and also depended on a considerate husband. In her 1969 book *Marriage Irish Style*, Dorine Rohan included a quote from a woman who stated, 'We have had four children in five years, and we don't want any more for the moment – but my husband is very decent, he uses the withdrawal method'.[50] Alice (b.1944) and her boyfriend sometimes used condoms but often 'he just used the *coitus interruptus*. That's the most dangerous thing, my God'. As well as being risky, Alice felt that the method was 'inhuman as well. It really just interferes with kind-of...'. Similarly, Teresa (b.1946) described the withdrawal method as 'that was an awful thing' and that she 'knew the risk was very high'. Alice and Teresa's comments perhaps could be read to be alluding to how the withdrawal method interfered with sexual pleasure. In her study of the birth control practices of men and women in England and Wales born in the early twentieth century, Kate Fisher found that some women reported that use of the withdrawal method diminished their sexual pleasure.[51] Yet, in the Irish context, there were few other options. Irene (b.1942) and her husband also used the withdrawal method to try and space their pregnancies because 'There was nothing else, like, you know?' The withdrawal method may have been used by couples who did not mind an unplanned pregnancy. Jacinta (b.1954) and her husband used the withdrawal method to space their second-last and final children. Aware of the risks involved with this method, Jacinta stated, 'We didn't mind if it didn't work because we didn't mind getting pregnant again, you see'.

Breastfeeding was another natural form of birth control, however, it only worked as a method of family planning for as long as the mother was feeding the child. Writing to the *Sunday Independent* in 1966, a mother of five from Limerick advocated breastfeeding as a method of family planning, stating 'If a mother nurses her baby for nine months (and what better method exists for both child and mother?) there is a time lag of twelve months almost. I know – it happened to me with five of them!'.[52] However, a response to this letter, while congratulating the mother of five 'on her ability to nurse her family' stated that 'unfortunately, a great many mothers, much as they would like to, find it impossible to do this'.[53] Similarly, as Caitriona Clear notes, Irish mothers consciously turned away from breastfeeding in the 1940s and 1950s, due to the

[50] Dorine Rohan, *Marriage Irish Style*, p. 67.   [51] Fisher, *Birth Control*, pp. 171–2.
[52] 'Mother of five replies', *Sunday Independent*, 24 July 1966, p. 17.
[53] 'Birth control...', *Sunday Independent*, 7 August 1966, p. 15.

constraints of work (particularly for farming women) and home life.[54] However, oral history evidence from one of her informants born in 1928 in Mayo suggests that some women were aware that breastfeeding might suppress ovulation and practised it to space their pregnancies.[55] A small number of interviewees in my study recalled using breastfeeding to space their pregnancies. Mary Margaret (b.1945) from a city, had four children with four years between each. She explained that she 'never in·my life, practised safe sex. I never took a pill, never had a condom, never in my life did I take to anything like that. Never. Not even once'. Instead, she explained, 'I breastfed my children, and it gave me space. And then I was careful. I knew I was ... I knew you could get pregnant so. And I was careful and I had four years between each one of my children'. In this instance, the use of 'careful' by Mary Margaret inferred that she was aware of her cycles and the days she was fertile, and avoided sex on these days.[56] Jacinta (b.1954) from Dublin also found that breastfeeding helped her to space her children but when she wanted to have a longer space, she needed to switch to another method:

I had Niamh when I was twenty-three. I didn't even know that your periods stop when you're pregnant. I knew nothing really. Whatever I'd read. I knew very little. Now, I know your periods can come back when you are breastfeeding. Mine didn't. So I would have breastfed her for a year and a half and that worked for us contraception wise without us even knowing it. Then I realised this works. So we had Mary at twenty-five, Susan at twenty-seven, and Paula at thirty. But I was actually breastfeeding as contraception.

After the birth of their four children, Jacinta and her husband decided they needed to take a break and used the withdrawal method for five years before the birth of their fifth child. Edward (b.1950) who lived in a city in the west of Ireland explained that his wife breastfed their second child 'for over a year and then a few months after that she got pregnant'.

For respondents born in the 1940s, it is evident that there was a wider range of family planning methods used, and family sizes were on average smaller than the respondents born in the 1930s. Table 3.2 illustrates

---

[54] Caitriona Clear, 'The decline of breastfeeding in 20th century Ireland' in Alan Hayes and Diane Urquhart (eds.), *Irish Women's History* (Dublin: Irish Academic Press, 2004), pp.187–98, on pp. 193–7.

[55] Clear, 'The decline of breastfeeding', p. 195.

[56] The term 'being careful' could sometimes refer to the withdrawal method but in this case, Mary Margaret was clear that this meant she monitored her cycles.

the persistence of calendar methods such as the safe period, temperature method and Billings method, but also that many individuals used a range of methods during their reproductive years. Natural methods remained popular; 21 out of 45 respondents born in the 1940s (46%) mentioned using calendar methods with 7 (15%) mentioning use of the withdrawal methods. Artificial methods were more popular among this cohort: 14 (31%) used the pill, 9 (20%) used condoms, 5 (11%) used the coil.

For respondents born in the 1950s and who mostly married in the 1970s and 1980s, it is evident that a wider range of methods were used, with higher rates of the pill, male and female sterilisation and condoms and reduced use of natural methods. As Table 3.3 illustrates, respondents born in the 1950s onwards tended to use artificial methods more than natural methods of contraception in comparison with the older interviewees. In particular, the contraceptive pill, which will be discussed in Chapter 4, was more widely used among women in the cohort born in the 1950s. Of the 33 respondents born in the 1950s, 18 (54.5%) reported using the pill during their marriage and 11 (33%) reported using condoms. Only 7 (21%) mentioned using calendar methods. This increase in the use of artificial methods was likely due to increasing availability, but also, as Chapter 5 will show, decreasing adherence to Church teachings among younger respondents. Permanent methods of contraception such as vasectomy and tubal ligation were also more common among the younger cohort; these methods will be discussed more in Chapter 9.

3.4   Access to Artificial Contraceptives

Class and location inevitably had an influence on individuals' birth control options. In 1973, an article in *Woman's Way* by Monica McEnroy stressed that 'rich women make their own arrangements and have no trouble getting a prescription for the pill signed regularly, or a diaphragm fitted by a gynaecologist. In rural Ireland difficulties are frequently solved by travelling to the nearest area where medical practice is competitive'.[57] Similarly, a woman writing to Mary Kenny's newspaper column in 1970 alluded to the difficulties faced by women who were less well-off, stating 'Because we have Medical Cards we cannot demand these things, but we know for a fact there are some well-off women able to get

---

[57] Monica McEnroy, 'Family planning prohibited', *Woman's Way*, 9 November 1973, pp. 12–13.

them without any bother and they snigger when they see us pregnant so often while they themselves pretend to be goody-goodies'.[58]

It is clear, that for the majority of men and women living in Ireland in the 1960s and 1970s, access to artificial contraception was difficult and depended significantly on class and location. Carmel and Martin (b.1952) who both lived in a small town explained:

MARTIN: We didn't know people who would be bringing in that sort of thing.
CARMEL: So, I mean –
MARTIN: It's not that would have been objected to, we just genuinely didn't know anybody-
CARMEL: You just wouldn't have known where to get your hands on something like that.
MARTIN: You may as well have been looking for cocaine, or something.

Martin's comparison of contraceptives to cocaine highlights the illegality and illicit nature of artificial contraceptives such as condoms. Similarly, Maria (b.1957) who married her husband in 1976, expressed the problems they had in getting access to contraception:

Because of the whole contraception thing, the difficulty around that. It was so hit and miss. Even when we were a few years married it was still so difficult, the availability of contraception, unless you were on the pill. That was the only thing. I mean, condoms were only available maybe in the family planning clinic.

As Maria's testimony shows, access to contraception was challenging, and this meant that those without the means to obtain artificial contraception, often had to resort to natural methods if they wanted to engage in family planning. Class, without doubt, was an important factor for oral history respondents' choice of family planning method, but location also had an important bearing.

As Chapter 1 has shown for the early twentieth century, there was a trade of contraceptives between Ireland and the UK. More broadly, the UK, as a result of its proximity to Ireland, was a market for reproductive healthcare and support, since at least the early twentieth century.[59] From 1968, with the introduction of the Abortion Act, Irish women also began to travel, primarily through 'abortion corridors' such as Liverpool and London, for terminations.[60] Oral history evidence also

---

[58] 'Woman's Press,' Irish Press, 9 November 1970, p. 8.
[59] See: Earner-Byrne, 'The Boat to England'.
[60] See: Earner-Byrne and Urquhart, The Irish Abortion Journey; Ann Rossiter, Ireland's Hidden Diaspora: The Abortion Trail and the Making of a London–Irish Underground, 1980–2000 (IASC Publishing, 2009); Deirdre Duffy, 'From feminist anarchy to decolonisation: Understanding abortion health activism before and after the repeal of the 8th amendment', Feminist Review, 124 (2020), pp. 69–85.

highlights the reliance of some individuals on friends posting them supplies over or they themselves smuggling back supplies from the UK. Dennis (b.1937) explained that access to condoms was 'from England or ... Put it this way. You got them through dodgy sources. You didn't know what you were getting'. Richard (b.1954) from the rural west of Ireland remembered 'one of the guys in school used to supply them in secondary school. Yeah and he had to do a demo one day and (laughs). That was it. But um yeah. That was – it was – that's how it was at the time'. Ted (b.1951) who lived in a rural area in the west of Ireland, also reflected on the challenges he faced in getting access to condoms. He explained at one point his wife Maria would cycle 'fifteen miles each way to a distant village to get the condoms from a friend. Possibly her friend's husband, who was American, had got the condoms from the States or through his job, as he worked at the airport'.

Indeed, several interviewees recalled the dirty humour that tended to surround condoms. This may have contributed to a sense of stigma and shame around their use. Jacinta (b.1954) explained:

It was more the lads going up north or over to England or something like that. That's when it was all ... Then there's all smutty talk about it, really, when you get them that way. Send the lads and they'd come back with condoms and be delighted with themselves. It made things worse, didn't it?

Martina (b.1955) told me that 'And I mean, at that time, condoms were a joke. Do you know what I mean? They were treated as a joke rather than something serious. Because people were so ... I don't know what the word is. Ignorant. There was a lot of ignorance around, you know?' Martina and Jacinta's testimonies suggest that the use of humour perhaps enabled individuals to talk about a secretive issue but that this helped to further stigmatise the problem. Ellen (b.1949) remembered the first time she heard about 'French letters' as a young woman:

I remember working in the hotel, and we had a French guest staying, and when they went away they wrote to one of the women, and the lads were having her 'Oh miss, you got two French letters in the post this morning'. All this. And I didn't know what French letters were, but I knew by the way they were talking about them that they were something. I wouldn't go home and ask my mother about it, so it was a long time before anybody told me what they were. I used to hear... You learned a lot from, as we said, from dirty jokes. The way these double meaning kind of jokes, and you kind of started thinking. You'd say 'What did they mean by that?' And you'd probably put your own interpretation and things were maybe not always the right way.

In addition, a number of respondents joked about condoms in the oral history interview itself.[61] Rosie (b.1938) told me 'a lot of people didn't like con – the, you know, just going to bed with your shirt on. I hear people saying that, or your pajamas's on, or whatever (laughing)'. Similarly, Colm (b.1940) recalled a conversation with a friend, stating:

COLM: And he would've said to me it's ... You probably heard it, there's an old' saying. 'It's not the same', he says. 'It's the same', he says, 'as washing your feet with your socks on'.
LAURA: Oh. (laughs) Okay, right.
COLM: (laughs). That's the way he put it.

These jokes perhaps allude to the idea that condoms in some way inhibited sexual pleasure by reducing sensitivity. The respondents' laughter also perhaps is indicative of an emotional response to an uncomfortable topic.[62] One respondent, also felt that condoms were unsatisfactory because they reduced the spontaneity of sex. Edward (b.1950) told me 'We'd use them but like you know, it's kind of – oh hold on a minute, you know. [...] And you start you know and then you realise this is going to go a bit further tonight, you now, hold on and that kind of kills it you know. So, we didn't really want that'. He later had a vasectomy which he and his wife found more satisfactory as a form of family planning.

Caps or diaphragms were less commonly used methods of contracep tion among oral history respondents, with some commenting on the interruptive nature of these devices. Mairead (b.1953) who grew up in Dublin, used a cap which she obtained from the Well Woman centre in the late 70s before she got married. She explained to me how the method was not entirely suitable because 'it was a messy old thing' and that because you had to put it in before intercourse, it meant that 'It would be kind-of elective. (laughs). Elective sex, like elective sections'. Similarly, Julie (b.1947) from the rural west of Ireland, also used a combination of the diaphragm and condoms with her husband, but found these methods unsatisfactory, stating, 'It's a strain on a relation-ship in a way. Because it seems to be the time that you're fertile that you're actually more receptive to the relationship'. Intra-uterine devices were also less common across the whole cohort. Úna (b.1946) had a coil

---

[61] Kate Fisher's respondents also utilised similar humour in relation to condoms. Fisher, *Birth Control*, p. 171.
[62] Stephanie Panichelli-Batalla, 'Laughter in oral histories of displacement: "One goes on a mission to solve their problems"', *Oral History Review*, 47:1, pp. 73–92, on p. 88.

fitted in her late thirties when she had completed her family. Two other respondents expressed that they had a coil fitted but found it uncomfortable and had it removed. Ann (b.1948) had a traumatic experience with an IUD which she had fitted in 1986. As a result of an infection, she had to have a hysterectomy. Two other respondents had concerns that these methods were abortifacients and stated that this put them off using them.

In addition to class, location also had an important bearing on access to contraception. It is clear that individuals who lived in urban areas with family planning clinics which emerged between 1969 and 1978 could more readily access artificial contraception. However, this really depended on class, as Chapter 6 will illustrate, and the majority of clients at the family planning clinics in their early years tended to come from middle-class backgrounds. Arguably, cities would have also had a higher number of GPs meaning a better chance of finding one who would prescribe the pill.

For those who lived in the border towns, it was possible to obtain contraceptives from chemists in Northern Ireland. As Nuala O'Faolain wrote in her 1996 memoir, *Are you somebody?*:

When Edna O'Brien's first books came out they were a catalyst for women to exchange confidences, and I learnt that quite a few people went to Belfast to get condoms. Condoms, hats, cheap butter: that was the extent of it.[63]

Maurice (b.1942) who grew up in the north of the country, married in 1971. He recalled going up to Northern Ireland to buy condoms, stating that 'there was no trouble buying them in the North. You only had to find a Protestant pharmacist. (laughs)'. However, he reflected that the condoms were not openly displayed and that 'You had to work up the courage to ask. But once I was married it was easy to work up that courage'. David (b.1948) and his wife Jean (b.1953) lived in a small town close to the border. David explained:

But you were lucky in that you had Derry, Strabane available for condoms and things like that. It's really what you could do. And yeah, people would have made use of the fact that they lived convenient to Derry and Strabane.

Diane (b.1949) also grew up and lived in a small border town. Diane felt that it was widely known that contraceptives could be obtained in the north, stating 'Well, when you live where we live in a border town, you shop in the north so easily that it was very common knowledge'. She explained that her husband used to go over the border to purchase condoms from a chemist there:

---

[63] O'Faolain, *Are You Somebody?* p. 60.

Oh, I think it was a very common pastime, yeah. I think it was a common pastime, and a common place to go and get them. I think lots of people went over to Northern Ireland.

Jim (b.1933) from Dublin, who lived in a border town, travelled to the north in the early 1980s to obtain condoms, stating, 'I mean, going over the border was very easy'. Northern Ireland's reproductive health services were also used by the Irish Family Planning Association in its early years when women were sent to the Royal Victoria Hospital in Belfast for IUDs.[64] Moreover, when David (b.1948) from a border town decided to have a vasectomy in the 1990s, he obtained this in Northern Ireland.

3.5   England: 'A Heathen Place'

The UK, and particularly England, was generally viewed as being more permissive in relation to sexual matters than Ireland. As Jennifer Redmond has suggested, 'The perception that Britain was a sexually advanced place in which looser morals were common appears to have been widespread, if inaccurate'.[65] Emigration from Ireland to the UK had a long history. It increased during the twentieth century and became an issue of moral and political concern after the foundation of the Irish Free State in 1922.[66] Colm (b.1940) from the rural Midlands, was one such migrant. He went to London in 1961 for a few years where he worked in a car factory. He said to me that in London, he felt that in relation to attitudes to sex, 'over there, it was anything goes. Do you know? And, and looking back on it, they were right,' and that his time in London had a significant impact on his knowledge. 'Let's put it this way, you came back a lot wiser than you went over'. Several of the respondents who spent time in England also reflected on the freedom that anonymity in England gave them. Rosie (b.1938) who grew up in the rural Midlands, emigrated to London in 1958, aged twenty:

Loved it, because I tell you something, you could be free. You could stand on your head and nobody would care a damn. Where Ireland it was so restrictive in those years. It was the '50s. And very restrictive.

Rosie found that attitudes were more permissive in England, mentioning that there were unmarried mothers in her office workplace. Moreover,

---

[64] 'Ireland's only family planning clinic', *Woman's Choice Weekly*, 9 June 1970, p. 55. Courtesy of Susan Solomons.

[65] Jennifer Redmond, *Moving Histories: Irish Women's Emigration to Britain from Independence to Republic* (Liverpool University Press, 2020), p. 130.

[66] Redmond, *Moving Histories*, p. 19.

it was in London that she found out about contraception for the first time. When asked whether she had heard anything about contraception before she moved to England, she said, laughing, 'Not at all. I heard it in London'.

Respondents who spent time in England reflected on the difference in attitudes. Jacinta (b.1954) worked in England for a summer and reflected on how attitudes to sex were different there among people of her age group:

I was working all summer over in England and it was a completely different attitude, they were all using them. While we were trying not to do it, they were all using condoms. Nineteen, twenty, whatever age we were. That age. They were all using condoms in England. Ireland was inclined to think: look at England, going down this awful route.

However, reflecting on these attitudes today, she expressed, 'England was a much better country at the time when you think about it. We were so held back when I think about that'. Marian, (b.1935) from the rural north of Ireland, described the difference between Ireland and emigrants' destinations:

England was different to Ireland. As a friend of mine said when she went to America she said the things that were a sin in Ireland weren't a sin in America … As regards family and family planning and all that.

Ann (b.1945) from a town in the southwest felt that in her home town:

they were more worried about what the neighbours would say. They governed their lives like, 'Don't show that. Don't tell that'. Whereas in England you were anonymous. And I think that's why people liked it so much because they could be more themselves without being judged all the time.

As Jennifer Redmond's work has shown, life in British cities was depicted as having 'a deleterious effect on both male and female emigrants because, as they came mostly from rural backgrounds, they were thus ill-equipped for the freedoms and pitfalls it contained.'[67] Angela Macnamara's views on England are typical of such ideas. In an article which appeared in 1963 in *Woman's Way* she wrote: 'Many an Irish girl abroad has been introduced to the evils of contraception under the guise of "the modern way of life". Her innocence and ignorance are mocked and exploited. Without realising it, she falls victim to a way of life leading insidiously away from God and everything she valued at home'.[68]

[67] Redmond, *Moving Histories*, p. 112.
[68] Angela Macnamara, 'Science and Control', *Woman's Way*, 30 November 1963, 55.

Clodagh, (b.1940) from the rural Midlands, went to England aged 18 to work for a period as a teacher in a private Church of England school. The nun principal from her old secondary school, 'was very upset that I went to England to – a heathen place, it wasn't good anyway'. The nun 'got me a job at home, a substitute again for someone on maternity leave' in her old secondary school so Clodagh returned home before completing a full year in England. Carmel (b.1952) remarked that people viewed England as 'a bad place to have to go to, and bad things happened there. The majority of the population being Protestant then didn't help. They didn't seem to think there was any Catholics there at all'. Similarly, her husband Martin (b.1952) reflected that 'People thought it was a location of sin'. Carmel and Martin found attitudes to be different in England and even lived together, something which they felt they would have been unable to do at home. Yet, the pretence that they were living separately had to be maintained when Carmel's mother visited from Ireland.

Some interviewees also reflected on the perception that there were more permissive attitudes to sex and contraception among English women. Dennis (b.1937) who grew up in a village in the south-west of Ireland, recalled a friend of his who went to England in 1955, telling him:

DENNIS: 'Do you know what?' He says, 'The girls in England, when they go out with you, they carry a condom in their handbag'. He said, 'Jesus', he said. (laughs).
LAURA: It must have been shocking.
DENNIS: That was a shock for him to find that she was ready for it and he was kind-of scratching his head, 'What have we missed on this', or whatever.

There was also a sense from some female respondents that being in England changed others' perceptions of them in relation to morality and family planning. Alice (b.1944) who grew up in the rural west of Ireland, for instance stated:

I remember going to England, and I came back, people thought that if you were in England you were game for anything.

Similarly, Hannah (b.1950) from a small town in the west of Ireland told me:

And of course, if you're in England, people automatically assumed... I remember meeting the mother of one of my close friends, still friends with her today, 'Oh you were one of the cute ones'. She said to me. I said, 'What do you mean?' 'Oh, you never got pregnant'.

Of course, in England, contraception was legally available. However, it was not always straightforward for women to obtain the pill from their doctor, particularly if they were unmarried.[69] Nevertheless, with regard to condom access, England appeared much more liberal. Elaine (b.1950) from the rural west of Ireland, spent five years in England, marrying her husband over there in 1972. She stated, 'You could be going up the street at night and the newspaper shops would be open and you could buy anything you wanted. We used to buy a bundle and bring them home'. Similarly, Richard (b.1954) recalled visiting the UK in the late 70s and expressed his amazement at seeing 'condom machines everywhere'. He said, 'I kind of said, "oh God. I can't believe this!" I said "Look at all this uh... Johnnies – you just throw in a coin and off you go!" (laughs). So it was, it was, very different'. Indeed, in England, condoms were readily available through slot machines from the late 1920s. As Claire Jones has shown, at least 166 machines were placed all over London between 1929 and 1950, providing consumers with access to condoms at any time of the day and meaning no personal interaction between the seller and consumer.[70]

3.6   Smuggling Contraceptives

Condoms were commonly brought back from England by Irish emigrants and holidaymakers. Clare's (b.1936) husband bought condoms in England which they used for contraception. Clare was concerned about the health risks of other types of contraception and felt that with condoms 'at least you were sticking as close to nature as possible'. Hannah (b.1950) grew up in a small town in the west of Ireland and worked in England in the 1970s. She brought condoms back for a friend of hers:

I do remember a girlfriend who was married and had, maybe she had three children at this time, but she asked me to bring ... you couldn't obviously get the pill for her, but to bring Durex home for her and I'd never bought them before and I remember going in and buying them, and I used to have a free flight home and I looked very young, so they never asked to look into the suitcase. Full of these condoms.

Sally (b.1956) from the rural east also recalled friends bringing condoms back from England for her:

We always knew, if say if one of the girls was going over to England to visit her sister, and this is about from 16 to 18. We never had much money, but whatever

---

[69] Cook, *The Long Sexual Revolution*, pp. 273–88.
[70] Jones, *The Business of Birth Control*, pp. 178–81.

we had, we'd give them money to buy condoms, to bring them back. To try and keep ourselves safe.

Paula (b.1955) and her husband, who lived in a city in the west of Ireland, used condoms after they got married in 1976 before they had their first child in 1978. Paula described the process of obtaining condoms from her friend's husband:

At this stage, we were using condoms which were not available. So, '76, '77. Yeah. So, I'd say it to my friend that I'd gone to college with, I'd say, 'Listen, we don't have any condoms. And I don't know how to get them'. … Her partner, he orders them. He'll sort it out for you. So he was sending away, I think to the UK for them … Then there was no mobile phones then obviously and hardly house phones. So, I'd meet up with my friend and she said, 'We'll meet you outside the corner of High Street'. And he'd give him the packet. It was an exchange.

Paula explained that the handover of the condoms occurred between the two men, rather than the women and 'very discreetly the package would be handed over. Then we'd go off to Dublin to their flat and have a nice weekend with the condoms that they had provided via courier service, of course via the UK'.

Condoms were also sent by post from England, however, until 1973 and the McGee case, these could be intercepted by customs officers. Ann (b.1945) from a town in the southwest of Ireland recalled asking a good friend of hers in England to 'send me on some French letters'. She explained:

I got them a couple of times, okay? But this particular time I got a letter from the customs stating, 'Under section something of the something something Act, we have confiscated your parcel'. And would I like to be at the opening of it in Dublin. So, I'd say there was a lot of lads had a good time. (laughs).

Daithi (b.1950) from a small town in the west of Ireland worked in England in the early '70s and would bring condoms back for his friends. He recalled one occasion where:

I was stopped once, and I did actually have them in my car in the boot, and I'm not too sure what happened to them. I don't know if they were taken off me, or, but they were certainly spotted by the guys.

Myra (b.1947) from a small town in the south-east of the country explained that her sister-in-law would post over condoms to Myra and her husband. Prior to that the couple had relied on 'minding ourselves'. However, her sister-in-law sent over such a large supply that Myra asked '"How long does she think we want them for?" We used to be giving them to the rest of the family, that's what we used to be doing'. However, access to condoms did not mean that individuals necessarily knew how to use them. Margaret (b.1954) and her husband obtained condoms on their honeymoon:

And so when we went on our honeymoon to Jersey, we came home with the case half full of condoms. (laughs). Every other day I was sitting, either him or me was going into another chemist. We didn't know what they were or how you use them properly.

Christopher (b.1946) was over and back to England for work during the 1960s and 1970s and would purchase condoms there and bring them back. He also brought back supplies for his neighbour. He recalled his neighbour asking him if the condoms could be washed and reused. None of the respondents who brought condoms back from England remarked on feeling afraid about possible prosecution. It was not just condoms that were obtained in England. Siobhan (b.1942) from a town in the Midlands, who worked in Dublin, recalled hearing about some women who obtained the cap in England. However, doing so was a secretive practice and not something that people publicised:

Well, people went, a lot of people, you know you'd hear them say that, 'She went over to England to get that'. But it was always kind of hush, hush. You know, there was no major discussion about it.

Moreover, a number of respondents reported on knowing women who travelled to England for abortions in the 1970s and 1980s. Evidently, Ireland's proximity to the UK meant that those with the means or contacts could obtain birth control there.

3.7   Responsibility for Family Planning and Decision-Making

In a 1979 interview, Frank Crummey, one of the founders of Family Planning Services, suggested that it was women who were predominantly taking responsibility for obtaining contraception from family planning clinics:

The big change I see is among the women in Ireland. It's they who are doing all the getting, who'll come and ask, who'll say if they have a problem. Men still won't come into the clinics. Also Irish women are beginning to insist on getting something out of sex which their mothers didn't. In some ways this shocks their husbands.[71]

---

[71] Rosita Sweetman, *On Our Backs: Sexual Attitudes in a Changing Ireland* (London: Pan Books, 1979), p. 157.

Crummey's statement here is revealing in that it suggests not only that it was women, rather than men, who were taking responsibility for family planning, but also alludes to a generational shift in terms of attitudes to sexual pleasure. Fisher has suggested that from the 1920s to the 1950s in England and Wales, birth control was seen as a male duty, with some men in her study viewing the management of family limitation as an expression of their dominance within all spheres of the marriage.[72] However, studies of birth control practices in other contexts for the later period have complicated this picture. For instance, Caroline Rusterholz has shown that in Switzerland from around 1955 to 1970, birth control was rarely viewed as solely a male responsibility within married couples. Instead, birth control was either a shared spousal responsibility or a female responsibility, depending on the knowledge each spouse had.[73] However, in her study of Ukraine for the same period, Yuliya Hilevych found that while couples in both cities in the study conformed to the idea of women being sexually ignorant and men taking responsibility for family planning, there were regional differences.[74]

The oral history evidence for this study suggests that as with knowledge around sex and reproduction, information on family planning was spread between women and responsibility for family planning largely lay with the female partner. Jeremiah (b.1942) from a small town in the north of the country explained that it was his wife who 'got whatever had to be got ... I never bought any of that, no'. He believed that his wife 'was better informed than I was', remarking that in general 'I think girls generally, you are a bit more, alert and alive to do it'. Similarly, Ellen (b.1949) from the rural south-east, who had six children, had responsibility for obtaining condoms, however, she would not go into her local chemist to buy them.

It may have been that owing to a lack of contraceptive options, and given that female-centred methods were most commonly used, that women ended up being the ones to take responsibility. Eugene (b.1939) from the rural Midlands, for instance, indicated that it was his wife who was knowledgeable:

Sure, we knew nothing – well Ann knew all, when it was safe, she knew the details yeah about the periods you know she knew about the safe period, you know she knew, knew all that.

---

[72] Fisher, *Birth Control*, pp. 189–237.   [73] Rusterholz, 'Reproductive behavior', p. 56.
[74] Yuliya Hilevych, 'Abortion and gender relationships in Ukraine, 1955–1970', *The History of the Family*, (2015), 20:1, pp. 86–105.

Siobhan (b.1942) also alluded to the fact that it was up to her to find out information on family planning. She said: 'We went to a few [talks on the safe period]... well, I went, Jim wouldn't'. She felt 'it was up to me, but the thing is that if I hadn't decided myself after the fourth, the fifth ...', implying she would have continued having children. This attitude appears to have persisted among some of the younger respondents. Noel (b.1952) from a city in the west of Ireland felt that the issue of family planning was his wife's responsibility: 'It's like everything else, the men stayed back and stayed out of it and put all the responsibility on the women. Generally'. Similarly, Nicholas (b.1953) also from a city in the west of Ireland expressed 'I always ... I, I would have said ... I've thought about this of course, there was a lot, a strong, very much an onus on the woman to family plan'. Nicholas' wife went to her GP to obtain the pill after the birth of their three children. Nicholas maintained 'The reality is that a man did not involve himself in family planning'.

Respondents who discussed pre-marital sex suggested that it was the man in the relationship who took responsibility for birth control. Paula (b.1955) from a city in the west of Ireland, explained how she went away for a weekend with her boyfriend, who was not from Ireland 'And he had known about the situation in Ireland. So he had come armed. Okay? He brought his condoms'. Similarly, Evelyn (b.1940) who grew up in Dublin, said that with regard to relationships she had before marriage, the 'men that I had sex with, they took precautions. So I hadn't had to bother my head'. However, she felt that after marriage, it was a joint responsibility.

Decision-making around how many children to have was a complex matter and depended on the dynamics of the individual relationship and the personalities of the individuals involved. In some cases, this was negotiated between the couple, who then came to an agreement. Marian (b.1935) who lived in a city in the west of Ireland, had three children, and used the term 'we' to describe the use of contraception in her marriage:

MARIAN: Yeah we went on the pill and we used condoms as well at one time or other.
LAURA: Yeah. And did you talk much with your husband about it or did you decide yourself that you wanted to space the ...
MARIAN: He didn't want ... I suppose we agreed to it between us.

Similarly, Myra (b.1947) from a small town in the south-east of the country recalled a discussion with her husband:

when I had the third one, he says to me, 'You're not having any more'. I said, 'I'm not Charlie, because I don't want any more'. But he didn't mind, but some fellas were still that way, you will have how ever many children you will have. I have friends that have seven and eight children.

In Myra's case, while her husband suggested that she shouldn't have any more children, she saw it ultimately as her decision. Such testimonies illuminate Irish women's growing agency around contraceptive practices.

3.8   The Impact of Lack of Access to Contraception

Writing to Mary Kenny's column in the *Irish Press* in 1970, a 26-year-old woman with three children under the age of three from Killarney explained the strain that lack of access to contraception was having on her marriage. The woman had consulted her doctor about the safe period and was told that her periods were too irregular to use this method effectively. She then asked for the contraceptive pill but 'was refused in no uncertain terms'. The woman's dilemma was representative of that of many mothers of this generation. She wrote:

I love my babies dearly, but simply cannot face another pregnancy for two or three years at least. My husband is a very good husband and father and we love each other very much, but the way things are right now I feel like walking out and never coming back. I am sleeping in the babies' room for the last three months. I am simply terrified of getting pregnant again. Now please don't think my husband is a sex maniac. No he is not and neither am I, but our love life (I prefer the word love to sex) has always been wonderful. Now whenever he comes near me or gets tender or loving in any way I walk away from him, what else can I do? Oh! If only we could have love even now and again without fear of pregnancy how happy our marriage would be. The tension is driving us both mad and I dread what will happen if things go on this way.[75]

Lack of access to reliable contraception had a profound impact on men and women in Ireland of fertile age in the 1960s and 1970s. More widely in this period, there was an increasing public acknowledgement of the ways that lack of access to contraception could jeopardise the harmony of a marital relationship. Without reliable contraception, the fear of pregnancy was a regular concern for couples. Worry from month to month and the impact of this anxiety on individuals' sex lives were common themes in the oral history interviews and in the contemporary press. After having five pregnancies, Siobhan (b.1942) explained that 'I didn't want any more children' and told me 'I just didn't like sex anymore. I was put off it completely'. Siobhan said she would refuse to have sex with her husband. She viewed this as her decision stating, 'Well it was up

[75] 'Woman's Press,' *Irish Press*, 9 November 1970, p. 8.

to me ... I made the decision and I said this, 'I would refuse or whatever'. Siobhan expressed that she did not mind being pregnant or giving birth, but found the balance of childrearing which fell to her to be a strain, 'because in those days, men, it was all left up to you, really, you know?'

Pierce (b.1948) who lived in Dublin after getting married, remarked on how lack of access to a reliable form of contraception caused significant stress for he and his wife. Pierce and his wife had four children. He recalled that with 'the first ones you'd want to have the family anyway like you know? Two or three, or maybe four. But then the trouble starts, you see. When you want to stop ... there's no stopping'. He and his wife used the rhythm method to try and space their pregnancies and to avoid having any more children after the birth of their fourth child, but Pierce remembered these periods when they were trying to avoid pregnancy as 'being fairly stressful because we were never sure whether, em, this – this rhythm worked or not, you know?' He described these periods of time as 'difficult' stating 'But I remember a lot of stress at the time, and Mary being worried about getting pregnant'.

Similarly, Maria (b.1957) summed up the anxiety she felt about getting pregnant as follows:

After our third child because, really, I mean, I was neurotic, I'd say, really, about not becoming pregnant. And as I said, knicker watching, watching for spots of blood with the period.

She told me:

And then you'd go to the loo and you'd be expecting your period and then the toilet paper would say, 'Oh, God no'. I remember times going out into the kitchen and we would be saying, 'Is it pink? Is there a sign of red in it?' This kind of thing, you know? Like when people ... when I hear people nowadays complaining about period cramps, they were the most fabulous feeling I ever got. Because I knew it was a period coming quickly.

Colm (b.1940) from the rural Midlands similarly explained the stress and worry experienced by women without access to contraception: 'Going from one month to the other. You know? One month, "Oh, thank God I'm not pregnant." Do you know? It's a terrible way to live'. Lizzie (b.1946) from the rural west of Ireland, had one daughter at the age of 39, followed by a number of miscarriages afterwards. She had no access to contraception. She alluded to the impact that lack of adequate contraception had on her marriage stating: 'I think there would have been a lot more happier marriages if people had contraceptives and a lot better'. She felt that had individuals had access to contraception:

They would have concentrated on the relationship instead of having always this worry and you felt the pressure, not that you were pressurised, because you let your body go, but you still had this in the back of your head in case I become pregnant. And yet you couldn't take the pill because it was against your religion. How silly were we?

In comparison to her experiences of sex during her marriage, Teresa (b.1946) felt that post-menopause her sexual experiences differed because 'it's great now at this stage in my life that we can be sexually active and not worry about pregnancy'.

A study by Karl Mullen, a Dublin gynaecologist, in 1967 surveyed 500 cases of marital stress found that 20% of stress in marriage was 'clearly associated with fertility control'. According to the article in *Woman's Way*, 'Dr. Mullen described a typical case: 'the wife who dreaded the nights and slowly became isolated from her husband. She became a very lonely person'. Mullen believed, however, that by 1972, women were less guilt-ridden than they had been when he undertook the study five years previously.[76] The impact of worrying about pregnancy was also referred to in the contemporary press. A father of five writing in the *Sunday Independent* in 1966 outlined the impact of lack of contraception on women's mental health, suggesting that the major cause of mental stress in many young Irish mothers was the fear of pregnancy and the impact that subsequent pregnancies would have on running the house. In the author's view:

She doesn't want any more children, yet, she lies in dread from month to month. If she does become pregnant, there is a complete escalation in the problems in the home. Trying to cope with six children while almost physically fit is one thing. Trying to cope while carrying a seventh is a completely different matter. And so it goes on to the eleventh and twelfth.

The man and his wife had practised the rhythm method but in their case it had not worked, meaning they had five children in seven years.[77] Margaret Lynch from Cork, writing to the *Sunday Independent* in 1966 in response to this letter stated 'Mothers of growing families do grumble about the little time there is to relax, but all the young mothers I know agree that this tension would be almost non-existent if the fear of pregnancy could be eliminated, for a time, at least.'[78] The strain of the 'safe period' was frequently discussed in *Woman's Way* magazine too.[79] In addition, a man interviewed by Dorine Rohan in 1969 suggested that fear of pregnancy led to marital infidelity. He told Rohan that 'A lot of

---

[76] Tom Myler, 'Women who live in fear', *Woman's Way*, 7 December 1973, p. 44.
[77] 'Family planning', *Sunday Independent*, 17 July 1966, p. 8.
[78] 'Birth control...', *Sunday Independent*, 7 August 1966, p. 15.
[79] For example, 'Marriage guidance: the safe period', *Woman's Way*, 6 October 1967, p. 45.

the lads who are married are out every night with girls because their wives won't let them near them for fear of more kids, and I don't blame them. We've been on the pill for three years and only for it I'd probably be out after the women too'.[80]

Betty Hilliard's study of married women in Cork similarly found that the fear of pregnancy had an important impact on the respondents' enjoyment of sex.[81] Likewise, Dolores, a district nurse in a Cork town in the mid-1950s who was interviewed for Máire Leane's study, spoke of the impact of lack of contraception on the women she met and how fear of pregnancy inhibited sexual enjoyment.[82] Similarly, Kate Fisher's study of England and Wales found that some respondents linked their 'fear of pregnancy and the inadequacies of contraceptive methods to their lack of sexual satisfaction'.[83] *Woman's Way* regularly published on the impact of lack of access to contraception on 'ordinary' women. In one article in 1972, a woman called Joan was featured. Joan stressed the anxiety she felt as a result of her fear of repeated pregnancies:

Another child would be disastrous because we just cannot afford it what with the high cost of living, not to mention being too busy to think. Because of the fear of pregnancy, we don't even sleep together. Consequently we are not living a normal married life, a natural life. It's as simple as that.[84]

The article also included the testimony of Esther who was described as a young mother with five children under the age of six, who stated, 'Frankly, I am waiting for the day when I can go into a chemist shop or a family planning centre and get just what I want'.[85]

Oral history testimonies also allude to the stress experienced by women with a lack of effective contraception. Helena (b.1945) worked as a hairdresser as a young woman. She said that contraception 'was one of the subjects that was nearly always on the go' with her customers 'and you see when they're coming in pregnant again, and there would be such anger in them. (laughs). Oh, they would be so angry. Geared towards the church and the husband. Yeah'. Sally (b.1956) from the rural east of the country told me that in order to prevent pregnancy she 'just tried avoiding having sex, or if anybody was going to England, you'd give them money for condoms. It was just horrible'. The anxiety took its toll on Sally. She told me 'We lived from month…[to month]. I nearly would grow old with a hump on my back, waiting and seeing if I'd get a period'.

[80] Rohan, *Marriage Irish Style*, pp. 99–100.
[81] Hilliard, 'The Catholic Church', pp. 36–7.   [82] Leane, 'Embodied sexualities', p. 45.
[83] Fisher, *Birth Control*, p. 213.
[84] Tom Myler, 'Women who live in fear', *Woman's Way*, 7 December 1973, p. 44.
[85] *Ibid.*, p. 44.

Sally felt that her first marriage broke down largely as a result of the strain caused from a lack of access to contraception. Sally did not feel that her experiences were unusual. She stated:

but life did revolve around it. Like you know, I'm sure there was many a woman sitting at the table having her breakfast, or her dinner, and these thoughts, 'Am I pregnant?' And I know from some of the girls that lived up on the council estate at the back of our house, up in the park, the father from England and the father, some of the fathers came home for two weeks in August, and say the month of September, October, the women were always worried whether they were pregnant or not. The husbands were gone back and wouldn't see them for another year. But if they got away with it and weren't pregnant, it must have been the most joyous occasion.

3.9   Conclusion

This chapter has outlined the key family planning practices of oral history respondents born in the 1930s–1950s. Due to the lack of legal access to contraception as well as the condemnation from the Catholic Church of artificial methods of family planning, the majority of men and women born in the 1930s and 1940s who were interviewed as part of this study, tended to rely on natural methods of birth control. Class and location had a significant impact on choice of contraceptive method. Ultimately, this chapter has shown the endurance of natural/calendar-based methods during the period. With artificial contraception being illegal up until 1979, and the majority of those interviewed identifying as Catholic, this was the main method available to individuals. However, for participants born in the 1940s and 1950s, it appears that while these methods persisted, individuals were gradually beginning to exert more resistance in relation to contraception. In particular, individuals exercised ingenuity in obtaining contraceptives from England, or as the following chapter will show, through obtaining the contraceptive pill from a sympathetic doctor. The reliance on England for contraceptives such as condoms which could be ordered by post, but the characterisation of England as a 'permissive' society, highlights the hypocrisy of the Irish situation in relation to contraception. Women, rather than men, were for the most part responsible for family planning within the married couple.

From the 1960s, women's magazine, pre-marriage courses and booklets were sources of information on family planning, however, these forums tended to focus on natural methods for the most part. Information was also passed on by word-of-mouth. Discussions around the satisfaction of various types of contraceptives also reveals that by the 1960s and 1970s, although there wasn't a sexual revolution in Ireland, individuals were beginning to recognise the importance of a healthy sex life to marital harmony. The chapter has also emphasised the impact that lack of access to contraception had on individuals, particularly women. While many respondents had a stoic attitude towards having children and accepted this as being part of the purpose of marriage, many women suffered considerable stress and anxiety over the issue. Many of these patterns persisted into the 1980s. Chapter 9 will show how, even after the legalisation of contraception in 1979, individuals still struggled to gain access to effective contraception, in spite of the increasing availability of artificial methods and permanent methods such as sterilisation.

4   The Pill, Women's Agency and Doctor–Patient Relationships in the 1960s and 1970s

Writing in *Woman's Way* magazine in 1966, journalist Monica McEnroy drew attention to the plight of many Irish women who were unable to avail themselves of contraception. She wrote that she had received letters from women all over Ireland 'who had asked their doctors for the Pill and had been refused'.[1] One woman, writing to McEnroy, explained:

I am thirty-eight. I have five lovely children. The eldest is eight and I have just lost another baby before its time. I have high blood pressure for the past two years. I asked my doctor could I not try the Pill as I want to try and look after the children. The worry of another miscarriage is always hanging over me, but he told me I would have to wait until they got word from Rome.[2]

McEnroy argued that women like the author of this letter should be allowed to decide for themselves with regard to birth control, and that the religious aspect was 'a matter between me and God'.[3]

This chapter builds on important recent accounts of the contraceptive pill in other predominantly Catholic countries with similar restrictions in place.[4] I will focus on three key themes: first, contemporary attitudes to the contraceptive pill in Ireland in the 1960s and 1970s, the experiences of Irish women who chose to take the contraceptive pill and the role of medical authority surrounding the pill. I seek to show here that, through

---

[1] Monica McEnroy, 'The contraceptive pill in Ireland', *Woman's Way*, 23 September 1966, p. 9.
[2] *Ibid.*   [3] *Ibid.*
[4] See, for instance, Teresa Ortiz-Gomez and Agata Ignaciuk, 'Pregnancy and labour cause more deaths than oral contraceptives: The debate on the pill in the Spanish press in the 1960s and 1970s', *Public Understanding of Science*, 24:6 (2015), pp. 658–71; Agata Ignaciuk, 'Paradox of the pill: Oral contraceptives in Spain and Poland (1960s–1970s)' in Ann-Katrin Gembries, Theresia Theuke and Isabel Heinemann (eds.), *Children by Choice?* (Berlin: DeGruyter, 2018), pp. 95–111; Tiago Pires Marques, 'The politics of Catholic medicine: "The pill" and *Humanae Vitae* in Portugal' in Harris (ed.), *The Schism of '68*, pp. 161–86. For a broad history of the contraceptive pill, see Lara Marks, *Sexual Chemistry: A History of the Contraceptive Pill* (New Haven, CT: Yale University Press, 2010).

negotiating access to the contraceptive pill, Irish women were also negotiating both their marriage dynamics and relationships with the medical
profession. Ultimately, the loophole regarding the prescription of the
contraceptive pill as a cycle regulator in the period before 1979 placed
Irish GPs in a position of significant power over women's access
to contraception.

4.1   Women's Accounts and Doctors' Authority

The contraceptive pill was available in Ireland on prescription from
1963 and marketed as a cycle regulator and, as Mary E. Daly has argued,
'played a crucial role in opening a debate on contraception'.[5] Users of the
contraceptive pill could circumvent the ban on contraception in Ireland
by asking for the pill as a cycle regulator rather than as a contraceptive. In
Spain, where contraception was banned until 1978, the contraceptive pill
was also marketed as an 'oral cycle regulator' or as an 'ovulostatic', and
during the 1970s, marketing materials and package inserts continued to
inform patients that these drugs 'should be used to allow for "periodic
rest of the ovaries"'.[6] Similarly, in Ireland, a 1967 advertisement for oral
contraceptive Lyndiol 2.5, which appeared in the *Journal of the Irish
Medical Association*, advertised the drug 'for a menstrual cycle as regular
as clockwork'.[7] The advertisement (Figure 4.1) shows a woman's hand
with a watch; the woman is wearing a wedding ring. As Elizabeth Siegel
Watkins has illustrated, by the mid-1960s, the use of contraception by
single women was frowned upon by some 'because it implied,
correctly, not only that these women were having sex but also that they
were planning ahead for it'.[8] There were similar attitudes in the UK;
and in the first years of its introduction there, the contraceptive pill
was restricted to married women.[9] Furthermore, GPs who did provide

---

[5] Daly, *Sixties Ireland*, p. 146.
[6] Ortiz-Gomez and Ignaciuk, 'Pregnancy and labour', p. 660.
[7] Advertisement for Lyndiol 2.5, *Journal of the Irish Medical Association*, volume LX,
no. 365, November 1967, no page number.
[8] Watkins, *On the Pill*, p. 2.
[9] Family Planning Associations only provided contraception to married or engaged
women, while the 118 government-funded local authority clinics restricted the
provision of contraception to married women who required it on 'medical grounds',
while many GPs believed that contraception should not be part of their medical practice.
From 1964, the contraceptive pill was available in Britain to unmarried women through
Brook clinics. In 1968 the Family Planning Association gave permission to their
branches to prescribe the pill also to unmarried women; their branches were required
to do so from 1970. Cook, *The Long Sexual Revolution*, pp. 272 and 287–91.

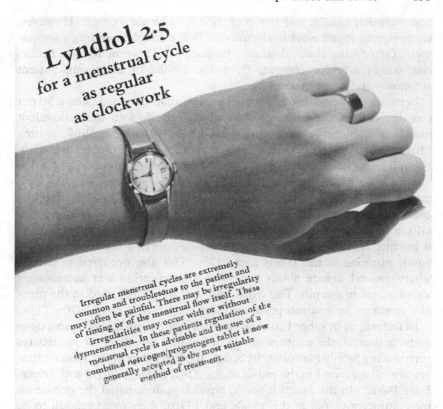

Lyndiol 2·5
for a menstrual cycle as regular as clockwork

Irregular menstrual cycles are extremely common and troublesome to the patient and may often be painful. There may be irregularity of timing or of the menstrual flow itself. These irregularities may occur with or without dysmenorrhoea. In these patients regulation of the menstrual cycle is advisable and the use of a combined oestrogen/progestogen tablet is now generally accepted as the most suitable method of treatment.

Lyndiol 2·5 provides completely effective regulation of the menstrual cycle with the correct balance of low doses of oestrogen and progestogen.

Lyndiol 2·5 is particularly useful for regulating the menstrual cycle during the puerperium. It can be used with confidence during breast feeding and does not adversely affect any aspect of lactation.

Side-effects with Lyndiol 2·5 are minimal even during the first cycle.

A very stable resting type of endometrium is produced, which sheds reliably at the end of the course of tablets.

Spotting and breakthrough bleeding during a cycle are very rare.

Lyndiol 2·5 is presented in a 22 tablet pack which not only ensures 28 day cycles but is also significantly easier for the patient to remember. Each tablet is marked with the day on which it should be taken.

Lyndiol 2·5 costs less than other available preparations.

Each tablet contains
lynestrenol 2·5 mg, mestranol 0·075 mg.
In wallets of 22 tablets (one month's supply).

Organon Laboratories Ltd · Crown House · Morden · Surrey · England
Sole agents in the Republic:
Evans Medical (Ireland) Ltd · Distillery Road · Dublin 3

Figure 4.1 Advertisement for Lyndiol 2.5, *Journal of the Irish Medical Association*, volume LX, no.365, November 1967.
Courtesy of the National Library of Ireland.

contraception usually did not prescribe it to single women. However, some women found ways to circumvent this, through attending a sympathetic GP or lying about their marital status.[10] This practice was occurring within a wider context, from the 1960s, of increasing patient autonomy and consumerism.[11]

Between 1966 and 1967, it was estimated that there had been a 50 per cent increase in the usage of the pill in Ireland, with four anovulent brands available in 1966 and at least ten in 1967.[12] In 1967, Syntex Pharmaceuticals, the manufacturers of more than half of the contraceptive pill brands, estimated that 12,000 Irish women (three out of every hundred) were taking the pill, and by the following year, this was estimated to have risen to five out of every hundred.[13] Given that the contraceptive pill was the only artificial contraceptive available from GPs in Ireland pre-legalisation, albeit through the use of coded language, it became an important emblem in debates around the legalisation of family planning in the 1960s and 1970s. This also occurred in Britain where general debate about access to contraception was increasingly about access to the pill. The word 'pill' was frequently used in the press as a synonym for contraception and vice versa by the early 1970s.[14]

In Ireland, as in other Catholic countries with similar legal restrictions on birth control, the contraceptive pill featured heavily in media debates surrounding family planning. In Spain, the first references to the contraceptive pill appeared in the publications *ABC*, *Blanco y Negro* and *Triunfo* from 1964.[15] In the Spanish press, physicians dominated the debate on the contraceptive pill in the 1960s and 1970s; their focus tended to be on the side effects of the pill.[16] In Poland, where there was no ban on contraception, information about the pill had circulated in popular magazines such as *Przyjaciolka* since 1960.[17] In Portugal during the same time period, debates over the contraceptive pill highlighted the dissatisfaction of a significant proportion of Portuguese elites towards Catholic authority over matters relating to sexuality.[18] In Ireland, magazines such as *Woman's Way* played an important role in illuminating the experiences

---

[10] Eva-Maria Silies, 'Taking the pill after the "sexual revolution": Female contraceptive decisions in England and West Germany in the 1970s', *European Review of History (Revue européenne d'histoire)*, 22:1 (2015), pp. 41–59, on p. 43.

[11] Alex Mold, *Making the Patient-Consumer: Patient Organisations and Health Consumerism in Britain* (Manchester: Manchester University Press, 2016), pp. 18–19.

[12] Mary Maher, 'A short history of the pill in Ireland', *Irish Times*, 14 March 1968, p. 8.

[13] 'The pill in Ireland: A short review of the facts', *Irish Times*, 1 August 1968, p. 6.

[14] Cook, *The Long Sexual Revolution*, p. 290.

[15] Ortiz-Gomez and Ignaciuk, 'Pregnancy and labour', p. 662.   [16] *Ibid.*, pp. 662, 664.

[17] Ignaciuk, 'Paradox of the pill', p. 108.

[18] Marques, 'The politics of Catholic medicine', p. 180.

of 'ordinary' Irish women and their views on the ban on contraception, as well as the importance of marriage dynamics, sympathetic doctors and the Catholic Church.[19] There was also widespread coverage in popular Irish television programmes. Indeed, several respondents recalled hearing about the pill on television. Christopher (b. 1946) remembered the pill being discussed on The Late Late Show, while Ellen (b. 1949) recalled the pill being publicised in 'an Irish programme [most likely The Riordans] and one of the women in the programme she was going to take the pill, and it was a big thing, you know, they made a big storyline out of it'.

In an article on women's experiences of family planning in Woman's Way magazine in 1968, Monica McEnroy interviewed a woman called Mrs Kearney, the mother of three children, who had been refused the contraceptive pill by her doctor. According to McEnroy, Kearney wanted 'to have the same facilities for living her married life in peace and harmony with her husband and three children as her sister in England', and she argued, 'No hospital has the right to make me obey these regulations. I am the one to decide what is necessary for my family.'[20] Similarly, in a subsequent article, McEnroy drew attention to the fact that 'a hopeful percentage of doctors are prescribing anovulants. They could help desperate women in the less enlightened areas.'[21] McEnroy advised readers to contact her with the names of sympathetic doctors so that she could devise a list of doctors who 'the women who send the sad fan mail to this page can be advised to contact'. Readers were encouraged to ask their doctor if they would 'help Woman's Way to help readers whose family life or health is suffering from lack of reliable conception control' with the understanding that their name would never appear in print.[22]

Women's accounts of the contraceptive pill thus were an important element of debates in the printed media around contraception in the 1960s and 1970s. This was in part because the fact that the contraceptive pill was dissociated from the act of sexual intercourse meant that it became an easier vehicle for discussion, unlike, for instance, condoms

---

[19] See Caitriona Clear, Women's Voices in Ireland: Women's Magazines in the 1950s and 1960s (London: Bloomsbury, 2016), pp. 46–8. Woman's Way magazine appeared every fortnight from 1963 until August 1966, when it began to be published weekly. The magazine was aimed at women of all ages and covered a range of themes, from cookery to fashion to current affairs. See Clear, Women's Voices in Ireland, p. 65.

[20] Monica McEnroy, 'Family planning', Woman's Way, 1 March 1968, p. 19.

[21] Monica McEnroy, 'Family planning and the law', Woman's Way, 15 March 1968, pp. 40–41.

[22] Ibid..

that continued to have an association with sexually transmitted diseases.[23] Alluding to this, Professor Dermot Hourihane (1933–2020), a professor of pathology and one of the founder members of the Fertility Guidance Company, explained:

What the pill did was, first of all, it was a first class contraceptive, and most of all, you took it orally, so you didn't have to put anything in or out, so there was no intrusion into your body. That made it acceptable to all Irish people. There was no feeling of this horrible, dirty thing, and putting on, or whatever. It was socially acceptable ... so then, of course, what happened was the church said the pill was okay for regulating irregular periods, so all the well-to-do women that could pay the doctor said, 'I'd like the pill, please, my periods are very irregular', and he would say, 'Right', with a nod and a wink sort of thing. That was an unstated contract almost between the doctor and the ... So it just made it more and more unfair, but it made contraception – it changed it from being alien into being more acceptable to an Irish woman or man.

As Hourihane's testimony suggests, oral contraceptives often appealed to women because of their reliability and independence from the act of sexual intercourse, while they were not interruptive or messy compared to other forms of artificial contraceptives.[24] In feminist magazine *Wicca*, published in 1977, Ann O'Brien discussed how she had decided to go on the pill after moving into a flat and deciding 'that I wanted to enjoy myself and feel safe'. In contrast to other forms of contraception, such as condoms and the cap, she felt that the pill had an advantage of reliability and 'because the Pill is oral it is inclined to be separated from sexuality, which in part explains its success in a sexually repressed country like Ireland, but also it means there is no temptation not to use it involved, it's just a matter of remembering to take it all the time whether active sexually or not'.[25] Similarly, writing in her 2013 memoir, a founder member of the Irish Women's Liberation Movement, Mary Kenny, explained how, in a conversation with her mother many years after the 1971 Contraceptive Train protest, she realised her mother 'wasn't against the Pill; I think this was because the Pill was discreet, and clinical, and removed from the act of sexual intercourse'. On the other hand, her mother 'couldn't talk about condoms' because of their association with venereal disease.[26] Moreover, the popularity and acceptability of the

---

[23] As the author of a letter to the *Irish Times* in 1970 explained, for instance: 'Because of the ban on information, the "pill" has become synonymous with contraception in this country. Diaphragm seems to be a dirty word and the I.U.D. unheard of'. 'Contraception: what do you think?', 22 December 1970, p. 6.

[24] Watkins, *On the Pill*, p. 54.

[25] 'One woman's experience', *Wicca*, 1977 [RCAPA, UCC, BL/F/AP/1498/3], p. 8.

[26] Kenny, *Something of Myself and Others*, p. 156.

contraceptive pill must be understood within the broader historical context where new pills were becoming available on prescription to treat a variety of health issues.[27] The pill could also be bought in six-month supplies and potentially taken without the male partner's knowledge.[28]

Although the contraceptive pill became available in Ireland from 1963, access remained difficult for the majority of Irish men and women. As John Horgan, in an article in *Fortnight* magazine in 1970, surmised:

[T]he fact that the pill is much more freely available to the fee-paying middle-class patients of doctors in private practice than to the working-class mothers who have no option but to attend Church-controlled maternity hospitals, introduces an ugly element of class distinction into a situation already reeking of contradiction and hypocrisy.[29]

Working-class women were most likely to be severely affected by a lack of access to the pill; if their local GP would not prescribe it, then these women were often reliant on public postnatal care at a maternity hospital where they might potentially obtain a prescription.[30] Two of the three major maternity hospitals in Dublin – the Coombe Lying-in Hospital and the National Maternity Hospital (NMH) – were Catholic hospitals, with Archbishop John Charles McQuaid acting as governor of their boards.[31] From 1963, the NMH in Dublin established a family planning service to provide advice 'in conformity with Catholic moral teaching'.[32] In his 1964 report on the Family Planning Clinic of the NMH, Dr. Declan Meagher stated that the clinic had been set up as a result of 'an increasing awareness of the real personal problems which uncontrolled fertility presented to many patients'. Patients attending the clinic in its early years were solely advised on methods 'related to those of the infertile period' and were given a forty-five-minute educational talk on responsible parenthood and the infertile period, which included a short educational film. Meagher estimated that almost 4,000 patients 'mostly from the lower socioeconomic groups' had attended the talks.[33] In his 1966 report on the work of the NMH Family Planning Clinic, Meagher acknowledged that while the safe period 'meets the needs of

[27] Andrea Tone, 'Medicalizing reproduction: The pill and home pregnancy tests', *Journal of Sex Research*, 49:4 (2012), pp. 319–27, on p. 321.
[28] Ursula Barry, 'The movement, change and reaction: The struggle over reproductive rights in Ireland' in Ailbhe Smyth (ed.), *The Abortion Papers* (Dublin: Attic Press, 1992), pp. 107–18, on p. 112.
[29] John Horgan, 'Sugaring the pill', *Fortnight*, no. 6 (4 December 1970), p. 9.
[30] Foley, 'Too many children?', p. 145.   [31] *Ibid.*, p. 144.
[32] Daly, *Sixties Ireland*, p. 148.
[33] Declan Meagher, 'Family planning' in NMH Clinical Report for the Year 1964, *Irish Journal of Medical Science* (February 1966), p. 94.

many couples, it is inadequate in serious medical and social cases'.[34] The Coombe Hospital also provided advice through a 'Marriage Guidance Clinic' from 1965.[35]

The Rotunda Hospital was not Catholic but the vast majority of its patients were Catholic owing to its location.[36] It appears to have referred some patients to an appropriate consultant for family planning advice but its 1962 report stressed that this was only in cases with extreme socio-economic factors; patients were also 'given the opportunity of discussing such problems with the Hospital Chaplains'.[37] A formal Family Planning Clinic was established at the Rotunda in January 1966, with Eleanor Holmes of the Social Work department stating 'the guidance it gave was much sought for and needed by patients with severe social problems, as well as on medical and obstetric grounds'.[38]

Women's accounts of the contraceptive pill often contrasted it with natural methods of birth control such as the rhythm method. Máire Mullarney, a founder of the Fertility Guidance Company, asked her doctor for the pill in 1964. Writing in 1992 she said 'I asked our doctor for the Pill right away. I did not consult anyone with a Roman collar. I might not have picked one who read the more adventurous journals'.[39] Her memoir expands on the benefits of the pill in contrast with the natural methods she had previously been using:

We agreed that with this blessed Rhythm, by the time the 'safe period' arrived we wished sex had never been invented. You see, if you were well-informed, as we were, you knew that, not only must the husband not ejaculate, but the wife must not allow herself to experience orgasm. This while sharing the same bed. So different with the magic Pill; I could say, "Well, not tonight, if you don't mind, but tomorrow will be fine.' And it would be. Formerly there used to be the waiting and wondering, would a period ever happen? And a husband depressed for months when, after all our care, I was pregnant again.[40]

For Mullarney, the contraceptive pill provided a much-needed respite from the anxiety of worrying about falling pregnant, in contrast with the rhythm method, which restricted sexual intercourse to infertile days. She was not unusual in finding the rhythm method problematic. As Dr. Dermot MacDonald and Dr. Declan Meagher, the two doctors who ran the family planning clinic at the NMH in Dublin, explained in a 1967 article, the rhythm method required couples who had recently had a baby

---

[34] Ibid., 95.   [35] Daly, Sixties Ireland, p. 148.   [36] Foley, 'Too many children', p. 147.
[37] Clinical Report of the Rotunda Hospital, 1st January 1962 to 31st December 1962, p. 68.
[38] Clinical Report of the Rotunda Hospital, 1st January 1966 to 31st December 1966, p. 70.
[39] Máire Mullarney, What About Me? A Woman for Whom 'One Damn Cause' Led to Another (Dublin: Town House, 1992), p. 159.
[40] Mullarney, What About Me? p. 161.

to abstain from intercourse until regular menstruation returned, which could be 5–6 months after birth in some cases.[41] This combined with the fact that couples were also advised to refrain from intercourse in the last two months of pregnancy, meant that the rhythm method imposed 'an intolerable strain on many marriages'.[42] They explained that by this point, the policy of the clinic was to prescribe "the pill" as a contraceptive 'for selected medical and social cases' and emphasised that advice on family planning should be freely available to all mothers, with fear of pregnancy being detrimental to marital harmony.[43] Dr. Niall Tierney, writing in response to the article, asked for further elucidation on the comments made by Meagher and MacDonald, particularly as the prescription of artificial contraception such as the pill was 'directly opposed to the official view of the Catholic Church'. In response, Meagher and MacDonald insisted that they did not advocate the pill. In their view:

The issue for doctors is not the morality of taking the pill but rather the morality of refusing to provide it for patients who feel entitled, in conscience, to take it. It is our duty to treat the patients; it is the patients who make the moral decisions. In this situation we have concluded that to deny the 'Pill' to couples who need it, is at variance with the dictates of justice and charity.[44]

Contemporary newspaper accounts suggest that the contraceptive pill was also being readily prescribed by general practitioners in Ireland – this involved doctors making a private agreement with patients. In 1968, the marketing director of Syntex Pharmaceuticals, Ronald Levin, stated that from 'the conversations we've had with doctors in the Republic [...] the majority of general practitioners in Ireland are prescribing the Pill for social reasons'.[45] One Dublin gynaecologist explained to journalist Mary Maher in March 1968 that 'more and more general practitioners are prescribing it, and very few doctors would refuse it now to any woman who asks for it'.[46] Another pharmaceutical company representative stated that he believed that 25 per cent of Irish women taking the pill were doing so for 'medical reasons', and 75 per cent for 'social reasons', with the firm's spokesperson joking 'Either that or there's a great increase in menstrual difficulties'.[47] However, the spokesperson quickly added that the company was strictly adhering to Irish legislation around

---

[41] Declan Meagher and Dermot MacDonald, 'A hospital family planning service', *Journal of the Irish Medical Association*, December 1967, pp. 443–5.
[42] *Ibid.*   [43] *Ibid.*
[44] 'Contraception policy', *Journal of the Irish Medical Association*, 61:368 (February 1968), p. 73.
[45] Mary Maher, 'A short history of the pill in Ireland', *Irish Times*, 14 March 1968, p. 8.
[46] *Ibid.*   [47] Maher, 'A short history', p. 8.

contraception and that 'chemists are just as strict about following pre-scriptions exactly', stressing that 'the great majority of doctors are deeply concerned and very anxious for a decision from Rome'.[48] Indeed, as Lara Marks notes, 'the widespread expectation of imminent change during the early 1960s had in itself led many Catholics to decide to use the pill before the encyclical was published'.[49] Dr. Kieran O'Driscoll, master of the NMH, stated that 'It is no exaggeration to say that our position in continuing to withhold this most effective and now widely accepted method, particularly in ill women, causes a serious problem of con-science for me and for other members of our medical staff. One can only hope that clear guidance will not be much longer delayed'.[50] However, with the publication of *Humanae Vitae* in 1968, the NMH no longer prescribed the pill. In a July 1968 letter written by Dr. Kieran O'Driscoll, master of the hospital to Archbishop John Charles McQuaid, O'Driscoll assured the archbishop that the 'Papal Encyclical is accepted as an explicitly clear directive on the subject of birth control, which will be adhered to'.[51] As Deirdre Foley has argued, 'While the behaviour of Catholics was increasingly related to personal conscience, rather than Catholic dogma, the influence of this teaching at Catholic maternity hospitals was, however, a hindrance to those who sought access to the pill'.[52]

Following the introduction of the encyclical, some Irish doctors now faced a new dilemma. *Humanae Vitae* came at a crucial moment in terms of the history of birth control – the question of contraception had become the topic of heated debate, particularly with the advent of the contracep-tive pill in Europe from the early 1960s, but now that Church guidance was clearly against contraception, doctors had to make a choice over whether they felt they could prescribe it. According to one article in the *Irish Times* in 1968, 'for a number of years now, since the introduction of the pill, the doctors have been unwillingly carrying a certain moral responsibility'. The piece stated:

on the one hand they were attacked for being reactionary, for not prescribing the pill more freely; on the other hand they had to defend themselves against the charge of opening the flood-gates by prescribing the pill at all. The doctors' attitude always was that the moral decision was one for the patient to make: he

[48] *Ibid.*   [49] Marks, *Sexual Chemistry*, p. 232.
[50] 'Ireland: Anticipating the Pope', *The Tablet*, 20 May 1967, p. 566.
[51] Letter from Kieran O'Driscoll, master NMH, 30 July 1968. [DDA: McQuaid Public Affairs, 20/9–10].
[52] Foley, 'Too many children?', p. 147.

would look after the medical problems and thus while Catholic doctors did not suggest using the pill as a contraceptive, they usually prescribed it on the patients' request.[53]

However, now that the moral position was made clear and Catholic couples were forbidden from using artificial contraception, the article asked, 'has the responsibility of the Catholic doctor changed?'[54] As a result of the lack of other contraceptive options, some sympathetic general practitioners prescribed the pill to women who had experienced numerous pregnancies. Writing in the *Journal of the Irish Medical Association* in 1969, Dr. Declan Meagher highlighted the difficult position that the Irish ban on contraception posed for doctors. He argued that the role of the doctor was to bring 'sympathy and understanding' to couples with problems controlling their fertility. Meagher believed that the primary responsibility of doctors was to decide on the best medical treatment for the patient. He argued that for some Irish patients and doctors, *Humanae Vitae* was not an infallible statement.[55] In Meagher's view:

It may be difficult for them to see it is immoral for man to deliberately induce a condition which nature itself produces constantly throughout the infertile days, or to turn a deaf ear to the over-burdened generous mother with five children under 7 at loggerheads with husband, children and religion who pleads 'But doctor, is it for the good of the family?'[56]

Meagher's testimony highlights the difficult dilemma faced by some Irish doctors. The use of a case of a woman with multiple children as an example, was typical of evidence put forward in favour of the legalisation of contraception at the time. Many doctors, however, were conflicted. At a Medical Union conference in 1971, for instance, one doctor asked, 'Am I to condemn a woman to Purgatory in this life by refusing her the Pill? Or am I to condemn myself to Purgatory in the next life by prescribing whatever contraceptive she asks for?'[57] Others such as Professor William Dwyer, a kidney specialist at Jervis Street Hospital, stated at a meeting organised by the Irish Family Planning Rights Association in 1971, that for some doctors 'it would be morally and professional irresponsible to recommend the safe period or rhythm as a total protection to

---

[53] 'Doctors' dilemma about prescribing', *Irish Times*, 30 July 1968, p. 7.   [54] *Ibid.*
[55] *Journal of the Irish Medical Association*, 62: 382, April 1969, pp. 124–5. Similarly, as Agata Ignaciuk's work has shown, in Spain, *Humanae Vitae* was largely irrelevant for doctors who supported family planning and who were involved in early birth control clinics. See: 'Love in the time of El Generalisimo: debates about the pill in Spain before and after Humanae Vitae' in Harris (ed.), *The Schism of '68*, pp. 229–50, on p. 243.
[56] *Journal of the Irish Medical Association*, 62: 382, April 1969, pp. 124–5.
[57] 'Dilemma: report on family planning', *Woman's Way*, 22 January 1971, p. 25.

any woman against any pregnancy in the future'.[58] For many doctors the issue was a delicate one. At the Medical Union conference in Sligo in 1973 two motions which were put forward with regard to contraception, firstly, to ask the Minister for Health to establish family planning clinics in the health board areas, and secondly, to ask for the lifting of the Irish law forbidding the sale of contraceptives, allegedly descended into chaos.[59] The union failed to come to an agreement on the issue and was criticised in the *Irish Medical Times* for 'shirking its responsibility' to members of the public who looked to doctors for guidance and help.[60] In any case, the situation with regard to the pill placed Irish doctors in a unique position of power.

4.2   Attitudes to the Pill

Oral history evidence suggests that there was significant stigma attached to taking the pill and negative attitudes towards women who were being open about taking it. Martina's (b.1955) testimony, for instance, highlights both of these points:

But I do remember one time we were at some function. And this lady, who was married to a guy from [large town in southwest of Ireland], she was American. I remember her saying that she was on the pill. And I mean, we were all, 'Oh my God, she's out there saying she was on the pill'. It was like saying she was out there robbing a bank. It was that strange. What kind of person is this? She's on the pill.

When I asked why people were so shocked by this behaviour, Martina explained, 'I supposed what shocked us about it was that she was open about it. I mean, this wasn't something you were going to say in company that you were on the pill. You'd keep it to yourself if you were on the pill'. Similarly, Alice (b.1944) from the west of Ireland stated that 'We thought that going on the pill was just unbelievable. There was one girl that came to live in our place, and she was on the pill. It was nearly the same as having leprosy, we thought so'. Likewise, in a 1968 article by Monica McEnroy, thirty-six-year-old Angela, who was described as married with six children and living on a farm, explained 'I went on the pill in England this time last year. I was over in Devon with my sister. It is a nuisance having to go to Dublin every six months to get a check-up but sure it is only twice a year after all. I would not say a word about it around here'.[61]

[58] 'Ireland: call to change family planning law', *The Tablet*, 4 December, 1971, p. 1182.
[59] Monica McEnroy, 'Family planning prohibited', *Woman's Way*, 16 November 1973, p. 12.
[60] 'Attack on Irish doctors over birth control', *Evening Herald*, 5 October 1973, p. 4.
[61] 'The sex life of the Irish', *Woman's Way*, 2 August 1968, p. 35.

There appear to be significant generational differences in terms of attitudes to the pill. Some interviewees asserted that women of their generation did not take the pill, implying that it was a practice of younger generations. For instance, when I asked Nuala (b.1935) from Dublin if she had ever heard of anyone taking the pill, she commented: 'Not in my day, definitely not. No. Would have maybe years after, but would be younger people then of course. Not in my day, no. There was no talk. [...] No. It was a different world.'

Similarly, when asked about whether she knew of anyone taking the pill in the 1960s and 1970s Úna (b.1944) told me: 'I don't think so. Not in my day. I don't think the pill was available. [...] Just behaved yourself.' Úna's comment 'Just behaved yourself' is revealing because again, it suggests that the pill brought sexual freedom to younger women, but also implies that she and her contemporaries led more chaste lives. Moreover, the above accounts resonate with Kate Fisher's findings that many of the women she interviewed maintained ignorance or naivety around the issue of birth control, because 'ignorance implied moral purity, innocence and respectability'.[62]

Several respondents also referred to their mothers' attitudes to the pill and how this impacted on their own views. Ellen (b.1949) from the southeast of Ireland, reflected 'my mother being so religious, she told me if even when I got married, she said if I was taking the pill that I wasn't to come home anymore'. Similarly, Catherine (b.1953) from the southwest of Ireland, took the contraceptive pill before she got married in 1975. She recalled a heated conversation with her mother after she got married. After Catherine told her mother she was on the pill, her mother stated 'Oh, you'll be condemned, weeping and gnashing your teeth. It's a mortal sin!' Other mothers had a different attitude and reflected on how different things were for their daughters than their generation. Marian (b.1935) who came from a large family from a rural area in the north of Ireland, told me:

My poor mother, I remember her saying to me, 'Well if I had had them pills I would have took them by the handful', when the contraceptive pills came out. Now she wouldn't have given any of us back if you know what I mean but she had one baby after another. There's only 18 months between some of us.

Some respondents also recalled their concerns around the side effects of the pill. Indeed, as Lara Marks has shown, medical experts in the UK and United States vigorously debated the side effects of the pill, in particular, thrombosis, during the 1960s and 1970s.[63] Professor John Bonnar,

---

[62] Fisher, *Birth Control*, p. 27.   [63] See: Marks, *Sexual Chemistry*, pp. 138–57.

professor of obstetrics and gynaecology at TCD, who conducted research into thrombosis and the pill, explained in an oral history interview 'I think the pill was a major advance. But we've an obligation, when it's being taken by young, healthy women, to see that it's as safe as possible. And its history, in that regard, is not anything to be proud of.' Moreover, it is evident from oral history testimonies, that concerns about the side effects of the pill seeped into the consciousnesses of many women. Audrey (b.1934) from Dublin recalled that when the pill came out in the 1960s, 'you heard horror stories of girls dying from it and all'. Indeed, discussions of the side effects of the pill had an influence on women's attitudes to family planning options. Winnie (b.1938) from a small town in the north of Ireland, explained that she would not have taken the pill had it been available to her because 'I wouldn't interfere with my body in that respect. I would have been too scared'.

Given the stigma attached to the contraceptive pill, women who decided to take it tended to keep this information to themselves. Cathy (b.1947) decided to take the pill before she got married in 1974. She told me:

I went on the pill a couple of months before I got married, and I used to go to the family planning clinic in Mountjoy Square [in Dublin]. That's where they were. But I remember, I'd go to the door and I'd be looking over my shoulder before I'd go in, making sure nobody saw me. Because I told nobody I was on it. Joseph knew, and my immediate friends would have known. But I never told my mother, I never told anybody in work. Like, they were all very religious, and you'd be seriously judged, like, if they knew you were doing something like that. Lads I worked with.

She believed that she would 'be vilified, I'd say if they thought I was doing that. Desperate, like'. Similarly, when asked if she knew anyone who had taken the pill, Julia (b.1936) explained to me 'Well, I would say that in those days, even if they were, they weren't going to … Say it. No I wouldn't think so, no'. Likewise, Judith (b.1950) who went on the pill before she got married aged 25, told me 'It wasn't something you'd advertise or go around telling'. Similarly, Brigid (b.1945) explained 'people were very reticent to talk about it at the time. People wouldn't admit at all to doing anything remotely like that'.

In addition, as one young woman writing into *Nikki* magazine in 1973, commented 'getting the pill is not an easy thing'.[64] Women who wished to obtain the pill were reliant on a sympathetic doctor, or could have obtained it at one of the urban-based family planning clinics. Annual reports from the IFPA illustrate the prevalence of the contraceptive pill as

---

[64] 'Feedback', *Nikki*, (November 1973), p. 68.

a family planning method for IFPA patients at Dublin clinics, as will be discussed in further depth in Chapter 6. Doctors therefore had significant authority in deciding who could be prescribed the pill. Similarly in Spain, the circulation of the pill in the 1960s and early 1970s helped to 'reinforce the doctor's technical and gender power position'.[65] According to Monica McEnroy, *Woman's Way* magazine received letters every week 'asking where a doctor can be found who will prescribe the Pill'.[66] Knowledge was disseminated between women about which doctors would prescribe the pill and which would not, as well as what to say in order to obtain it. Myra (b.1947) for instance, explained to me:

Well I remember oh, there was, I think Dr. Smith used to do it, because he was more liberal. I don't know, I think – I don't know, was he a Protestant? I'm not quite sure, because there was a different doctor I went to. But they gave it to you if you wanted to regulate the periods, you got the pill to regulate your periods so that I suppose ... But no, I'd say there was a lot of people who got the pill off of him.

Similarly, Christopher (b.1946) from a rural part of south-east Ireland told me 'You would have, it would be diagnosed for not contraception but for, for other reasons, for supposedly some other reason ... You would get an understanding GP who would say – "Ah yes, I can see this now and this will fix that" and it would be nod, nod, wink, wink'. There is also evidence to suggest that some women from working-class backgrounds possessed knowledge of how they might gain access to the contraceptive pill. Marian Larragy, a member of the Contraception Action Programme, an offshoot of feminist group Irishwomen United, recalled visiting the residents of flats in Ballymun, one of Dublin's most underprivileged areas, in order to gain signatures for a CAP petition. She recalled meeting a young mother who had been in her class in primary school who 'signed the petition and told me that everybody in the flats was getting the pill "to make their periods regular"'.[67]

Other respondents recalled 'shopping around' for a doctor who would prescribe the pill. Nicholas (b.1953) who lived in a town in the west of Ireland, explained that his wife initially went to a doctor who refused to give her the pill. In Nicholas' words 'he frowned totally on the idea'. However, his wife found another GP who in contrast 'was well on board

[65] Agata Ignaciuk, Teresa Ortiz-Gómez, Esteban Rodríguez-Ocaña, 'Doctors, Women and the Circulation of Knowledge of Oral Contraceptives in Spain, 1960s–1970s' in Teresa Ortiz-Gomez, María Jesús Santesmases (eds.), *Gendered Drugs and Medicine: Historical and Socio-cultural Perspectives* (Farnham: Ashgate, 2014), pp. 133–52, on p. 141.

[66] 'The Papal Encyclical', *Woman's Way*, 13 September 1968, pp. 44–5.

[67] Marian Larragy cited in Ann Rossiter, *Ireland's Hidden Diaspora*, p. 146.

towards prescribing the pill ... And there was a good engaged team conversation with my wife and her doctor. I thought that was good at the time, looking back on it now ... But he was a progressive doctor'. Similarly, Noel (b.1952) believed it was 'just a case of you just finding the right person'.

Andrew Rynne, who worked as a doctor doing vasectomies for the IFPA, noted in his memoirs that during his time in general practice, female patients regularly asked him if was 'morally all right' for them to use contraceptives. In other words, he felt that 'doctors were sometimes looked upon as kind of surrogate priests, a role that I for one thought quite absurd'.[68] Doctors had significant authority, and as with priests, as will be outlined in the next chapter, there was a sense among some respondents that women could not question their judgement. Maud (b.1947) for example explained 'In those days you didn't question the GP really. Like today you go in there now and you look on the internet and you're reading up and stuff'. Similarly, Ellen (b.1949) asked her GP for the pill after the birth of her fourth child in 1976. She said, 'when I went to the GP, he just said "I don't like giving the pill." But I think if I had pressed him for it, he would have given it to me. Because I think some GPs at the time did give it.' Indeed, some respondents believed that doctors would only give out the contraceptive pill in extreme circumstances. For instance, when I asked Colm (b.1940) from a rural area in the Midlands, about whether women would have had access to the pill in Ireland in the 1960s and 1970s he replied: 'Jaysus, you couldn't. Well I suppose you could go to the doctor and get a, go to the doctor and get a, a cert ... to say that if this woman, then ... You know the type of thing, or endanger her life, like this'. Similarly, Ellen (b.1949) whose GP refused to give her the pill, explained that some doctors did prescribe it, but only in extreme circumstances:

They would give it to you, see, if you were kind of said 'I'm going to kill myself if I have any more children'. Or you know, if they thought having another child would have been bad for your health, that you wouldn't have been able for a child or something like that. They would have had to have reason for giving it. They just wouldn't have given it out willy-nilly I'd say.

Aoife (b.1947) explained how she really had to justify her need for the pill to her doctor. She said, 'I was saying, you know, if you don't help me, I'm in a mental hospital and so are all my children that's it because I cannot cope with this, you know. And I'll disgrace you if you don't you know and kind of threatened him and this is what I did – I had to fight. [..] I had to learn to fight'.

[68] Andrew Rynne, *The Vasectomy Doctor: A Memoir* (Cork: Mercier Press, 2005), p. 120.

Doctors clearly had considerable power in choosing whether they would prescribe a woman the contraceptive pill. For some doctors, their status as 'sympathetic' was undoubtedly lucrative. It is also clear that women also exhibited agency in finding a sympathetic doctor. Knowledge of sympathetic doctors, and information on what to say, was usually spread through word-of-mouth. Similarly, Leanne McCormick's important work on abortion in Belfast has shown the significance of women's networks in the transmission of knowledge about illegal abortion and the restriction of such networks of knowledge within Protestant dominated neighbourhoods.[69] For instance, as Irish feminist campaigner Ruth Riddick, who would go on to establish the Open Door Counselling service for women experiencing crisis pregnancies, explained in an oral history interview to me:

Now, needless to say, the Irish solution to an Irish problem was in place long before Charlie Haughey ever mentioned it. I remember being told by girlfriends what it is you said to which doctor to get put on the pill. That was relatively common knowledge. The pill, at this point, had been introduced since 1960. Now that we had television, now that our communication systems were working bigger and better we knew about the pill. The question only became where to get it.

Similarly, Fine Gael politician and member of the Irish Women's Liberation Movement, Nuala Fennell wrote in her 2009 memoirs that 'women who identified understanding and helpful general practitioners passed on the word to other women.'[70] Jean (b.1953) from a small town in the northwest explained that 'And then you would have known there was a GP here, not necessarily your own – one particular GP and you could have gone to him and he would give you the contraception'. Similarly, Sally (b.1956) from a rural area in the east of the country, told me, 'And there were certain doctors in their area, that would give them, and other's that wouldn't. So amongst us, we all knew, just say it was Dr. Riordan who would, and Dr. Murphy wouldn't. But you dare didn't tell your mother you were going to Dr. Riordan, because she'd know immediately. But there again, your medical records were not being followed through'. Alison (b.1953) from a Church of Ireland background, referred to the importance of women's networks in circulating information about the pill. She explained:

Now at that stage, obviously the pill wasn't widely, or wasn't, wouldn't have been legally. You wouldn't have been able to buy it over the counter or anything. But,

[69] See: McCormick, 'No sense of wrongdoing'.
[70] Nuala Fennell, *Political Woman: A Memoir* (Dublin: Currach Press, 2009), p. 79.

again, there was a hostel in Baggot Street, called the YW, where a lot of the Church of Ireland people who came up to Dublin to work would've lived there ... You know, so there was a network of women ... my age group who kind of knew the scene. So if you wanted to go on the pill, I had a friend who lived in there, she told me where to go. So there was a doctor out in [suburb], a lady doctor out in [suburb], who looked after people who wanted to go on the pill, and she looked after your gynaecology as well.

However, as Joanne O'Brien, a member of feminist activist group Irishwomen United explained, while 'There was information shared between women about who you could go to or whatever ... I think you had to have a fair amount of self-confidence to go in and ask for something like that'. For women who decided to ask their doctor for the pill, this was an admission that they were having sex. Martina (b.1955) recalled 'the fear of going to the doctor and asking him to put me on the ... To get the pill'. She explained 'I mean it's so silly, it's almost you're going in and you're imagining he's thinking you're now having sex ... And asking for the pill means that you're admitting you're actually having sex'. Lizzie (b.1946) was afraid to ask her doctor for the pill for fear of moral judgement. She explained:

No, because you wouldn't have the courage to go in and ask. You wouldn't. Mentally, you just would not be able ... I would not be able. I would not have been able to go in and say, because I would have felt that I was an easy person. What do you say, what do they call it? A loose person.

Similarly, Alice (b.1944) recalled believing as a young woman that it was a worse thing to be on the pill than to have sex outside of marriage. She went out with a man 'for a good while, and imagine, I never went on the pill or anything ... It was a bigger sin to go on the pill than to have sex'. Women who obtained the contraceptive pill did not necessarily go to their own GP due to fears that they would be refused or that their family would find out about it. Mairead (b.1953) who grew up in Dublin explained, 'You wouldn't go to your family doctor. You'd be afraid, they probably wouldn't tell your parents but you would be afraid, you know that they would'. Mairead instead obtained the pill from the Well Woman Centre. Similarly, Carmel (b.1952) explained that a lot of women would go to a different GP than their regular one because 'The doctor would know you and your parents, and everything else'.

Several oral history respondents, did however, mention more compassionate general practitioners who put them on the pill without them having to emphasise their personal difficulties. Clodagh (b.1940) from a rural area in the southwest, for instance, got married aged 22 in 1962, having her first child one year later. By 1968, she had six children under the age of four and ten months. Following the birth of her seventh child in 1972, she went on the pill:

In between the twins and the next lad because definitely I couldn't, no way could I be having another baby you know. And then when he was born, say four years after that was in 1972, I think my period went very irregular anyway like you know and I was with the doctor and this was a really old doctor like a very nice doctor now but he put me on the pill but for to regulate the periods but I think it was really maybe so that I wouldn't be pregnant as well I'd say.

Similarly, Nora (b.1940) had a positive experience with her GP in a rural area in the southwest of Ireland. Nora had married in 1967. Her first child was born in 1969 but died two days after being born. She went on to have another child two years later, followed by a traumatic miscarriage, and then another child two years afterwards. She explained that she was offered the pill by her GP in 1974: 'The doctor gave it to me because he said, seeing as I'd had the miss and all that, he said, "I think you've had enough for a while anyway"'. Nora explained to me that she was 'surprised' to have been asked if she would like to take the pill 'because I never expected to get it. I didn't even ask him for it'. She believed that her doctor 'felt that I needed it'. Similarly, Evelyn's (b.1940) general practitioner in a small town in the northwest 'didn't think twice' about giving her the contraceptive pill, however, her testimony suggests that she had to initially mention her personal difficulties in order to convince him: 'He didn't even question it   I just said to him, "I just don't know what I'm going to do…The kids are lovely but…". He said "I'll give you a prescription for the pill now." That was it, there was no discussion, no discussion at all'.

Elaine (b.1950) similarly had a positive experience with her female doctor in a small town in the west of Ireland. Elaine's marital life was difficult and her doctor was aware of her personal challenges. She recalled her doctor saying, "Here," she says, "take this. You don't need that hassle at all." Elaine explained that she "didn't know the first thing" about contraception, "all I knew was it would stop me from having kids. That's all she told me, really. Take that down." Elaine's experience was markedly different to Martina's (b.1955). Martina, from a rural area in the southwest of Ireland, had two children by the age of 20, and was in an abusive relationship where she regularly experienced violence and rape. She felt that, knowing her situation, her doctor should have suggested contraceptive options to her, but he never did:

No doctor said to me, 'Look, you should go on the pill'. And they knew … And I mean, my own GP knew the situation at home. He knew all of that but he never said, 'You should prevent having more children'. And it was when I had my fourth child, the gynaecologist, he said … I was 25 when I had my fourth child. And he said, 'Let that be the last'. And something clicked in me, I said, 'Yeah, this is sensible'. Just and that was my last. And from there on then I used contraception. And eventually got my tubes tied. But nowhere along the line did anyone say, 'You know, you should prevent getting pregnant'.

Martina felt 'You were left to fend for yourself. I mean that help wasn't even there. It wasn't forthcoming. Maybe if he'd been another doctor maybe he would have but not the doctor that I went to, anyhow. And he used to say to me things like, "Did you get rid of that guy yet?"'

Some women reflected on negative encounters with their GPs regarding contraception. Mrs C.W. from Kildare, writing to *Woman's Way* in 1971, remarked that 'every couple should at least expect a sympathetic and understanding hearing from their doctor' if they were seeking advice on family planning. She felt that this was not the case at that present moment, however, and that 'one is liable to hear the riot act read if the doctor does not approve of contraceptives'.[71] Cathy (b.1949) recalled her cousin who had six children being refused the pill by her GP:

… she had six kids, she didn't get married until she was 35 and she had six children in a few years. And she got to a point and I remember she went to the doctor one day and he said to her, 'You could be having them until you're 55'. And she said, 'Well, I don't want to be having them until I'm 55, can you give me something?' He wouldn't give it to her. Imagine that.

Although Cathy remarked that her cousin was religious, 'she wouldn't have asked for it only, she just had enough. She just thought six was enough and she didn't want to get pregnant again'. Such experiences were not unusual or restricted to Ireland. Maud (b.1947) emigrated to the UK from the west of Ireland in the 1960s. She had a similar experience with her Irish GP in England who refused to give her the pill for religious reasons:

I registered with my local GP over there obviously, he was Irish. This is what they did in England, they always stuck with the Irish people. So he was very Catholic, very stern. Very stern. So at that particular time when I got married, he wouldn't give you the pill, it went against his religion, so he lost a lot of his patients, young people, like the likes of me. English people.

Amongst her Irish friends in England, however, Maud believed 'A lot of people I knew were on the pill. Oh yeah. And they weren't with the Catholic doctors'.

[71] 'Over to you…', *Woman's Way*, 11 June 1971, p. 6.

Single women may have had particular difficulty in gaining access to the contraceptive pill from general practitioners in Ireland. Indeed, Eimer Philbin Bowman's 1977 study of first time visitors to a Dublin family planning clinic showed, some doctors were in general unhappy about prescribing the pill for any length of time to an unmarried woman, with one respondent explaining, 'He said he would give it to me for three months for irregularity but if I wanted it again I would have to go somewhere else'.[72] Some women also perceived that contraception was not available to single women. Annette, interviewed by Emer O'Kelly about her experiences of travelling to England for an abortion, explained that at the age of 24 in 1968, she 'was so green, that I didn't think a single girl could go to a doctor and ask for a contraceptive'.[73] As well as perhaps having difficulty finding a GP that would prescribe the pill, some chemists also refused to stock it, even after legalisation in the 1980s, as will be discussed more in Chapter 9. One GP who practised in a city in the west of Ireland in the 1970s told me: 'It was illegal, you know. So ... but then there were ways and means, you know. I remember that I had a very friendly pal who was a drug rep for one of the companies, you know, who did – I can't remember which one it was. And he'd always leave you a few boxes, you know, sample boxes. So, there was never a problem'.

Furthermore, there were cases where husbands interfered in women's access to the contraceptive pill. Aoife (b.1947) told me her husband 'discovered the pill and he threw it into the fire because that was against our religion and that was his excuse'. One mother of four, writing to *Woman's Way* advice column in July 1968 explained that her doctor had stopped prescribing her the pill because her husband had 'called in to object ... on the grounds that "you have to take what is before you in life"'. The agony aunt stated 'I think that both your doctor and your husband have forgotten that you are the person to decide. I suggest that you make this point quite firmly and cheerfully'.[74] Other women did not tell their husbands they were taking the pill for fear of causing an argument or tension in their marital relationship.[75] One such woman was twenty-eight-year-old Clare, married for six years with four children, and who had been taking the pill for almost a year. She had not told her husband so as to avoid rows and tension in their relationship, as she believed he would not approve. She had tried the safe period but found it

---

[72] Eimer Philbin Bowman, 'Sexual and contraceptive attitudes and behaviour of single attenders at a Dublin family planning clinic', *Journal of Biosocial Science*, 9:4, (October 1977), pp. 429–45, on p. 435.
[73] Emer O'Kelly, *The Permissive Society in Ireland?* (Cork: Mercier Press, 1974), p. 17.
[74] 'Marriage guidance', *Woman's Way*, 5 July 1968, p. 27.
[75] 'Undercover on the pill', *Woman's Way*, 1 June 1973, pp. 8–9.

to be 'utterly useless…in fact, my last two children were born while we were using this method'. Clare expressed her relief now that she was taking the pill, stating, 'It's wonderful to know that I won't become pregnant. I was very ill and had a difficult time carrying all my children. I think that I'd have had a nervous breakdown if I'd found myself pregnant again'.[76]

4.3   Conclusion

Evidently, debates around the contraceptive pill in 1960s and 1970s Ireland were complex. As in England, the contraceptive pill became a synonym for contraception more generally, and a means for the press to discuss the issue. The fact that some women could obtain the contraceptive pill through lying about their menstrual difficulties, illustrates the significant hypocrisy of the Irish ban on contraception, but also shows how some women found ways to resist the ban. Moreover, some doctors, through lack of other options, were prescribing the pill to women who might have been better suited to an alternative form of contraception. Women who took the contraceptive pill evidently displayed considerable agency and resistance in gaining access to it, and the circulation of knowledge regarding how to get access, and from whom, shows the importance of women's networks in helping women to circumvent the legislation. Nevertheless, attitudes towards women who were taking the pill indicate significant stigma towards individuals who used birth control, and women who took the pill were often forced to keep this secret. Finally, and as will be discussed more in the next chapter, the decision to take the contraceptive pill could sometimes result in a dilemma with regard to conscience for Catholic women, however, such women often justified taking the contraceptive pill for economic reasons.

[76] 'Undercover on the pill', p. 8.

In his 1967 poem, 'The Redemptorist', the Irish poet Austin Clarke (1896–1974) depicted the experience of an Irish woman in the confession box:

'How many children have you?' asked
The big Redemptorist.
                         'Six, Father'.
                               'The last,
When was it born?'
                    'Ten months ago'.
'I cannot absolve your mortal sin
Until you conceive again. Go home,
Obey your husband'.
                     She whimpered:
                               'But
The doctor warned me...'
                          Shutter became
Her coffin lid. She twisted her thin hands
And left the box.

We learn in the remainder of the poem that following the woman's death after another pregnancy, her children were left weeping in the orphanage. The priest in this poem is depicted in a negative light, 'proud of the Black Cross on his badge', and absolute in his adherence to the Catholic Church teachings on contraception.[1]

Important oral history research has highlighted the influence of Catholic beliefs on individuals' family planning practices in the contexts of England, Quebec, Spain, the Netherlands and Switzerland respectively, while work by Betty Hilliard and Máire Leane has illuminated the power of the Church over sexual behaviour in the Irish context.[2] Other

---

[1] Austin Clarke, *Old-Fashioned Pilgrimage and Other Poems* (Dublin: Dolmen Press, 1967), pp.35–6.

[2] See: Geiringer, *The Pope and the Pill*; Gervais and Gauvreau, 'Women, priests, and physicians'; Marloes Marrigje Schoonheim, *Mixing Ovaries and Rosaries Catholic Religion and Reproduction in the Netherlands, 1870–1970* (unpublished Ph.D. thesis,

151

scholars have shown the influence of Catholicism on family planning advice and services in Poland and Belgium.[3] Moreover, through correspondence from 'ordinary' Catholics regarding *Humanae Vitae*, Alana Harris has shown, how the debate 'ventilated diverse renderings of male sexuality and spousal responsibilities'.[4] Building on this work, and drawing on oral history interviews, letters to Archbishop John Charles McQuaid from Irish men and women, as well as correspondence in women's magazines, this chapter will explore the significance of religious influences on individuals' attitudes to family planning in the period following Pope Paul VI's encyclical *Humanae Vitae* in 1968.

The majority religion in Ireland at the time was Catholicism, so this chapter will focus primarily on the influence of Catholic teachings on individuals' experiences, but the experiences of those from other faiths who were interviewed as part of this project will also be referred to in brief for comparison.[5] I will suggest that Catholic teachings had an enormous impact on individuals' family planning practices but that this influence was beginning to wane by the late 1970s. In addition, this chapter draws attention to the power of priests as permission granters and shows that while the Catholic hierarchy continued to be unequivocal in its support of *Humanae Vitae*, there were some dissenting voices in the priesthood as well as sympathetic priests who were beginning to challenge the status quo by providing individuals with absolution for sins relating to contraception.

5.1   *Humanae Vitae* and Responses from the Church Hierarchy and Laity

The papal encyclical *Humanae Vitae* was published by Pope Paul VI on 25 July 1968. For many Catholics, it was hoped that the pope's encyclical would constitute a more relaxed approach to the issue of birth control. Austin Clarke's 1967 poem 'Our Love is Incorruptible' illuminated the

Radboud Universiteit Nijmegen, 2005); Rusterholz, 'Reproductive behavior'; Hilliard, 'The Catholic Church and married women's sexuality'; Leane, 'Embodied sexualities',.

[3] Agata Ignaciuk and Sylwia Kuźma-Markowska, 'Family planning advice in state–socialist Poland, 1950s–80s: Local and transnational exchanges', *Medical History*, 64:2, (April 2020), pp. 240–66; Anne-Sophie Crosetti, 'The "converted unbelievers": Catholics in family planning in French-speaking Belgium (1947–73)', *Medical History*, 64:2, (April 2020), pp. 267–86.

[4] Alana Harris, 'A Magna Carta for marriage: Love, Catholic masculinities and the *Humanae Vitae* contraception crisis in 1968 Britain', *Cultural and Social History*, 17:3, (2020), pp. 407–29, on p.423.

[5] As noted in the introduction, the Lambeth conferences of 1930 and 1958 indicated an acceptance of contraception in the Anglican Church.

anxiety felt by couples waiting for the decision from Rome prior to the announcement of the encyclical: 'Now that the Cardinals are rubbing/ Hands, will they permit us to be rubbered?' while his poem 'The Pill' expressed a similar sentiment: 'Pessary, letter, cap. What can/ We do until they have decreed/Their will, changing the ancient creed,/But lie awake on a separate pillow?'[6] However, to the disappointment of many Catholics, *Humanae Vitae* reinforced the Church's views relating to the purpose of marriage and condemned all methods of artificial contraception.[7] As journalist Dorine Rohan wrote in 1969 in relation to the encyclical, 'Anger, sadness, astonishment, relief have been felt and expressed in every sphere of the community'.[8] Rohan felt that the pope's decision on contraception would divide Irish Catholics into three groups: those who would adhere to the Church's teachings; those who would use contraception and cease going to the sacraments, and those who would continue to use contraception 'and endeavour to keep up their religion without going to confession'.[9] The testimony of Clodagh (b.1940) is perhaps representative of how many Irish men and women felt about the encyclical:

The pope brought out the encyclical, *Humanae Vitae*, well, I was so disappointed when I read that, they weren't allowing contraception or nothing like for a married couples like, I could understand it if they were, you know, banning it for people who weren't married but people who were married like and like that now as I said to you maybe in the beginning when we got married, the first four or five, you kind of think, that's why I got married having kids and blah, blah and that's okay but then as time went by like and you know you realised and then you had to abstain and that caused rifts as well, you know…

Clodagh believed having children to be part of the purpose of marriage, however, after feeling she had done her duty with her first five children, could not understand why she was not entitled to contraception. Her testimony also highlights the impact that abstention as a form of family planning, in line with Church teachings, had on her relationship with her husband.

The pope had been delayed in making his pronouncement on birth control which had given rise to hope that there would be some change in the Church's stance. By the time he released the encyclical, it was well-known that he was going against the majority opinion of his

---

[6] Clarke, *Old-Fashioned Pilgrimage*, p. 34.
[7] For more on the history of *Humanae Vitae* and how the encyclical was received and engaged with in a variety of countries, see: Harris (ed.), *The Schism of '68*. On reactions from the medical profession in Dublin, see: Foley, 'Too many children'.
[8] Dorine Rohan, *Marriage Irish Style* (Cork: Mercier Press, 1969), p. 92.
[9] Rohan, *Marriage Irish Style*, p. 100

commission.[10] Writing to Archbishop John Charles McQuaid in July 1968, for instance, a man from Cork stated 'The manner in which the statement was made is to be regretted after the public had been prepared for the opposite decision by statement of experts and theologians etc for the past two years'. The man asserted that the majority of the members of the special commission 'favoured a different line of thought'. He concluded his letter by saying 'to those burdened with huge families and low incomes this encyclical is a big blow'.[11] Similarly, a Dublin mother of nine, wrote to McQuaid to express her 'gratitude and admiration' for the recent encyclical but expressed regret 'that the statement was so long delayed and that the direction and guidance given by our priests, even here in Dublin was so divergent'.[12] Indeed, the pope's pronouncements may have come as a surprise to members of the clergy themselves. Father Bernárd Lynch attended the Dromantine House Society of African Missions seminary in Newry, Co. Down in the mid- to late-1960s. As a young seminarian, Father Lynch and his contemporaries were so sure that a more flexible statement on birth control would be forthcoming from Pope Paul VI that the seminarians christened him 'Pope Pill'. In Lynch's view, this was because 'we all thought... now, remember the sixties were something else, even in a seminary. We all thought and believed that he would allow that, it made such sense – we all came from big families'.

The encyclical sparked debate worldwide and Ireland was no exception. Letters sent to Irish newspapers indicate the problems individuals faced in trying to adhere to its guidelines. One mother of four, from New Ross, Wexford, wrote to the *Sunday Independent* in August 1968 to say that the rhythm method 'is impossible in my case because my periods are hopelessly irregular'. She explained that 'without the Pill, which I have been taking since last November, I would have to abstain totally from sexual relationships with my husband. Surely this would make a mockery of our marriage, which is, after all, a sacrament'.[13] A mother of three wrote that she felt 'rather bitter' about the encyclical, stating 'We are condemned to have many children because we love in our marriage'. Likewise, another woman from Greystones, Co. Wicklow, wrote of the impact of the encyclical on mothers, stating that numerous children resulted in 'overworked, worn-out mothers. Strain and tiredness are killers of happiness and dignity for the mother, children and husband'.[14] As Deirdre Foley

---

[10] Fuller, *Irish Catholicism*, p. 199.
[11] Letter to Archbishop McQuaid, 29 July 1967, [DDA, xx/8/2(1–3)].
[12] Letter to Archbishop McQuaid, 1 August 1968, [DDA, xx/8/12].
[13] 'It's a mockery of marriage', *Sunday Independent*, 11 August 1968, p. 14.
[14] 'I feel bitter' and 'Kills happiness', *Sunday Independent*, 25 August 1968, p. 8.

has argued, '*Humanae Vitae* created a temporary obstacle for many Irish Catholics, particularly the less well-off, in accessing artificial methods of contraception (primarily the pill) in Ireland'.[15]

Following the introduction of the papal encyclical in 1968, *Woman's Way* published a series of letters received on the subject of 'The Pope and the Pill'. These letters provide further insights into attitudes towards the encyclical among Irish women readers. Mrs. R.H. from Cork, who was almost thirty, explained that she had married at nineteen and had six children in eight years. She had been told by her physician 'that I am almost certain to keep having children for the best part of the next twenty years if I am not careful.' R.H. asked 'is it any wonder that there are so many women suffering from mental breakdown due to the strain of trying to manage on their incomes and living from month to month?' Mrs. M.B.D. from Tullamore stated that the safe period caused 'stress and strain that marriage in this day and age is unable to withstand' and argued that 'we all have our lives to live and the right to exercise our free will'. Mrs. Maura Hann from Arklow stated that the encyclical 'was a bitter disappointment to the majority of Catholic couples' with lack of access to contraception being 'the chief cause of the unhappiness and apathy so prevalent in Irish homes to-day.' Others were more positive about the pope's proclamation and perhaps, as a consequence of their religious views, agreed with the encyclical. 'Widow and mother of five sons' stated that the whole world should thank Pope Paul 'for the wonderful job he has made of the white paper on birth control.' Mrs. F. O'Sullivan asked 'what is all the fuss about?,' stating that Catholics had never been allowed contraceptives before and the Church should not be expected to engage in 'bending over backwards to keep them Catholic by every means in her power that those who want to have their cake and eat it feel that the Pope should give his blessing on their promiscuity.'[16] Evidently, there was a range of polarized views on this topic. The print media, in particular women's magazines, was an important vehicle for women to express their views on the matter.

In Ireland, as Peter Murray has argued, 'the encyclical enabled authoritarian forces to reassert themselves and paved the way for the adoption of the hard-line conservative positions that were subsequently asserted, to gradually diminishing effect, on issues of State law change'.[17]

[15] Foley, 'Too Many Children?', p. 160.

[16] 'The Pope and the pill', *Woman's Way*, 6 September 1968, p. 2–3.

[17] Peter Murray, 'The best news Ireland ever got? *Humanae Vitae*'s Reception on the Pope's Green Island' in A. Harris (ed.), *The Schism of '68: Catholicism, Contraception and Humanae Vitae in Europe, 1945–75* (Palgrave, 2018), pp. 275–301, on p. 294.

Archbishop John Charles McQuaid described the encyclical as an 'essential document' which reiterated the teaching of the Church.[18] Some went further in their condemnation of artificial contraception. The bishop of Galway, Rev. Dr. Michael Browne, in a letter following the pope's pronouncement, focused particularly on the dangers of the pill:

there is also the publicity and the commercial drive of the big industry engaged in the manufacture and sale of expensive pills. We should remember how the thalidomide pill, which produced terrible deformities in the children, was put on sale. Another pill has now been produced, the long-term affects [sic] of which on mother and child are not certain.[19]

Browne's letter here, which refers to the thalidomide disaster, focuses on the potential side effects of the contraceptive pill as a means of warning people from using it. Indeed, the side effects of the pill had sparked considerable discussion among medical experts in the UK and US in the 1960s and 1970s, and as Marks has argued, the links between the pill and thrombotic disease were particularly concerning in the wake of the thalidomide tragedy which had been especially catastrophic in Europe.[20] More widely, it was not uncommon for religious elites like Browne to selectively draw on concerns about the side effects of the pill in order to bolster their arguments against it. Agnieszka Kościańska has shown how in the Polish context, Zbigniew Lew-Starowicz, a devout Catholic and popular sexologist, mobilised 'the intellectual cover and scientific rhetoric of contemporary medical knowledge' in his arguments against the pill, also alluding to the mistakes of the thalidomide tragedy.[21]

The Irish bishops issued a statement in October 1968 in which they affirmed their confidence that the Irish people would accept *Humanae Vitae* and reminded the laity that 'the pope speaks not as one theologian among many, but as the Vicar of Christ who has the special assistance of the Holy Spirit in teaching the universal Church'.[22] Louise Fuller has suggested that this statement was 'more humane than statements of less than ten years previously' particularly as there was a recognition of the 'delicate personal problems and intellectual difficulties to which this

---

[18] 'The encyclical: first Catholic reactions', *The Tablet*, 3 August 1968, p. 766.

[19] 'Galway hears its bishop', *Irish Times*, 5 August 1968, p. 11.

[20] Lara Marks, *Sexual Chemistry*, p. 138.

[21] Agnieszka Kościańska, 'Humanae vitae, birth control and the forgotten history of the Catholic Church in Poland' in Alana Harris (ed.), *The Schism of '68: Catholicism, Contraception and Humanae Vitae in Europe, 1945–75* (Palgrave, 2018), pp. 187–208, on pp. 199–201.

[22] Statement issued by the Irish hierarchy on the encyclical, Humanae Vitae, Maynooth, 9 October 1968, *Furrow*, 19/11 (November 1968), pp. 661–2, cited in: Fuller, *Irish Catholicism*, p. 200.

teaching may give rise for some'. The bishops expressed their hope that 'priests especially in the confessional will show that understanding and sympathy which Our Divine Lord himself always displayed'.[23] However, the problem of contraception did not simply go away. As Diarmaid Ferriter has asserted, Archbishop McQuaid and his colleagues spent much of the early 1970s 'under siege' as the contraception issue was discussed so frequently on the radio and television.[24]

5.2   Dissenting Voices

Humanae Vitae generated considerable anguish for some priests.[25] There were some dissenting, progressive voices within the Irish priesthood, but there were significant consequences for those who spoke out.[26] Father James Good (1924–2018), a lecturer in medical ethics at UCC, and Father Denis O'Callaghan (1931-), professor of moral theology at Maynooth, and chairman of the Irish Theological Association, were not afraid to criticise the encyclical.[27] James Good had entered Maynooth in 1941 and was ordained in 1948 before undertaking a doctorate at Maynooth and teaching at All Hallows College. He then went to Innsbrook, Austria to undertake a doctorate in philosophy before returning to Cork and teaching at UCC. In an oral history interview recorded as part of a series of interviews with individuals in Cork in 2002–2003, Good stated that in relation to *Humanae Vitae* 'I felt very strongly from the beginning that where it was necessary married couples could limit their family. I taught that in my medical ethics class'.[28] Good explained, 'I rejected *Humanae Vitae* publicly the day it was promulgated'.[29] His views on the encyclical were published in *the Tablet* where it was stated that 'he could not accept the Encyclical and thought that most theologians and lay people would reject it'. He called the pronouncement 'a major tragedy'.[30] Nora (b.1940) remembered Father Good's church being 'packed' because he

---

[23] Statement issued by the Irish hierarchy on the encyclical, Humanae Vitae, Maynooth, 9 October 1968, Furrow, 19/11 (November 1968), pp. 661–2, cited in Fuller, *Irish Catholicism*, p. 200.

[24] Ferriter, *Occasions of Sin*, p. 415.   [25] Tentler, *Catholics and Contraception*, p. 268.

[26] On 'rebel priests' in Britain, such as Father Paul Weir, who opposed the encyclical, see: Harris, pp. 419–21. On opposition by priests in the United States, see Tentler, pp. 269–72.

[27] Fuller, *Irish Catholicism*, p. 199.

[28] Life and Lore oral history interview with Father James Good by Maurice O'Keeffe Recorded as part of series on Cork city, 2002–2003. Accessed via: www .irishlifeandlore.com/product/father-james-good/

[29] Life and Lore oral history interview with Father James Good.

[30] 'The Encyclical: first Catholic reactions', *The Tablet*, 3 August 1968, p. 766.

was known to be sympathetic to the use of contraception. Good felt that his position as a university member enabled him to publicly denounce the encyclical, in contrast with his fellow priests and theologians:

I had a matter of conscience actually, I felt so strongly about it and I was aware that a lot of my fellow priests, particularly the theologians, they felt the same. But you see, professors of theology, Maynooth, had no right of tenure against the bishop, they could be dismissed overnight. And several of my friends who were professors in Maynooth, they got warnings: 'If you continue to say this, you will be dismissed' you know, and ordered to withdraw. So I wouldn't blame them for not coming out in the open as they would be goners. But I knew I couldn't be touched as a university member, you see. The only control bishops, or Bishop Lucey, had over me was that he could not recommend my appointment as professor of theology.[31]

As a result of his outspoken views and the fact that he was known to be giving women who were using birth control absolution in confession, Father Good was called before Bishop Cornelius Lucey. His right to exercise his priestly duties was suspended in mid-August 1968, meaning he was banned from giving mass or hearing confession.[32] In an interview with the *Irish Times* in 2018, Good said, 'the process took less than an hour and I was given no opportunity to defend myself'. He recalled 'it became increasingly embarrassing for me to be saying parish Masses on Sundays and not being allowed to preach. Being banned from the confessional was also distressing'.[33] Writing in 1969, Dorine Rohan expressed the view that 'many men and women are deeply in sympathy with Dr. Good'. She wrote of one woman she interviewed who had been helped by him with her marriage problems saying to her in tears that Father Good "really cares and knows about our problems'.[34] Father Good sent his letter of resignation from the position of professor of theology to Bishop Lucey in 1970. He recalled Lucey's response:

He sent me a little note via the chaplain of the university saying that he got my note of resignation and "I am now enclosing your salary of professor of theology". The cheque enclosed was for £40 (laughs) for thirteen years salary at £200.[35]

Good remained a UCC staff member working in Education and continued to contribute to newspapers and broadcasts in the late 1960s and early 1970s.[36] He elaborated on his views in *The Tablet* in April 1969 in

---

[31] Life and Lore interview with Father James Good.
[32] Murray, 'The best news', p. 278.
[33] 'Humanae Vitae and the suspension of the priest opposed to it', *Irish Times*, 22 January 2018.
[34] Rohan, *Marriage Irish Style*, p. 96.
[35] Life and Lore oral history interview by Maurice O'Keeffe with Father James Good.
[36] Murray, 'The best news', p. 279.

an article entitled "Humanae Vitae', a Platonic Document'. He argued in the article that 'the reaction from the married laity shows that the ideal of *Humanae Vitae* cannot be translated into real life as it stands'. Good felt that 'the message has come clear and strong that for the normal couple the alternatives of abstinence or continued procreation are totally impracticable'. Good also disagreed that the rhythm method was a viable method of family planning in a real-life context. Good suggested that *Humanae Vitae* 'has to be substantially modified' to be transformed from an ideal to a 'norm of practical living for real people'.[37] Good later moved to Kenya in 1975 to work as a missionary there.[38] The fact that he moved to Kenya was interpreted by some parishioners as being a punishment for his outspoken views. Nora (b.1940) recalled the affair:

There was a Fr. Good, he was up in the Lough. And there used to be loads of people go to confession with him because he believed in ... and then Connie Lucey said to him, he was the bishop at the time, he sent him out foreign, out to the missions. To Turkana Desert, or something like that. He went out there then and he retired himself, the bishop. He must have been sorry for sending Fr. Good there. He only died there some time a couple of years ago. He was very much in favour of the pill or whatever. Of trying to regulate your family.

Another outspoken voice on *Humanae Vitae* was Father Denis O'Callaghan. It is important to note that O'Callaghan's later career was not without controversy and he was singled out in the 2011 Cloyne Report for failing to respond appropriately to allegations of child sex abuse against priests within the diocese from 1996 to 2008.[39] Earlier in his career, O'Callaghan contributed to the birth control debate through the publication of articles in Catholic newspapers and journals in the late 1960s.[40] In 1970 he spoke publicly at a meeting of the Medical Union on the subject of family planning alongside three gynaecologists and Senator Mary Bourke (later Robinson). At the meeting, he stated that there was no simple answer to the problem of whether it was morally right or wrong for Catholic doctors to prescribe contraception, arguing that 'because in each situation you have four very intractable people: the doctor, the priest, the husband and the wife, and these four will very seldom agree',

---

[37] James Good, '"Humanae Vitae", a Platonic Document', *The Tablet*, 19 April 1969, pp. 386–7.

[38] 'Humanae Vitae and the suspension of the priest opposed to it', *Irish Times*, 22 January 2018.

[39] See: Report by Commission of Investigation into the handling by Church and State authorities of allegations and suspicions of child sexual abuse against clerics of the Catholic Diocese of Cloyne (2011). www.justice.ie/en/JELR/Pages/Cloyne-Rpt

[40] Fuller, *Irish Catholicism*, pp. 202–3.

adding that 'We are within a changing and developing situation' and that he 'would hate to lay down what sounded like rigid guidelines at this stage'.[41]

Archbishop McQuaid was incensed by these comments and had his secretary write to O'Callaghan asking him for a full copy of the statement made at the meeting.[42] In his letter to McQuaid, O'Callaghan acknowledged the 'confusion in the community conscience caused by varying interpretations of *Humanae Vitae* on the part of Hierarchies in the Catholic world and by the divergent approaches in medical and confessional practice'. O'Callaghan felt that his comments at the meeting were meant 'to show that the principles of moral theology can help to find a way out of the impasse and can take account of all the factors in the situation'. He did not want to be identified with 'any extreme position and felt that his comments had been 'disjointed' in the *Irish Times* report of the meeting.[43] O'Callaghan asked to meet with the archbishop to discuss further but this request was not granted.[44]

In order to clear up the confusion that had been caused by O'Callaghan's statements, McQuaid had a letter read at all masses in the Dublin diocese on 29 November 1970 in which he reiterated the teachings of *Humanae Vitae*. While O'Callaghan was not named in the letter, it is clear that it alluded to his recent statements. McQuaid stated 'Any writer or speaker who wishes to venture into the area of the doctrine of moral law is gravely obliged to understand correctly and to state accurately the objective moral law as the teaching authority in the Church explains that law'. The remainder of his letter went on to affirm that within the diocese, the bishop was the only teaching authority. McQuaid reiterated that 'any such contraceptive act is wrong in itself'.[45] McQuaid received numerous letters from laypeople congratulating him for the pastoral and for his courage and clarity. One Dublin couple wrote to the archbishop in November 1970 to thank him for his pastoral letter stating that they had 'been often pained by the misleading statements given prominence by the news media and the failure to point out the necessity of prayer and trust in God in coping with the difficulties of responsible family planning'.[46] Another Dublin woman, wrote to say 'it is wonderful to hear the full teaching of the Pope set out with such clarity

---

[41] 'Birth control concession by theologian', *Irish Times*, 14 November 1970, p. 1.

[42] Fuller, *Irish Catholicism*, p. 203.

[43] Letter from Denis O'Callaghan to Archbishop McQuaid, 18 November 1970, [DDA, xx/54].

[44] Fuller, *Irish Catholicism*, p. 204.

[45] 'Archbishop speaks on birth control', *Irish Times*, 30 November 1970, p. 1.

[46] Letter to Archbishop John Charles McQuaid, 29 November 1970, [DDA, XX/64/1].

for the faithful'.[47] Other letters highlighted the despair felt by some Catholics. One woman from Dublin writing to McQuaid in December 1970 explained 'I am sadder now, I think, than at any other time in my spiritual life.' She felt 'greatly troubled by this teaching because, not only do I not personally understand the grounds for it (altho' up to now my husband and I have adhered to it) but I also am afraid that most of the sincere Catholics I know are equally troubled and four of the five priests I know best cannot, in conscience, subscribe to the teaching'.[48]

McQuaid's letter became the first of three pastoral letters he produced on the theme of 'Contraception and Conscience' with the subsequent two parts read at mass in Dublin in February and March 1971.[49] The March letter, which was also published in Irish newspapers, declared that if contraception was legalised, it would be 'an insult to our Faith; it would, without question, prove to be gravely damaging to morality, private and public; it would be and would remain a curse upon our country.'[50] McQuaid argued against the idea of contraception being a right, reiterating his previous statement that 'any such contraceptive act is always wrong in itself' and he suggested that the issue of making contraceptives available was one of 'public morality.' Moreover, he wrote that 'the public consequences of immorality that must follow for our whole society are only too clearly seen in other countries.'[51] A Dublin woman, writing to the Archbishop in March 1971 stated that 'it was like a breath of fresh air to hear your letter read at mass today'.[52] Other women wrote personal accounts of their experiences in their letters of support. A Longford woman writing to the archbishop in March 1971 apologised for writing to him 'like this' and provided a detailed account of her family's situation:

We have 12 boys and 2 girls and I lost 5. Nine of those were born and 4 dead since my kidney was removed up there in the Mater in 1951. The doctors warned me then not to have any more but what they didn't know I was three months pregnant during the operation, he will be 19 years in June. A few years later I lost 3 babies in one year. In 1960 I was unconscious for ages after a birth with a haemorrhage. Of course the doctors told me any more would be fatal but 2 years later, we had a boy. Seven years ago I was gravely ill and when the baby was born he had club feet and is now a confirmed epileptic. 13 months later we had a boy and I nearly went to the mental with nerves. I really thought we would have no

---

[47] Letter to Archbishop John Charles McQuaid, 29 November 1970, [DDA, xx/64/2].

[48] Letter to Archbishop McQuaid, 8 December 1970, [DDA, LVII/730/10].

[49] 'Alteration of law would be "a curse upon our country": Archbishop's pastoral', *Irish Times*, 29 March 1971, 11.

[50] "Alteration of law', *Irish Times*, 11.   [51] *Ibid.*, 11.

[52] Letter to Archbishop McQuaid, 28 March 1971 [DDA, xx/82/6].

more, but 2 years ago at almost 46 I was pregnant, 2 doctors refused to attend me and no home in Longford would take me in, so I spent 7 weeks in the Rotunda and had the first girl in 21 years by section operation. She is the most beautiful thing that ever came to this world.[53]

The woman wrote "Good for you' to have spoken out again about contraception and the pill'.[54] Although this woman had been through significantly traumatic experiences in relation to childbirth and pregnancy, it is clear that, like many others, she was unwavering in her support of the Church's position on contraception. Numerous other letters expressed their thanks to McQuaid for his pastoral and for making the Church's position on contraception clear, while others described the pastoral as 'courageous'. Others wrote of their loyalty to him in the face of the 'adverse publicity' his letter had received.[55] Yet, a number of letters also exist in the Dublin Diocesan Archive that were written in opposition to McQuaid's pastoral. One letter, from a male writer, explained that 'as a Catholic who intends to marry shortly, the subject of your pastoral is one of great concern to me. I am sad that I could find no consolation in your extreme and uncompromising statement'.[56] Another, from a Dublin woman, also soon to be married, commented on the negative tone of the pastoral and asked 'Why does His Grace frequently speak of contraception, for example? I'm getting married soon, - and at present working with housewives in the home daily, all over Dublin. Well I do think in conscience using God given reason, that planned children are the only children that should be brought into this world.'[57] This woman's account also highlights the tension between the Second Vatican Council's (1962–1965) ideas of 'responsible parenthood' and the lack of means to achieve this.[58] A Dun Laoghaire woman also wrote to McQuaid to express her 'despair' stating:

I do not belong to any groups or organisations, nor have I even written to anyone on such an issue before, but I have the gravest fears that should the Catholic Church in Dublin continue on this course it will soon cease to have any meaning for me, for my children, and for a large number of my friends.[59]

---

[53] Letter to Archbishop McQuaid, 30 March 1971 [DDA, xx/82/28]   [54] *Ibid.*
[55] *Ibid.*, 5 April 1971 [DDA, xx/82/42].   [56] *Ibid.*, undated [xx/106/14].
[57] *Ibid.*, 22 February 1971 [xx/106/1].
[58] In Spain, the Second Vatican Council's discussions about responsible parenthood led to broader discussions about family planning and contraception among Spanish Catholics. See: Ignaciuk, 'Love in the Time of El Generalísimo', pp. 229–250.
[59] Letter to Archbishop McQuaid, 29 March 1971. [DDA, xx/89/2]

At the top of the letter, McQuaid wrote to his secretary who was responsible for replying to the letters to 'Just acknowledge and hope she will see the truth'.[60] A letter from the mother of five children was also sent to McQuaid with no address or name attached. The woman wrote candidly of the difficulties she experienced during her pregnancies and as a result of a spine injury and kidney trouble she had 'to spend almost six of each nine months in bed before the birth of my children'. The woman's letter highlights the problems she faced in trying to follow the Church's teachings:

The rhythm method does not work for me and speaking as a trained nurse I assure you we made no mistakes. We tried total abstinence but my husband does not agree with this and says this is not marriage and that if he had wanted to lead a celibate life he would have chosen it.

The woman explained that she had had a major operation two years previously and had been told by her doctor not to have any more children. However, her situation was causing her great anxiety:

Have you any idea of the mental and spiritual anguish of a Catholic mother placed in this predicament!! and being told by Drs that I cannot use oral contraceptive methods? [...] Your pastoral letter yesterday had an appalling effect on my husband, he told me after Mass that he was sorry but that he shall not attend Mass any more and had come to this decision having listened to your pastoral letter!

The woman wrote that her marriage was 'ideal in every way except for this big problem' and stated that she was 'now in total despair of being able to carry on'. She asked for the archbishop to show more compassion in relation to the issue of contraception and to pray for her and her family.[61] Another woman from Dublin wrote to the Archbishop, as 'a young Catholic mother' and questioned how the 'enactment of such legislation would remain "a curse upon our country", this is hardly the language of temperance'. The woman closed her letter asking:

How can the Church in this country really condemn the woman who tries to elevate herself to a dignified level of womanhood. I think therefore the time has come when both Church and State must allow the women of Ireland to decide for themselves on this very personal issue.[62]

A series of letters from women responding to Archbishop McQuaid's pastoral were also published in *Woman's Way* magazine, and again, they

[60] *Ibid.*, [DDA, xx/89/2].
[61] Letter to Archbishop McQuaid, 30 March 1971, [DDA, xx/89/3].
[62] Letter to Archbishop McQuaid, 30 March 1971, [DDA, xx/89/6].

highlight the range of views on the matter. Mrs. T.D. from Kilkenny wrote to the magazine to state that she was 'very angry after having read Dr. McQuaid's letter criticizing contraception', stating that it was unfair that certain older rules of the Church such as fasting had been relaxed, while others had not. Similarly, Mrs. L. Morris from Fermanagh, expressed her disappointment in the clergy and their 'little faith in Irish mothers' and drew attention to the double code of morality in society that was 'to blame for a lot of promiscuity.'[63] Others were more support- ive of the pastoral. Mrs. M.L. from Laois, the mother of ten children, stated that she fully supported the Church's teaching on contraception and divorce and believed that the archbishop had 'every right to speak out strongly on such objective moral laws.' Other letters highlighted inter-generational tensions. According to Mrs. M.L., 'having success- fully reared my children in difficult and often poor circumstances I find it difficult to understand young couples nowadays and their comparatively easy way of living, their attitude towards their Christian way of life as regards marriage, marital rights and so on.' Arguments against the legal- isation of contraception often centered on fears around young people and promiscuity, suggesting that promiscuity was the next step along a slip- pery slope. Mrs. Geraldine Lynch from Dundalk stated that if contra- ceptives became legal, it would be 'an open invitation for young couples who have become tired of drink, smoking and everything else?'[64] Similarly, Mrs. Marie C. Dunne wrote to the magazine asking 'if contra- ceptives were to be sold over the counter legally what would happen to our unmarried youth who took advantage of it? It could be injurious to their health, apart altogether from the moral aspect,' adding that 'a permissive society is a sick society and what sane person wants a sick society?'[65]

McQuaid also received numerous letters from members of the clergy congratulating him for the letter. For instance, Bishop Cornelius Lucey in Cork wrote that the pastoral was 'thorough and yet concise; it was clear; and it was timely. God bless you for it'.[66] For many parish priests, the letter brought relief and clear guidance. A Dublin-based priest wrote 'personally I am comforted and gratified to have your guidance'. The priest explained that 'due to reading of so-called 'out dated theology' and to the loose conversation of the very many clergy I meet in my missionary

[63] 'Over to you…', *Woman's Way*, 14 May 1971, p. 6.
[64] 'Over to you…', *Woman's Way*, Friday, 28 May 1971, p. 6.
[65] 'Over to you…', *Woman's Way*, 4 June 1971, p. 6.
[66] Letter from Cornelius Lucey to Archbishop McQuaid, 30 November 1970, [DDA, xx/ 63/14].

life not excluding some of my own younger brethren, I was beginning to wonder if perhaps I was too old fashioned – maybe even a rigourist – both in the pulpit and in the confessional. You have set my mind at ease and with God's grace and many help I will with a soothed conscience remain "a Pope's man"'.[67] It is evident that some priests found the direct guidance useful in light of the ongoing debates in the media. Another Dublin priest wrote 'At present there are so many unusual things said by professors and others, that ordinary priests like myself begin to worry if we are just clinging on to our own prejudices or standing up for the teaching of Jesus Christ. Your Grace has done a great service'.[68]

However, there continued to be some voices of dissent among the clergy. A man from Rathdrum, Co. Wicklow, wrote to McQuaid in March 1971 to report 'a scandalous occurrence' that had taken place at mass in Rathdrum church that day. The celebrant, Rev. Fr. Deane, in introducing McQuaid's pastoral letter allegedly 'proceeded to give a sermon containing his own ideas about this matter, one at least of which was clearly at variance with your letter'. Father Deane apparently only read a shortened version of McQuaid's letter 'omitting parts that he apparently disagreed with' and remarking that the Church could not 'at present change the law on contraception, that a change in the law of the country would inevitably come, and that in his opinion the minority had a right to avail of contraceptives'.[69] McQuaid was clearly enraged by this act of dissent and contacted Father Joseph Callan, the parish priest in Rathdrum. Callan replied promptly to McQuaid's letter stating that he had discussed the matter with Father Deane, as well as making inquiries among parishioners, and that it was clear that Deane had introduced the subject of contraception at some length before reading the pastoral letter. Father Callan asked him why he did this and he replied that he wanted to give the people 'the context of the debate on contraceptives; to warn the people that these things would be here at some future date, that the pastoral was educational.' According to Callan, Deane admitted that he said that there were people who had a right to contraceptives but that his preaching 'was all in favour of the teaching of the Pastoral'.[70] McQuaid replied to Callan promptly stating 'I must take a serious view of the error expressed by Father Deane and would ask you to request him never again to speak in such a fashion or to act on the principle that anyone has a right

---

[67] Letter from Sebastian Agnew to Archbishop McQuaid, 29 November 1970. [DDA, xx/63/12]

[68] Letter to Archbishop McQuaid, 30 November 1970. [DDA, xx/63/16].

[69] Letter to Archbishop John Charles McQuaid, 28 March 1971, [DDA, xx/106/6].

[70] Letter from Father Joseph Callan to Archbishop McQuaid, 2 April 1971. [DDA, xx/94/10].

to contraception. His preaching could not have been "all in favour of the Pastoral". I shall see him myself later'.[71]

Some priests inevitably struggled with the Church's stance on contraception. As Leslie Tentler has suggested for the United States, *Humanae Vitae* had the effect of 'exacerbating an already corrosive crisis of priestly morale and identity'.[72] Father Bernárd Lynch explained to me how the Church's stance on contraception troubled him as a newly-ordained priest in 1968. Lynch was posted to Knock Shrine, Co. Mayo, in the early 1970s for a few months to take confessions with an older priest who had been one of his professors in the seminary. Many of the women who came to confession spoke of their issues in controlling their fertility:

After a while, I kept hearing confessions like, 'Father, I'm the mother of six children and still fertile, I can't afford to have another child.' 'Father, we've eight children, my husband is an alcoholic, comes home, demands his marital rights.' 'Father, I can't feed the children I have.' So, I'm sitting there – I'm coming from Disney World, which was the seminary, really, in this regard, Disney World – and this is the real world. And I'm supposed to be, without sounding ... I'm supposed to be an instrument of God and God's love, and this is what ... and I'm flummoxed, I'm completely ... it took me a while, and I can't be exactly, before I would say to a woman ... I mean, I suppose first of all I just listened, and then gave them absolution, give them whatever penance, three Hail Mary's. But then my conscience really began to trouble me, and I was only 24.

Father Lynch began to tell women to follow their conscience. Dorine Rohan suggested in 1979 that some priests were advising women who sought their advice to take the pill while others were, like Father Lynch, leaving the decision up to the person's own conscience. However, for other priests, the ruling of *Humanae Vitae* relieved them 'of the unenviable onus of decision which they had to carry when married people sought their advice'.[73]

It is evident that some priests were more sympathetic on the issue of contraceptives as a result of their experiences. Father Patrick Scott, for instance, wrote to Taoiseach Liam Cosgrave in December 1973. Scott was a Redemptorist priest based at St. Patrick's, Esker in Co. Galway. He explained that he agreed with the Bishops 'that the "contraceptive mentality" and the "permissive society" are socially undesirable'. However, Scott explained that he believed a change in the laws around contraception was necessary. He wrote:

---

[71] Reply to Father Callan, 2 April 1971. [DDA, xx/94/10].
[72] Tentler, *Catholics and Contraception*, p. 272. Likewise, in Quebec, some priests 'found themselves in an untenable moral predicament. Church doctrine and married life were irreconcilable.' (Gervais and Gauvreau, 'Women, priests and physicians', p. 307.)
[73] Rohan, *Marriage Irish Style*, p. 93.

I think this is true not for the sake of the minority just, but for all strands of the population. For the past year I have been giving missions in poorer class areas of Galway, Sligo and Waterford cities, and in rural areas too. Everywhere I have met women, in their thirties or early forties, with 5, 6, or more children, and in desperate situations. Many of them have husbands who will not or cannot practise abstinence or the safe period. Many of them cannot face the prospect of another child. Many of them are afraid to take the pill or have been forbidden by their doctors to take it. For such women I do not believe that to use a contraceptive would be a sin – it would at worst be the lesser of two evils. I do not believe that the state should forbid them. And although the law does not prohibit the use of contraceptives, it does make them unobtainable, at least in the south and west.[74]

While Scott wrote that he would not like to see contraceptives 'freely available', he felt that they should be 'available in a controlled way to people with genuine problems. I don't think that would necessarily spread the contraceptive mentality'.[75]

In contrast to the Catholic hierarchy's stance, in 1971, Dr. Alan Buchanan, Church of Ireland Archbishop of Dublin stated that he was in favour of relaxing the laws relating to contraception as long as there was some adequate control over the sale of contraceptives, while Presbyterian Church representatives expressed similar statements.[76] Alison (b.1953) who was brought up Presbyterian, did not recall the issue of contraception ever being discussed in Presbyterian Church teachings and told me 'basic- ally I did what I wanted'. She explained that in relation to the law on contraception in Ireland, which she viewed as 'coming from the attitude of the Catholic Church', she felt that 'being Presbyterian or Protestant or whatever, things like that, it was... I didn't feel any, under any, duress to be tied to those laws'.

Lily (b.1946) also grew up Presbyterian and did not recall hearing any teachings against contraception. She felt that with regard to the law against contraception in Ireland, 'You would have felt a bit, um... what is the right word? Um, that they weren't thinking of anyone else only their own religion'. Christopher (b.1946) who was brought up in the Church of Ireland, similarly felt 'I thought it was crazy, yeah, you know, it's a personal issue for couples to manage, let's say as their conscience guides them. And I have a feeling let's say that their conscience should not be guided by let's say a single person of either sex, you know'. Others found the dominance of the Catholic Church in Ireland to be frustrating.

---

[74] Letter from Father Patrick Scott to Taoiseach Liam Cosgrave, 10 December 1973, [NAI, 2004/21/461].
[75] Letter from Father Patrick Scott.
[76] 'Ireland: Church–State Controversy sharpens', *The Tablet*, 17 April 1971, p. 389.

Edward (b.1950) who grew up in Northern Ireland in the Protestant faith, but moved to the Republic of Ireland as a young man, explained:

I hated the role of the church you know and it used to do my head in like you know, you're watching the news at night and something would happen and they'd be getting the opinion of the local priest or something like that. It's none of his goddamned business. Like we're talking international politics here and we're getting the priest, you know, to state his opinion, you know.

5.3   The Confession Box and 'Sympathetic' Priests

As Chapter 2 showed, Church teachings had an important influence on individuals' attitudes to sex, in particular, reinforcing the idea that it was sinful or 'dirty'. A mother of six interviewed by Dorine Rohan in 1969, explained her inhibitions in relation to sex, stating, 'I'd like to have a better physical side to my marriage, but it's just hopeless. I was always taught that sex was dirty and sinful, and I have never been able to adjust. No, I haven't gone to see anyone about it. I feel it's too late, but I feel guilty for my husband's sake'.[77] Similarly, a husband interviewed by Rohan said, 'Sex is the only sin in Ireland. You can go to confession and say you got drunk or were uncharitable and it doesn't matter. You are just "a hard man". But anything to do with sex, and the gates of hell are wide open for you.'[78] Numerous oral history respondents felt similarly with regard to sex which was shrouded by feelings of sinfulness and guilt. The confession box was therefore an important realm for unloading these feelings. Ellen (b.1949) for instance, felt guilty when she first became pregnant within marriage. She said:

I remember going into confession the first time that I was pregnant. I went into confession, and I told the priest I'm pregnant, and he was laughing at me, and he said it's a natural act with your husband he said, there's nothing wrong with that. But I just thought I had to, and it was a sin even to be pregnant kind of.

Ellen's testimony here highlights the guilt felt by many Irish men and women in relation to sex, and even though she was following Church teaching in becoming pregnant within marriage, she still felt that she had done something wrong. She also recalled a time when she lost a baby and her mother advised her to go to see the priest to be 'churched'. Churching was a common practice from the nineteenth century where new mothers were considered 'unclean' after they had given birth and they were required to be 'churched' or purified by their parish priest.

[77] Rohan, *Marriage Irish Style*, p. 74.   [78] *Ibid.*, p. 75.

This process usually happened several weeks after the birth of the child.[79] While the practice of churching was beginning to die out by the 1960s, many were influenced by their mothers' attitudes and experiences. Clare (b.1936) felt that churching suggested 'It was nearly as if you had committed a sin by having a baby. Even in marriage' and she never went.

The confessional also became an important arena for priests to discourage women from using contraception. Siobhan (b.1942) from the rural Midlands told me the following about her friend Mary's experience. Mary had decided to use contraception after the cot death of her baby at six months old in 1972. Mary went to the priest for confession and told him that she had used contraception. Siobhan explained:

She went to the priest down here on Main Street in town, just down there. And she told the priest her confession and she said that she couldn't face having another baby, but she ended up having two more a good while after that. But she told the priest that she had used contraception. He told her, God, he wasn't going to give her absolution. And it broke her heart, she cried for weeks afterwards.

Siobhan's testimony about her friend is not unusual and highlights the turmoil that some women faced in deciding to go against Church teachings and use artificial contraception. For practising Catholics, the rite of confession was an important sacrament where they would confess their sins to a priest. Indeed, a four-volume survey undertaken by the Council for Research and Development in 1973–4 is testament to the enduring adherence to confession in the early 1970s.[80] It recorded that 89.8 per cent of Irish Catholics attended confession up to three times a year, 69.8 per cent about six times a year, and 46.5 per cent once monthly.[81] Confession has been an important element of other studies of Catholic family planning practices. Marloes Schoonheim's work on the Netherlands from 1870 to 1970 shows how there, 'confession was not only an effective way to check people's obedience to the reproductive rules of the Church but also coach them in 'proper' moral behaviour'.[82] Similarly, David Geiringer, in his study of the experiences of Catholic women in England, has shown how at the start of respondents' marriages, 'confession was an important part of the tactics they employed for negotiating sexual and spiritual demands'.[83] However, during the later

---

[79] Delay, *Irish Women*, pp. 183–5.   [80] Fuller, *Irish Catholicism*, pp. 120–1.
[81] Appendix I: Communion and Confession attendance by Irish Catholics, 1973–1974 in Fuller, *Irish Catholicism*, p. 275. Source: A survey of religious practice, attitudes and beliefs in the Republic of Ireland, 1973–1974, (Dublin: Research and Development Unit, Catholic Communications Institute of Ireland, 1975).
[82] Schoonheim, *Mixing ovaries and rosaries*, p.220. Accessed online: https://repository.ubn .ru.nl/bitstream/handle/2066/26915/26915__mixiovanr.pdf on 03-02-2021.
[83] Geiringer, *The Pope and the Pill*, pp. 140–1.

phases of their marriages, many of the women interviewed by Geiringer came to see their sexual behaviour as something which 'bore little relation to matters of faith', with confession having less significance for his respondents as it had done for their parents.[84] Caroline Rusterholz's study of family planning practices in Switzerland also illustrated that for the small number of women in her study who confessed using birth control 'The moral cost of using birth control for these women seemed to be high enough to lead them to confess but not high enough to eventually lead them to comply with the doctrine of the Church'.[85] In the Irish context, as elsewhere, the confessional was an important realm where women sought permission and forgiveness for contraceptive practices, but also, for the most part, as in Mary's case above, it enabled priests to reinforce Church teachings on the issue, impact on individuals' choices by encouraging large families and compound women's feelings of guilt.

Other scholars have found that the confession box was a unique space where women attempted to negotiate their use of contraceptives. As Betty Hilliard has suggested, many women in her study had a dread of going to confession and were faced with the choice 'to stop avoiding further pregnancies or be refused absolution'.[86] A number of my interviewees recalled encounters with priests in the confession box which clearly had a significant emotional impact on them. Ellie (b.1944) and her husband used the withdrawal method in order to try and space their pregnancies. She recalled 'going to confession and saying it was the withdrawal method. And I was told that I was committing the sin that I was depriving my husband out of his pleasure'. I asked Ellie how she felt after the confession, and she said, 'I felt dreadful. I felt dreadful and I remember, he kept me for bloody ages'. Bridget (b.1945) from a small village in the south-west of Ireland, recalled her mother telling her about her experience:

Well you were expected like to … you were expected to have a big family, like? Do you know? It was the thinking. And the Church was, that was the thinking in the Church and you were nearly praised for having this big family, do you know? Because I can even remember my mother saying that she went to confession and confessed that she only had two children. Do you know, that kind of way? And that was very hard to feel that, you felt guilty.

Bridget's view suggests that having a large family perhaps could be viewed as a form of social capital in Ireland but also highlights the guilt

---

[84] Geiringer, The Pope and the Pill, pp. 140–1.
[85] Rusterholz, 'Reproductive behavior', p. 52.
[86] Hilliard, 'The Catholic Church and married women's sexuality', p. 38.

that was felt by women who were unable to comply and produce large families. Indeed, many respondents felt that there was an expectation engrained in them from Church teachings that they should be having large families and that that the purpose of marriage was procreation. Colm (b.1940) from the rural Midlands alluded to this, stating, 'As the priest says, "You go forward, increase and multiply".' Likewise, Lizzie (b.1946) from a small town in the west of Ireland felt 'if you went to the priest in those days, your duty was... it was bred in us, increase and multiply'. Several respondents reflected on the unquestionable authority of the Church. Martina (b.1955) explained. 'Their whole teaching was procreation. It had nothing ... I mean, there was nothing to do with love or anything. It didn't matter whether there was love or not. You just produced children and that was it. And it didn't matter what set of circumstances you were in. That was your job. And you daren't say anything against it'. Similarly, Kate (b.1944) said, 'It was against the law of the church for contraception to be used. And if they said it you just didn't question it, just like that. If they said you don't do it, you just don't do it and that's it. But I suppose now you'd be questioning a lot of them. Back then we didn't'. Likewise, Jeremiah (b.1942) explained, 'You weren't encouraged to question the clergy, you know?' Indeed, Carol (b.1954) from Dublin felt that women did not have much of a say in their reproductive choices in the 1970s when she was a young woman. Referencing the Eavan Boland poem, 'The Famine Road', she said:

And it's the attitudes, the disdainful attitude, and the dismissive attitude of you know, 'Go home and grow your garden, you'll be fine'. You know. That that was very much part of the time, the place. You know, that you didn't have it... a say in things. You know.

This expectation was also reinforced in the confession box. Tessie (b.1938) recalled going to her local priest for confession in the late 1960s or early 1970s. She explained the encounter in the following way:

TESSIE: I would be going into confession and trying to disguise my voice and say, 'Bless me father for I have sinned' and he'd say, 'Is that you, Tessie?' And I'd say, 'Yes, Father'. And first thing he'd say to me, 'How many children have you got?'. And at that time I had two. 'Still two?' I'd say, 'Yes, Father'. Now, he never went any further than that, but still.
LAURA: You felt kind of...
TESSIE: Yeah, oh no, no, no. Go forth and multiply. They weren't bloomin' well coming to feed them, were they? Look at all the unfortunates that had eight and ten children.

Similarly, Helena (b.1945) said that 'talking to older women now at this stage of my life, and talking about that, and family planning and that and the one thing – the one greatest insult that is put on these women was when they went to confession, the priest would ask, "What age is your youngest child?" Inferring that if they didn't – they had to, you know, go home and make more, which is shocking'. Julia (b.1936) also recalled going to confession and telling the priest that she was abstaining from sex, 'I remember telling him in confession you know, and … I don't know what now he said, what it was, it was sort of your duty to …' Indeed, several interviewees felt that the Church was advocating the idea that it was part of their marital duty to have sex with their husbands and produce children. Ann (b.1945) felt 'It was just sheer lust and procreation like that the church would tell you, you know, "Oh, that's your lot in life kind of." That's what you were there for. It was terrible'.

Before 1990 in Ireland, a married woman did not have the legal right to refuse sexual intercourse with her husband.[87] Some respondents recalled priests interfering directly in their marital relationships and suggesting that women should be upholding their husbands' conjugal rights. Aoife (b.1947) for instance, experienced significant trauma during the birth of her first child who had severe disabilities. She then suffered a miscarriage a year later before giving birth to her second child the year after that. Owing to the severe stress she was feeling in her personal life and frequent experience of marital rape, she obtained the contraceptive pill from her GP, which her husband had discovered and thrown into the fire. In her words:

He said, 'If you won't provide me with my needs I'll have to go elsewhere'. So, he says that he went to the Jesuits to confession or advice to ask an unmarried fella who wears dresses, you know, about family planning. Oh my God, that made me so mad and that priest told him that I had to produce as many, provide him with his needs and provide him with any number of children, that God would decide how many children I was to have, and that was it. So, Eoin came home all holy and with permission from that pup of a priest that if I didn't satisfy his needs off he went.

Aoife's testimony here is shocking, but this was the lived experience for many Irish women, and shows not only the interference of priests in marital relationships but also how the Catholic religion was used by some men to justify their sexual behaviour. Sally (b.1956) also recalled hearing about priests making home visits because 'it would be that the husband would have gone to the priest to complain about not getting his marital rights'.

---

[87] Diver, *Marital Violence in Post-Independence Ireland*, p. 232.

Priests took a range of stances in relation to contraception. Father Michael Browne, director of the Irish Catholic Marriage Advisory Council stated in 1971 that there were very few priests who granted absolution to couples who used contraception but believed that some individuals 'shopped around' for a confessor who might understand them.[88] Mrs. E. W. from Dublin, writing to *Woman's Way* in 1971, explained how after having five children in a row, she 'plucked up courage and after making my Confession, decided to ask the priest's advice'. She explained her reasons for wanting to space her pregnancies to him, 'a 2-roomed flat, the ever-present fear of eviction, my husband's casual employment' and asked if 'anything could be done'. Mrs. E.W. was 'brusquely and unkindly' refused absolution and the priest told her to 'go home and get my husband to agree that in no circumstances would we do anything to control our family'. She then approached another priest 'who was kind, but who gave me the usual rigmarole about a large family being lucky, God's plan for me and all that.' In total, Mrs. E.W. had eleven children, nine of whom were alive. In E.W.'s view, 'the crimes perpetrated against my generation of women cannot be wiped out by allowing permissiveness to the present one'.[89] Maura, interviewed by *Woman's Way* in 1973, reported that her local priest was sympathetic to her personal dilemma about taking the contraceptive pill. Although he advised that contraception was against church teachings, he explained that 'he personally believed that it was a matter for her own conscience'. However, this may not have been a typical experience. Angela, the mother of four, went to her priest for advice and had a markedly different experience: 'He was furious. He gave me a lecture about the evilness of contraception and how I would be flaunting the authority of the Holy Father'.[90] Clare, a 28-year-old mother of four consulted her priest after difficulties using the safe period but found his attitude 'unfair and hard to accept. He just couldn't realise the emotional problems involved.' Clare's priest told her that the first duty of marriage was procreation and encouraged her to continue to use the safe period and that God 'would give us the strength to abstain'. Not seeing a moral difference between the safe period and the use of the pill, Clare decided to go on the pill.[91]

The moral qualms that women faced in relation to contraception were apparent to staff at Irish family planning clinics. Cathie Chappell, who

---

[88] Kate Kennelly, 'Dilemma: report on family planning', *Woman's Way*, 22 January 1971, p. 26.

[89] 'Over to you', *Woman's Way*, 18 June 1971, p. 6.

[90] 'Undercover on the pill', *Woman's Way*, 1 June 1973, pp. 8–9.   [91] *Ibid.*, p. 8.

worked at the Limerick Family Planning Clinic recalled in 1979 when the Pope came to visit Ireland that 'women came to the clinic to have their IUDs taken out for the duration of his visit. I remember that so clearly. A lot of women came. They weren't easy with the fact that they were disobeying the rules while His Holiness was with us, you know?' Anne Legge, an IFPA doctor, stated in 1971 that she 'would never prescribe the Pill or any other contraceptive method for anyone with religious scruples about accepting it', instead encouraging such individuals to go away and think about it further or 'help them come to terms with their conscience'.[92] Mary Fahy, a nurse at the Galway Family Planning Clinic also recalled a Franciscan priest who she and her colleagues would advise women with moral concerns about contraception to 'go and have a chat with him and see. He was more moderate in his views about what women should and shouldn't do'. Frank Crummey recalled advising a woman at a family planning talk at a ladies' club to go to Father Ralph Egan, a Passionist priest based in Mount Argus for confession. However, Crummey did not realise Egan's sister was present in the group, who went home and told her brother 'Your name is going all over Dublin'.

Martin (b.1952) and his wife Carmel (b.1952) compared sympathetic priests who would absolve individuals for using contraception with sympathetic doctors who prescribed the pill:

MARTIN: If you found a sympathetic priest, he'd probably give you your penance and off you'd go. If you had an unsympathetic priest, he'd give you your penance and tell you, you can't do it again. There was a difference between those who effectively turned a blind eye to the issue, and those that continued to take it seriously.

CARMEL: That was a bit like the doctors, I suppose, who were prepared to give you the pill. And then, you found him, so he obviously had a queue out the door. That was the same with the priests, you would know which priest to go to.

Indeed, on a practical level, many priests made up their own minds on the issue following the introduction of *Humanae Vitae*. Paula (b.1955) had a close relationship with her uncle who was a priest. She recalled that he worked in a deprived urban area and that women came to him 'crying because they were pregnant again, because they were using no method, no contraceptives'. She said her uncle was 'horrified' hearing about these women's experiences and he said to Paula that:

---

[92] Kate Kennelly, 'Dilemma: report on family planning', *Woman's Way*, 22 January 1971, p. 27.

his advice to the women would be, he'd use the phrase, 'Go get yourself a few smarties. Go do something. If your husband will not take responsibility, you go do whatever you have to use contraceptives because another child for you is just … ' They're living in poverty. The women are suffering. The men are having their pints with this back then. So he would have told me that he felt very grieved by it.

Paula felt that her uncle was seen by his parishioners 'as someone they could confide in. And women who could talk to a guy who understood the situation and who would give them empathy and empathise with their situation, just give them practical advice'.

Father Paddy Gleeson, who had been ordained in 1964, was appointed as an emigrant chaplain in Luton, Bedfordshire in England a couple of weeks after *Humanae Vitae* had been published. In his words, 'Now to say that all hell broke loose after that would be an understatement'. Father Gleeson recalled that priests at the time were being phoned by newspaper reporters to get their opinion on the new encyclical. In contrast to the 'hard-line approach' of some Irish bishops, Gleeson found the approach of the Bishop of Northampton Charles Grant to be refreshing. Grant called all of the priests in the Northampton diocese together and addressing the group said, 'There have always been hard priests and easy priests', and then he paused and he said, 'I would always want to be considered an easy priest', and he sat down. The priests present at the session were advised that 'if people came with their conscience troubled seeking forgiveness they were to be forgiven, they weren't to be as Pope Francis says, "Put through an interrogation"'. Father Gleeson found this guidance to be reassuring and stated that he 'always treasured it'.

It is possible that some Irish priests in England were more flexible on the issue. Catherine (b.1953) who lived in England, recalled her local priest, who was Irish, telling parishioners to follow their own conscience in the mid-1970s. She said, 'I suppose because he was living, I suppose, in a society where it was more acceptable, he was listening to women talk about these contraception issues they had'. Some Irish women felt that Archbishop of Westminster Cardinal Heenan had a more compassionate approach to the issue than his Irish counterparts. A woman writing to Archbishop McQuaid in 1971, for instance, contrasted Heenan's attitude with that of McQuaid's, stating, 'But for the fact that Cardinal Heenan spoke at that time and said keep going to the Sacraments I don't know what I would have done'.[93] In 1969, in response to an article on Cardinal Heenan and the question of conscience, a writer named Sheila Kerr, based in Belfast, said, 'I hope that all Irish priests

---

[93] Letter to Archbishop McQuaid, 30 March 1971. [DDA, xx/89/3]

will take their cut from Cardinal Heenan and show a little human kindness and charity, particularly in the confessional'.[94]

Information on sympathetic priests was likely circulated by word-of-mouth among women. Nuala Fennell, who had been a member of the Irish Women's Liberation Movement wrote in her 2009 memoir that:

... there was a small network of understanding priests to whom to confess. A Dublin acquaintance of mine who was on the pill for years, travelled the three hundred and twenty-mile round trip every month to confess to a priest in Cork.[95]

Some of the interviewees in Máire Leane's study also reported a priest in Cork City (likely James Good) who was willing to provide absolution to women taking the contraceptive pill.[96] Similarly, as Diane Gervais and Danielle Gauvreau found in their study of family limitation in Quebec, 1940-1970, some women there 'shopped around' for an understanding priest who would not refuse them absolution at confession, while Leslie Tentler has discussed similar practices in the United States.[97] Clodagh (b.1940) told me her doctor, advised her that if she had moral qualms about going on the pill, to 'have a chat with your confessor like and don't be going to an old lad, go to a young person'. Her doctor's testimony seems to suggest that there was a perceived shift occurring within the priesthood with the older priests seen to be more likely to refuse absolution.

Frank Crummey, family planning activist and a founding member of Family Planning Services, believed that many Irish women simply did not tell their priests about their decision to use artificial contraception. Interviewed for Rosita Sweetman's book, On Our Backs, in 1979, he stated:

But this business about artificial contraception being a mortal sin, I think the women just don't tell the priest anymore. I mean are the 30,000 people on our mailing list all non-Catholics? And what about the 70,000 Irish women on the Pill, are they all non-Catholics? And if they're just using the Pill as a cycle regulator then we must have the unhealthiest women in the world.[98]

Women anticipated a negative reaction from the priest if they admitted using contraception. Cathy (b.1949) told me 'Oh my God, you'd be excommunicated. Well, probably not strictly speaking, but I mean if you went into confession and told them you were on contraception

---

[94] 'Over to you', Woman's Way, 28 February 1969, p. 2.
[95] Fennell, Political Woman, p. 79.   [96] Leane, 'Embodied sexualities', p. 43.
[97] Gervais and Gauvreau, 'Women, Priests, and Physicians', p. 313. Tentler, Catholics and Contraception, p. 244.
[98] Sweetman, On Our Backs, p. 157.

they'd absolutely rip your throat'. Indeed, oral history testimony confirms that many women on the pill simply did not tell their priest. When I asked Nora (b.1940) about whether she felt guilty about going on the pill given the Church teachings on the matter, she responded, 'No, I didn't really. I wasn't telling them either I was taking it, I suppose'. Similarly, Myra (b.1947) who used condoms, told me 'You know, like the contraceptives; we were all getting these but we were saying nothing'. She explained:

Oh you couldn't use it, it was a sin to use it. So if we were getting the johnnies from England, as we used to call them, we never told the priests inside of confession. I used to always say it was none of their business and well, I wasn't a bit – however I can put it. You know how some people, everything that the church says was law. I wasn't a bit like that. I did my own thing.

Siobhan (b.1942) also told me she didn't tell her priest in confession, 'No, I wouldn't. No. I know up here I know I didn't. I had sense enough. No, I wouldn't'. Others knew that the priest would be against their decision but felt it was not any of their concern. Colm's (b.1940) wife underwent tubal ligation, and in his words 'We didn't say nothing to no priest. I told them, herself and myself, "Lookit, go ahead". It's our business. Nobody else. That's it.' Similarly, Anne, a mother of four, who was interviewed by *Woman's Way*, had the tubal ligation procedure in 1987, aged 42. She explained: 'I realise that the Catholic Church is not in favour of sterilisation, but that doesn't bother me. I remain a practising Catholic. I go to Mass and the sacraments. I haven't mentioned it in Confession. I haven't discussed it with a priest. I feel it is between me and Him. It's my body. I believe I had the right to make the decision and that He will understand. It was right for me.'[99] Other women rationalised their use of contraceptives. Carol (b.1954) told me 'I think I was quite practical about things you know. I can sort of compartmentalise things. I mean I would have been uptight enough, I suppose about, let's say, certainly about getting, you know, pregnant outside marriage or whatever, you know, but no, I don't think it actually bothered me too much.' Likewise, when asked about whether she felt guilty taking the pill, Sandra (b.1951) replied. 'Not really, no, no, no. You might, at times, question yourself and say ... but then you'd say, "Well, look, I am not... I wouldn't be a good mother to a load of kids. I wouldn't be happy".'

However, other women expressed feelings of guilt and shame about using the pill. Ann (b.1945) from a small town in the southeast of Ireland, was prescribed the pill by her GP, however, she told me, 'I didn't stay on it

---

[99] 'The permanent contraceptive', *Woman's Way*, 18 March 1988, p. 6.

long. I think maybe I tortured myself that I was doing wrong.' Lizzie (b.1946) from a rural area in the west of Ireland, also explained that when she was younger, her long-term boyfriend 'pleaded with me to go on the pill and I just couldn't do it, it was very much against my religion'. Instead, she took risks and 'I sweated. I put myself through and I'd be like a briar'. The relationship broke up after eight years, with Lizzie telling me 'I often think we broke up because I wouldn't go on the pill'. Similarly, Virginia (b.1948) explained, in relation to condoms:

I still wouldn't have been... I'd have been, felt guilty about using it, you know, that sort of thing... It wasn't, it wasn't something that you enjoyed doing, because there was that, um, kind of residual guilt feeling, because it wasn't, it still wasn't allowed.

Maud (b.1949) who lived in England, had to have a major operation for a chronic condition and was advised by her consultant not to have any more children. During her surgery, she was also sterilised. Prior to having her operation, a priest came to see her and told her that by being sterilised she was committing a sin and he refused to give her absolution. She told me, 'I was so upset because I was going out for major surgery and he couldn't give me absolution'. The priest returned to her later on and apologised but stated there was nothing he could do as it was 'part of your religion'.

Feelings of guilt could persist for a couple's entire fertile years. Julie (b.1947) from the rural west of Ireland consulted with a chaplain before her husband had a vasectomy in the late 1980s. She explained: 'I actually felt very guilty even about Paul having the vasectomy done. I felt, I actually spoke to a chaplain inside the hospital actually, about it. I confided to him and I must say that he was very good'. She said that the chaplain told her, 'You've accepted the children you had and, he pointed out it was more like responsible parenthood, rather than ... so I found that was very helpful.' For couples who wished to use contraception, it could be difficult to reconcile their choices with Catholic teachings. In a response to a piece by an Irish priest on the theme of contraception in the *Irish Times* in 1970, one woman described about the personal conflict she felt in using contraception:

Many times I have been present at Mass in misery, staying away from Holy Communion and worrying about the bad example shown to my older children. I feel in my heart that it can't possibly offend God to show love for one's husband while at the same time trying to prevent conception, but after years of strict Irish Catholic upbringing, scruples are hard to overcome.[100]

---

[100] 'Contraception: what do you think?', *Irish Times*, 22 December 1970, p. 6.

Through disobeying the papal teachings on contraception, this particular woman felt particular emotional distress and guilt, and while she tried to rationalise her birth control practices, she felt that a life following Catholic teachings made it difficult to avoid these feelings. Other women were content to follow the Church's teachings. Breda, interviewed by *Woman's Way* in 1973, a 36-year-old mother of seven children, lived on a council estate and felt that having children was 'what marriage is all about'. She had never attempted the safe period because her husband 'wouldn't have anything to do with it, so what's the use? I'd only wear myself out fighting about it'. In her view, 'I don't know why there's so much fuss about contraceptives. The Church is against them, isn't it? Pope Paul has said so himself, so anyone who calls herself a Catholic shouldn't think any more about it'.[101] Similarly, Annie (b.1939) the mother of eleven children, explained to me how she was asked by her gynaecologist 'What kind of contraception would you like?' Annie, who was staunchly Catholic, explained, 'And I looked at him and I said "I don't need any." I mean, I didn't even think of such a thing. And that was it. I was kind of disgusted with him asking me'. Annie felt that the number of children she was to have was God's will and 'you know, when we got married, it was … you just had as many kids as God sends'.

For couples who wished to adhere to Church teaching on the issue of family planning, the only Church-approved methods were calendar methods such as the unreliable safe period, the temperature method, or later the Billings Method, which began to gain popularity from the 1970s. The safe period, or rhythm method, was critically referred to by some as 'Vatican roulette'. Maurice (b.1942) for instance recalled: 'The recommended […] was Vatican roulette, do you know? And we knew it was roulette because that's what we had been doing. (laughs)'. Christina (b.1935) and her husband used the safe period after having six children, for economic reasons, because they felt that they would not have been able to 'afford many more' but also because it was in line with Church teaching and 'being a Catholic, I don't think if there was [artificial contraception] I would've used it'.

Audrey (b.1934) from Dublin, who had four children, recalled of the 'safe period': 'Even the priest would say it to you. They'd say you were allowed to use the safe time if you…the so-called "safe time"'. Audrey married in 1957 and had her first child in 1958. She used the safe period to allow some space before her next child, stating, 'But we managed. I mean, I managed anyway. I don't know … managed to get over two years was

[101] 'Undercover on the pill', *Woman's Way*, 1 June 1973, p. 10.

grand.' She also recalled being told 'The Billings. You were told the Billings. Use the Billings. You'd want to have willpower like I don't know what'. Clodagh (b.1940) believed that her decision to avoid artificial methods was down to the influence of the Church teachings on her, stating, 'I'd say so because it was wrong, that's it and your conscience wouldn't let you do it because that's the way we were drummed into us'. Individuals' peers may also have helped to reinforce Church teachings. Marianne (b.1948) for instance, told her neighbour that she and her husband were using the withdrawal method. Her neighbour told her that this was a 'mortal sin' and that she would need to go to confession. Marianne said her neighbour told her '"Your soul is blackened." I lived with that, knowing that my soul was black'. Similarly, Bernadette (b.1947) decided in 1984 to undergo tubal ligation after the completion of her family. She recalled telling a friend of hers who visited her in the hospital before the operation. Her friend 'was big into the natural method and all that, and she more or less begged of me not to do it'. Bernadette felt that her friend believed the operation would be 'interfering with nature'.

Individuals were, however, starting to follow their own consciences on the issue. Other women were beginning to justify their decision to go against Church teachings on birth control for economic reasons. Marie Monaghan, aged 24, and the mother of six children, the youngest children being four-month-old triplets was interviewed by *Woman's Way* in 1969 and explained:

I certainly don't want any more children; I've had enough. My doctor has promised to put me on the pill and I won't have any qualms at all about using it. People can sermonise as much as they want to about what the Pope said in the encyclical and so on, but how do you look after your large family when your husband is unemployed and the bills are mounting up?[102]

Monaghan's account here justifies her going against Catholic doctrine and taking the contraceptive pill for economic reasons, and the pill was viewed as necessary in order to better her family situation. Such testimonies suggest that some Irish women were finding ways to navigate both the legislative and religious restrictions on contraception, and that they did not necessarily have misgivings about doing so.[103] The decision to use contraception therefore often came down to personal conscience and by the late 1960s and early 1970s, many women were beginning to believe that it was a matter for themselves to decide.

---

[102] *Woman's Way*, 28 March 1969.
[103] Rusterholz also found that some Swiss Catholic women justified their use of birth control for economic reasons. Rusterholz, 'Reproductive behavior', p. 51.

And, it appears that Church teachings regarding contraception were becoming less relevant to the lives and practices of the younger respondents I interviewed. Louise Fuller suggests that by the 1970s, Irish Catholics were 'by then picking and choosing which aspects of Catholicism (as preached by the official Church) they would give allegiance to and live out; and which they saw as irrelevant, and simply discarded'.[104] Cathy's (b.1949) testimony exemplifies this. She said to me that by the 1970s 'I stopped going to confession sometime around then. I just stopped. I haven't been to confession in donkeys years. I never saw it as I stopped, you know, the way I picked ... I probably cherry picked what I wanted to pick for a while. Then I kind of moved away'. Indeed, it appears that the younger members of the cohort of interviewees were more inclined to come to their own decisions on the matter rather than being as influenced by Church teachings as the older respondents. Barbara (b.1950) who brought condoms back from England with her husband explained: 'Now as the religious bit of it never bothered me because I figured this is my life'. Mairead (b.1953) also explained, 'No, I would have kind of made my own mind up. I would have had probably thought more as a health, you know, health reasons for not using it. I wouldn't, no, that would never have entered my, that it's against my religion, no. I don't think'. Likewise, Noel (b.1952) recalled that when he and his wife were getting married, they felt 'There's more to life than just this'. Noel explained that he and his wife discussed the issue of contraception and that his wife said 'Who dare to tell us what we, we should act in our own home'. David (b.1948) explained that he and his wife Jean (b.1953) 'made up our own minds', while Carmel (b.1952) said that she and her husband Martin (b.1952) 'just didn't take any cognizance of that at all. We just kind of did our own thing'. However, while some interviewees did not have significant qualms about going against Church teachings, they still felt guilty. In relation to using contraception, Ted (b.1951) for instance explained: 'we sort of felt a certain kind of guilt about that'.

Reflecting on the Church teachings of the 1960s and 1970s, many respondents expressed the view that they had changed their minds in recent years. Stephen (b.1943) explained, 'I was brought up with a Catholic background, and Christine was also, and we were church goers every week and still are but we have a different attitude towards things now than we had fifty years ago'. Similarly, Clare (b.1936) told me, 'I have a different idea about religion than I had when I was young', while Jean (b.1953) expressed the view:

---

[104] Fuller, *Irish Catholicism*, p. 229.

Well, I suppose the Church were very strict in certain things, sex outside marriage and all that, and you didn't have it until you got married. But then, and homosexuality, that was hardly mentioned at all. It's a terrible thing really. So I suppose you just as you got older, you read more and became more aware of what was going on. Whereas before you just listened to what was said and that was it. But I think as you got older, and a wee bit wiser and that, you came to your own conclusion about lots of things really.

Inevitably, the Church scandals of the 1980s and 1990s had an important impact on some individuals' faith. Áine (b.1949) for instance said, 'But what broke my heart about the Catholic Church was when all the abuse came out'. Noreen (b.1954) recalled the scandals of Father Michael Cleary and Bishop Eamonn Casey stating, 'You sort of … those are the kind of things you sort of start to say, "Well, there's a law for one but not for the other"'.

5.4   Conclusion

Mrs. T.F. from Dublin, writing to *Woman's Way* in 1971 felt:

The Catholic Church has always discriminated against women and if men were having the babies, contraception would not be a mortal evil. There is not a man alive who would go on childbearing for ten or twelve years or take his temperature and write up charts every morning for three months with six or seven children screaming in the background, yet we allow ourselves to be dictated to by these men. We hear a lot of talk about self-control but what about the woman married to an alcoholic or whose husband demands his biological rights on any day of the month? These men expect women to live a life of martyrdom while they make sure that life is pretty comfortable for themselves.[105]

By the 1970s, younger generations of Irish men and women, such as Mrs. T.F. were beginning to question the Church's teachings in relation to contraception, and many others were exhibiting resistance in their contraceptive practices. It is evident, however, that for the older generations, Church teachings had a significant impact on their family planning choices, and given that there was not only a religious ban on contraception, but a legal one too, Irish men and women who used artificial contraception may have had their guilt compounded, compared to Catholic men and women living in countries where contraception was legal.

Although it is clear that the encyclical *Humanae Vitae* caused considerable anguish for some members of the priesthood, speaking out against papal teachings could have serious consequences, as shown in the cases

---

[105] 'Over to you…', *Woman's Way*, 9 July 1971, p. 6.

of Father James Good and Father Denis O'Callaghan. Many priests toed the line and the confession box was an important sphere where priests could continue to exert power over women's family planning choices. Yet, it is clear that some priests were also beginning to follow their own consciences, and used the confession box compassionately to assist individuals who were troubled by their decision to use contraception. From the 1970s, it is evident that many Irish men and women were beginning to pick and choose the elements of Catholic teachings they wanted to adhere to, and for some, Church doctrine on contraception was one of the aspects being abandoned.[106]

---

[106] Fuller, *Irish Catholicism*, p. 229.

6   Family Planning Clinics and Activism in the 1970s

From the late 1960s to late 1970s, a number of family planning clinics were established across the country. The first of these, the Fertility Guidance Company, later the Irish Family Planning Association (IFPA), was founded in 1969. The name 'Fertility Guidance Co.' was chosen so as not to promote opposition, but to illustrate the group's aim 'to advise on the problems of infertility as well as the reverse'.[1] Others soon followed such as Family Planning Services (later FPS) (1972), the Cork family planning clinic (CFPC) (1974), the Navan family planning clinic (NFPC) (1975), the Limerick family planning clinic (LFPC) (1976), the Galway Family Planning Clinic (GFPC) (1977), and Bray family planning clinic (BFPC) (1978). The Well Woman Centre (WWC) was opened in Dublin in 1978. In order to get around the law, family planning clinics received a donation rather than a fee for their services, and 'their activities were strictly unlawful, in the sense of circumventing the law's purpose, rather than illegal in the sense of being explicitly prohibited by it'.[2]

Emilie Cloatre and Máiréad Enright's scholarship on illegality and the family planning movement has shown how the illegal practices of activists 'enacted critiques of the prevailing law' but also 'established new Irish modes of engagement with contraception, not yet provided by the state, which were no longer saturated by religious morality, or necessarily, by conservative medical power, but instead were characterised by solidarity with clients, care and even humour'.[3] Their work has also shown how Irish clinics helped to challenge the law around the sale of condoms from the 1970s to the 1990s.[4]

Drawing primarily on thirteen oral history interviews conducted with activists and staff involved in family planning activism in the 1970s, this

---

[1] Solomons, 'Dublin's first family planning clinic', p. 525.
[2] Cloatre and Enright, 'On the perimeter of the lawful', p. 473.
[3] Cloatre and Enright, 'On the perimeter', p. 499.
[4] See: Cloatre and Enright, 'On the perimeter' and 'Transformative illegality', pp. 261–84.

chapter further explores the work of the clinics through a focus on the IFPA, FPS the Galway, Cork and Limerick family planning clinics and the WWC.[5] It illustrates the personal risks that men and women took as part of their activism and their motivations for involvement. However, there was also a clear sense among many of the interviewees that the authorities would turn a blind eye to their activities. The family planning movement in Ireland must also be viewed in relation to the international movement. While the clinics primarily served the urban middle-classes, they nevertheless provided vital family planning services to individuals who could not access them otherwise.

The demand for the clinics across the country shows that many Irish men and women were beginning to exercise their own agency in relation to their reproductive choices. The stories of these family planning clinics, in particular the GFPC and LFPC, also show the importance of medical authority and how the medical model was seen to legitimise the work they were doing, but also enabled the clinics to provide a wider range of family planning options. While the clinics were independent of each other, it is evident that through regular meetings and correspondence, and in some cases, the sharing of supplies and legal advice, they created a community of family planning activists.

6.1   The Establishment of the Clinics

In April 1968, a Family Planning Study Group was founded by Dr. James Loughran, a GP in Skerries, to consider the question of family planning in Ireland.[6] During the summer and autumn of 1968, four private meetings were held in Dublin at Buswell's Hotel. Eight people attended the meetings: Loughran, Dr. Michael Solomons, Dr. Joan Wilson, Yvonne Pim, Dr. Robert Towers, Dr. Dermot Hourihane, and Máire Mullarney.[7] The final member of the group was 'a moral theologian at a Jesuit college' who provided the meetings with 'knowledge of Catholic doctrine coupled with advice and encouragement' in return for strict anonymity.[8] According to Yvonne Pim, the mixed range of religious backgrounds of the group was beneficial. She felt 'it was quite fortuitous that we were quite a disparate

---

[5] The Navan family planning clinic was opened by doctors Mary and Paddy Randles in 1975. The Bray Family Planning clinic was established by members of the Bray Women's Group in 1978. Unfortunately, I was unable to make contact with the founders of these two clinics for interview.

[6] Michael Solomons, 'Dublin's first family planning clinic', *Psychomatic Medicine in Obstetrics and Gynaecology, 3rd International Congress, London, 1971* (Karger, Basel, 1972), pp. 524–6, on p. 525. Courtesy of Susan Solomons.

[7] Solomons, *Pro-Life?* p. 24.   [8] *Ibid.*, p. 25.

group, because obviously mainly Roman Catholic, Jewish, Protestant, and so we brought in all the elements without being overtaken by anyone, well, obviously the Catholic Church being the majority'. Loughran would go on to play a crucial role in the 1973 McGee case, in his position as Mary McGee's GP. Yvonne Pim was a social worker who, with Dr. Joan Wilson, had been involved in providing sex education talks in Protestant secondary schools. Dr. Robert Towers was the editor of the *Irish Medical Times*. Dr. Dermot Hourihane, a pathologist, had been involved with the Catholic Marriage Advisory Service and was disillusioned by the inadequacy of the rhythm method. Máire Mullarney was a qualified physiotherapist and nurse as well as a theologian and the mother of eleven children.

Michael Solomons' wife, Joan Maitland, introduced him to Dr. Mary Redding who had been involved in the family planning movement in Britain. He sat in on a few sessions at the North Kensington Family Planning Clinic in 1959 and during this visit met Joan Rettie, secretary of the International Planned Parenthood Federation (IPPF). According to Solomons, Rettie had received a growing number of letters from women in Ireland who had obtained the address of the IPPF in women's magazines or by word of mouth. Following the meeting with Rettie, Solomons agreed that she could give his name and address to Irish correspondents writing to the IPPF. He could then advise them in Mercer's Hospital; Solomons believed 'this was the first time public, as opposed to private, patients had access to contraceptive advice'.[9] The study group continued to meet until February 1969 to plan the clinic and issues around training and the supply of contraceptives. The clinic would be funded by the IPPF on a continuing basis with the rest of the funding coming from voluntary subscriptions, philanthropic donors and organisations.[10] Legal advice was also sought from a barrister, Noel Peart, who suggested it would not be a contravention of the law if contraception was not sold, while the establishment of a company would lessen the possibility of any individual member being subjected to legal action.[11]

The FGC began seeing patients on 25 February 1969.[12] A report in the IPPF newsletter stated that 'so far there has been no adverse publicity, indeed the centre has been favourably commented upon in the press'.[13] A leaflet from 1970 summarised the aims of the clinic as being 'to assist married couples requiring advice on family planning, to deal with marital problems, including infertility, and to promote the interests of family welfare and community well-being'. Married couples were

---

[9] Solomons, *Pro-Life?* p. 17.   [10] *Ibid.*, p. 28.
[11] Solomons, 'Dublin's first family planning clinic', p. 525.   [12] *Ibid.*
[13] *International Planned Parenthood News*, No.184, (June 1969).

'encouraged to come and discuss their situation in complete confidence, in a relaxed atmosphere, where they can be assured of skilled medical advice. The individual's conscientious and personal convictions are respected in choosing a suitable method of family planning'.[14] In a letter sent to Irish doctors in 1969, inviting them to become members, it was stressed that the company was a 'non profit making concern' whose aims were 'to assist married couples in the planning of responsible parenthood and in problems of sterility and other marital difficulties'.[15] By 1970, the clinic operated on Tuesdays and Fridays from 7 to 8 p.m. by appointment, Tuesdays and Wednesdays, 2.30 to 4 p.m. and Monday mornings from 10.30 to 12.[16] By the end of 1970, the clinic expanded to six sessions a week with ten patients per session. The staff also increased, with the clinic acquiring eleven doctors, sixteen lay workers, an extra nurse and a financial administrator. The demand for services meant that there was a waiting list of three to four weeks.[17] In 1971, a second clinic was established at Mountjoy Square. The FGC officially changed its name to the Irish Family Planning Association in 1973.[18]

Family Planning Services, the next family planning clinic to emerge, emanated from The Irish Family Planning Rights Association (IFPRA) which was established in October 1970, and was concerned with the hypocrisy around the Irish laws on contraception.[19] The IFPRA described itself as a 'non-political, non-sectarian group formed to promote in Ireland the internationally recognised human right of family planning'.[20] The group aimed to have the law changed so that artificial contraception would be openly legal.[21] The committee members of the group included Jim Loughran from the IFPA, Michael Melville, Vincent McDowell, Brendan Walsh, Robin Cochran and Frank Crummey. The group held public meetings on the topic of family planning.[22] Frank Crummey, who would go on to play a key role in the Irish family planning movement, had campaigned on issues such as corporal punishment and been involved in the Language Freedom Movement, described this period as 'a very exciting time to be alive'. The idea for the creation of FPS emerged out of the discussions of the IFPRA and the feeling that while there was a family planning clinic in Dublin, it was necessary to

---

[14] Fertility Guidance Clinic leaflet, c. 1970. Courtesy of Susan Solomons.
[15] Letter to prospective members, dated 1969. Courtesy of Susan Solomons.
[16] Fertility Guidance Clinic leaflet, c. 1970. Courtesy of Susan Solomons.
[17] Solomons, *Pro-Life?* p. 30.   [18] *IFPA Annual Report 1973*, p. 3.
[19] Hug, *The Politics of Sexual Morality*, p. 91.
[20] 'Family planning', *Irish Press*, 16 October 1970, p. 14.
[21] Hug, *The Politics of Sexual Morality*, p. 91.
[22] 'Family planning "a necessity"', *Irish Examiner*, 23 October 1970, p. 24.

provide 'a more practical approach' and a clinic that would provide non-medical supplies.[23] While the IFPA provided a full family planning service to their clients, they did not distribute contraceptives beyond their own clinic, instead, providing prescriptions and order forms to clients who could then import items on their own, such as from the IPPF in England.[24] Indeed, the IFPA was, in the 1970s, 'considered more conservative in its approach to the law than FPS and its associated clinics'.[25] A group of eight individuals, Frank Crummey, Robin Cochran, Dr. D.J. McConnell, Dr. Brendan Walsh, E.M. Lee, Dr. James Loughran, A.B.D. McDonnell and Pat O'Donovan, decided to set up a separate company to import contraceptives in bulk, with the rationale that having a company that was separate from the IFPA would mean that the clinic's work would not be jeopardised if the group members were imprisoned.[26] According to Crummey, '[We] decided to set up another company called Family Planning Services where we would blatantly advertise our products in magazines and have a postal service'. FPS was therefore established in 1972 with the aim of providing non-medical contraceptives such as condoms, and family planning information, with the hope that in the future the group would be able to set up an educational department.[27] In April 1973, the FPS moved to their first premises in Lower Leeson Street, Dublin and later to a larger premises in Pembroke Road in April 1974.[28]

The Cork Family Planning Clinic opened in February 1975 with a staff of four doctors and four nurses, one of the doctors being its founder, consultant gynaecologist and obstetrician, Dr. Edgar Ritchie. The reception was manned by volunteer lay-workers.[29] Dr. Ritchie, who grew up in Abbeyleix, graduated as a doctor from TCD in 1958. He worked as a junior registrar in Oldham, Lancashire, alongside obstetrician/gynaecologist Patrick Steptoe, who would later pioneer IVF treatment. Dr. Ritchie then worked as a medical missionary doctor in Umuahia, Nigeria from 1960–1970, after which he returned to Ireland, securing an appointment as an obstetrician in Victoria Hospital, Cork, and later at the Erinville Hospital, which had links with the UCC medical school. The clinic received initial financial support from the IFPA and the IFPRA, and

23 Margaret Bolt, 'Who's who around the country: no.1 Family Planning Services', *Family Planning News*, 1:1, (August 1975), p. 7.
24 Cloatre and Enright, 'On the perimeter', p. 476.   25 *Ibid.*, p. 491.
26 Sweetman, *On Our Backs*, p. 156 and 'Free contraceptives from child lover', *Sunday Independent*, 19 November 1972, p. 12.
27 Bolt, 'Who's who', p. 7.   28 *Ibid.*
29 'Business as usual', *Irish Times*, 5 March 1975, p. 10.

started out offering consultations from 7–9 pm on Tuesdays, Wednesdays and Thursdays.[30]

Discussions around the establishment of a family planning clinic in Limerick began in 1975. A public meeting attended by over 70 people was held in Limerick in June that year featuring Laurine Elliott and Dr. George Henry of the IFPA and Dr. Walter Prendeville, who worked in a Dublin clinic. The meeting was chaired by Councillor Jim Kemmy who said that family planning was 'a basic human right'. Elliott claimed that there were more individuals from Limerick visiting the Dublin clinics than anywhere in the country. At the end of the meeting, 45 people who were present indicated that they would be willing to be members of a committee to set up a clinic in Limerick.[31]

Another public meeting was held in October 1975, chaired again by Jim Kemmy, and addressed by Margaret Bolt of FPS and Laurine Elliott.[32] At the meeting, the objectives were set out as being to obtain a premises for the clinic; to seek finance; to obtain a doctor. Obtaining a doctor was a particular challenge and Kemmy claimed, 'There have been some doctors with us in spirit, but the response has not been as forthright as we would have wished. Those of us who have lived in the real world know from experience, that some of the younger doctors are responding but do not want to be identified publicly'.[33] The clinic officially opened in mid-February 1976, a small announcement appearing in the *Limerick Leader* on Valentine's Day.[34] The clinic was initially run entirely by lay volunteers who provided non-medical contraceptives which were available through a telephone service or directly to callers at their premises at 6 Cornmarket Row, the office being manned on Tuesdays and Thursdays initially.[35]

The Galway Family Planning Clinic (GFPC) opened in July 1977. It emerged from two key groups. The first, the Galway Family Planning Association (GFPA), was a collective of individuals interested in setting up a family planning clinic. The second group was a collective who ran a postal service for non-medical contraceptives which was set up while the clinic project stalled.[36] The GFPA was established in late 1975 or early 1976.[37] The original subscribers of the GFPA included Brian Leonard

---

[30] 'Cork family planning clinic', *Evening Echo*, 4 February 1975, p. 5.
[31] 'Big numbers visit family planning clinics', *Limerick Leader*, 24 June 1975, p. 1.
[32] "Pill clinic' meeting', *Limerick Leader*, 18 October 1975, p. 1.
[33] 'Family planning clinic for Limerick', *Limerick Leader*, 20 October 1975, p. 1.
[34] 'Clinic', *Limerick Leader*, 14 February 1976, p. 4.
[35] 'Family planning service for Limerick', *Irish Times*, 12 February 1976, p. 11.
[36] Cloatre and Enright, 'On the perimeter of the lawful', p. 478.
[37] John Cunningham, 'Spreading VD all over Connacht': reproductive rights and wrongs in 1970s Galway', *History Ireland*, 19:2, (March/April 2011).

(university professor), Sheelah Duddy (teacher), Broddie Mannion Raftery (nurse), Michael Conlon (administrator), Anthony P. Crowley (medical representative), Padraig O'Carra (university teacher), Seaghan Ua Conchubhair (liaigh and croineir) and Frances Lenihan (doctor).[38] Plans to establish a family planning clinic moved slowly; in June 1976, a location was secured in Dominick Street, however, the GFPA was then told that because the premises was originally an architect's office, they would need to apply for planning permission for a 'change of usage'.[39] In the meantime, Evelyn Stevens, Emmet Farrell, and Pete Smith, decided to establish a postal service modelled on FPS, in order to distribute contraceptives by mail order, for a donation.[40] Following advice from FPS, Smith, Stevens and Farrell founded the mail order service in April 1977 out of Farrell and Stevens' home at 77 Ardilaun Road. After a few months, the group realised that there was a need for a clinic with involvement from medical professionals and they reconnected with the other group. The clinic finally opened on 21 July 1977. Evelyn Stevens secured John Waldron as a doctor for the clinic and Mary Fahy as the clinic nurse.

The WWC opened its doors on 17 January 1978 at 63 Lower Leeson Street, Dublin. Founder Anne Connolly had been heavily engaged in student politics at TCD, as deputy president of the Students' Union. She had been involved in the introduction of condoms for sale at the Trinity Student Union shop around 1974–1975. Connolly had been approached by the Marie Stopes Foundation in the UK about the potential of setting up a clinic in Dublin. The CEO of Marie Stopes had heard about Connolly as a result of her work in the Student Union, where she had begun a referral service for students who required the addresses of abortion clinics in the UK. In Connolly's view, 'very early on, one of the reasons the Marie Stopes approached me was because they wanted it to be a centre which would provide abortion counselling and referral on.' Connolly met with representatives of Marie Stopes. While she expressed to me her reservations at the time given the organisation's links with the IPPF, Connolly explained that 'overall it was an opportunity to do something really exciting in Ireland'. The WWC was arguably more politicised than the other clinics.

Formal and informal networks were crucial in the early years of the clinics. From an international perspective, the IPPF (founded in 1953),

---

[38] *Memorandum and Articles of Association: The Galway Family Planning Association Limited*, dated 7 January 1977. Courtesy of Dr Evelyn Stevens.
[39] 'It's all a question of planning', *Irish Examiner*, 23 June 1976, p. 16.
[40] Cunningham, 'Spreading VD'.

was crucial to the development of the FGC.[41] As Bibia Pavard has shown, the organisation had two key objectives: to advance the universal acceptance of family planning and responsible parenthood in the interest of the well-being of the family through education and scientific research, with family planning viewed as a human right.[42] However, for developed countries, there was an emphasis on the free will of couples, while for developing countries the emphasis was on the necessary reduction of population in order to allow for economic development.[43] Michael Solomons maintained contact with Joan Rettie during the sixties and in May 1968, he wrote to her for advice about setting up a clinic in Ireland.[44] Philip Kestelman, secretary of the IPPF European Regional Medical Committee met the family planning study group in the summer of 1968 and following this, Joan Rettie came to Dublin in August 1968 to provide advice and financial support, starting with a grant of £1000.[45] In Dermot Hourihane's view, 'in the contraceptive world, Ireland was an issue, so it would have been missionary work, so to speak' on the part of organisations such as the IPPF. The support of the IPPF in setting up the FGC may be viewed in the context of its wider efforts to establish family planning programmes globally, with much of this work focused on developing nations.[46] However, the support of the IPPF was critical to the endurance of family planning clinics in European countries such as Poland, in the case of the Society for the Conscious Motherhood, through the provision of financial support, expertise and international legitimisation, and in France where the IPPF provided the support necessary to set up the *l'association Maternité heureuse*.[47] Indeed, the financial backing of the IPPF would prove to be crucial to the survival of the IFPA in its early years. Janet Martin, writing in the *Irish Independent* in 1970 stated 'the Government's downright refusal to look at the question of contraception in this country means that an outside organisation – the International Planned Parenthood Federation – has had to take us under its wing

---

[41] IPPF was officially created in Stockholm in 1953 after several international conferences which had taken place since 1946, at which women doctors, such as Helena Wright, Joan Malleson, and Margaret Jackson and activists Margaret Sanger and Elise Ottesen-Jensen, had played leading roles. Rusterholz, *Women's Medicine*, pp. 169–78.

[42] Bibia Pavard, 'Du *Birth Control* au Planning familial (1955–1960): un transfert militant', *Histoire@Politique. Politique, Culture, Société*, n° 18, septembre–décembre 2012 [on line: www.histoire-politique. fr], p. 8. For more on the development of the idea of family planning as a human right, see Rusterholz, *Women's Medicine*, pp. 178–180.

[43] Pavard, Du *Birth Control*, p. 8.   [44] Solomons, *Pro-Life?* p. 26.   [45] *Ibid.*, p. 27.

[46] For a critical overview, see Matthew Connelly, *Fatal Misconception: The Struggle to Control World Population* (Harvard University Press, 2008).

[47] Kuźma-Markowska and Ignaciuk, 'Family Planning Advice in State-Socialist Poland', p. 9.

(along with all the other underdeveloped countries in the world) to finance a proper family planning clinic'.[48] According to Yvonne Pim:

We were very fortunate to have funding and a great deal of support from the IPPF and Joan Rettie, who was in charge there, had known Michael Solomons, so bit by bit then, they agreed to enable us to set up, and they funded us because obviously we'd no money at all. We had to get contraceptives, how do you pay for those? We wouldn't be able to charge patients, of course, because that would be against the law.

Clinics also shared advice and, in some cases, supplies and doctors, in their early years. National networks were also important in fostering a sense of community among activists. Mary Fahy recalled the GFPC receiving advice from the IFPA in relation to legal matters. Moreover, meetings attended by representatives of all of the family planning clinics were held four times a year and provided an opportunity to share information and advice. Dorothea Melvin (GFPC) recalled:

So, we met one another all the time really and talked to one another all the time and shared advice and information and, you know, if, say for instance, if I came back from the North with a big bundle of literature, I'd post off some to all of them. You know, just see what other stuff was available and that. Or posters.

Anne Connolly (WWC) also attended the regular meetings with the staff of the other family planning clinics across the country. In her view, 'it was good, it was very good collaboration'. She also recalled that Frank Crummey (FPS) 'was a regular visitor into us and he was a huge advocate'.

Some activists were keen to contrast their activities with those of feminist groups or individuals taking legal challenges, and there was a sense that there were two sides to the movement. Arguably, the WWC bridged both of these sides in that it provided a service but because of its abortion counselling, was more high profile and politicised. Evelyn Stevens (GFPC) stated, 'I know there was legal stuff going on. There were people in Dublin at different stages taking challenges to court because they wanted the legislation to change. But we were a bit more pragmatic and just getting on with it.' As Yvonne Pim (FGC/IFPA) explained, the clinics were providing a service 'with no fanfare at all'. In Pim's view, 'We had to go quite quietly, and I think that was very important.' Feminist campaigners in contrast:

They kept it in the front of the headlines. It's another way of doing it. Still it was like, in a sense, a relay race, handing on the baton to them. They could take it further. We were going along under the radar.

---

[48] 'The facts about women's wrongs', *Irish Independent*, 15 October 1970, p. 8.

Similarly, Dorothea Melvin (GFPC) explained:

And of course, the other side of it was that there were two sides, I suppose, to the movement. One was the mouth of the movement as I call it which was the girls and the Spare Rib and the Condom Train and all that kind of thing. The journalists didn't engage much with the clinics. It was like two completely separate legs of the same stool kind of thing. But everything worked in its own way.

6.2   Motivations

Family planning activists were motivated to set up clinics for a variety of reasons which often stemmed from personal and professional experiences. While some scholars of NGOs have dismissed 'foundation myths' as being 'marketing exercises' or 'disingenuous' I would argue, conversely, that in the case of the Irish family planning clinics, an exploration of the reasons why individuals set up these clinics is crucial to understanding the wider social and cultural climate.[49] The personal experiences of activists involved in such organisations are missing from the current historical narrative and oral history offers a way into understanding what underpinned individuals' motivations, as well as the personal impact of activism and legal risk-taking.

Dr. James Loughran and Dr. Joan Wilson, a Scottish GP, were motivated to become involved in setting up the FGC as a result of their experiences in general practice in Ireland.[50] Máire Mullarney, another founder member, was a practising Catholic but, like Dermot Hourihane, was disillusioned by the inadequacy of the rhythm method. In spite of the fact that she had used this method and later the temperature method, Mullarney and her husband 'had eleven children in sixteen years, which would seem to be rather more than would be likely if we had made no attempt to control production'.[51] Mullarney wrote that she and Robert Towers' motive 'was to help people to control their fertility and to know they could do so with a clear conscience'.[52] Mullarney read a 1964 book published in the US called *Experience of Marriage*, and could recognise similarities in the experiences of the couples featured in the book with her own.[53] She had also been inspired by a visit a family planning clinic in

---

[49] For a critical account of 'foundation myths' see: Matthew Hilton, James McKay, Nicholas Crowson, and Jean-François Mouhot, *The Politics of Expertise: How NGOs Shaped Britain* (Oxford University Press, 2013), pp. 56–63.

[50] Solomons, *Pro-Life?* p. 24.

[51] Máire Mullarney, *What About Me? A Woman for Whom 'One Damn Cause' Led to Another* (Dublin: Town House, 1992), p. 162.

[52] Mullarney, *What About Me?* p. 164.   [53] *Ibid.*, p. 161.

Lisbon which was organised by a priest and 'furnished like a comfortable family home'.[54] Yvonne Pim was motivated to get involved partly as a result of her own experiences in accessing contraception. She explained:

There was the pill, and there were diaphragms. There were condoms, then there were IUDs, none of which were available in Ireland. I was also conscious at a personal level that I had to travel out of the jurisdiction in order to have my own fertility needs met. I just thought that it was most unfair that women in general were being denied this opportunity.

Moreover, Pim was inspired by her experiences as a social worker at the Rotunda Hospital:

I had been a basically trained social worker, and when I had done a little bit of work at the Rotunda Hospital, I'd seen for myself at first hand the multiparas on the district, as they called it. Women with no control over their fertility whatsoever, and obviously no likelihood of it either. I was very conscious of my own situation. I belonged to a minority church, in other words, the Church of Ireland, which had no restrictions on fertility. Of course at that time, control of fertility was available, but not obviously by law in Ireland.

Dermot Hourihane, another founder member of the FGC, was also moved to action as a result of his personal experiences trying to follow the Catholic teachings on family planning. He explained to me:

My wife and I tried to follow the Church's teaching and found it difficult. Then I gradually ran Catholic contraception advice in London, not very successfully, I must say. My wife was one of the only people to get pregnant while I was doing it, and that was run by Catholic doctors, and then I gradually reached the conclusion that the argument about contraception was just hopeless, unconvincing, and the idea of following Thomas Aquinas, the genitalia are made for fertilisation and only for that, not for pleasure, is ridiculous. When the papal encyclical came out, *Humanae Vitae*, formally outlawing all contraception, I was absolutely disgusted. That tilted me into practising contraception myself and thinking that other people should have the opportunity to have it.

Hourihane obtained condoms by mail order from the Family Planning Association in England but was aware of his privilege in this regard, stating 'very few people would have the ability or the knowledge to do that'. He explained:

There was a lot of ignorance. I guess everybody who was married and thought they had enough children already or too many maybe would have known about it. There was ... It was easy to get talking about it, but it was very difficult to do anything about it. I felt like the people who needed the contraception the most were the least likely to get it. I was educated, and I was in a position where I could

---

[54] *Ibid.*, p. 163.

get ... I used to hand write the letters myself to the Family Planning crowd in Britain. It was a very shameful society, looking back on it, and to say they didn't care about the children, the fifteen children that were born to somebody with seventeen pregnancies, those were the kind of figures that were common, and you could only see that in poor people who were on public health services. It was just social injustice.

Dr. Michael Solomons was a gynaecologist, who like his father before him, Dr. Bethel Solomons, gave advice to his private patients on methods of birth control when they required it. However, he wrote that he was 'aware of the injustice of a situation whereby those who had the money could travel outside the state, to the North or to Europe, to obtain contraceptives. There was absolutely nothing one could do to help our public patients'.[55] Solomons was motivated by his experiences in medical practice and the problems patients had using natural methods of family planning.[56] Solomons' arguments in favour of family planning were typical of campaigners internationally who framed family planning as responsible parenthood, but also acknowledged the potential benefits to the physical and mental health of the parents. He also viewed artificial methods as more effective and having the advantage that they allowed the woman control of her fertility without having to depend on her partner.[57]

For Frank Crummey (FPS), his belief that individuals should be entitled to contraception stemmed from the idea that all children should be 'truly wanted, instead of being looked on as additional mouths to feed in a family'.[58] In an oral history interview with me, he also explained his sadness at the wider plight of women in Ireland, including his own mother. He said:

It's so sad. I mean, I could cry. I get very emotional. My mother was deserted at the age of 34, after four children. She spent the rest of her time rearing her children, done a wonderful job. But the idea of her going out with a man ... I know one man on the road asked her out. a widower, a lovely man ... She couldn't. That meant she was condemned, whether she liked it or not, to a life of celibacy for the rest of her life.

Dr. Edgar Ritchie's desire to establish the CFPC in 1975 emanated from his professional experiences:

Well, in the early 70s there was very limited advice available or in fact service available and it was obvious that there was a great need. I would have, having come back from Africa, I would have been aware of people who were at loss as to how to plan their family and so that was the kind of, and without going into

---

[55] Solomons, *Pro-Life?* p. 16.   [56] *Ibid.*, p. 21.   [57] *Ibid.*, p. 26.
[58] Frank Crummey, *Crummey v Ireland: Thorn in the Side of the Establishment* (Londubh Books, 2010), p. 98.

specifics, there would have been people that I would have known at that time who came for help and who in fact it was something of a matter of life or death, you know. It was serious as to whether they would endanger their lives by having another pregnancy and so on. So, it was quite a moral or ethical decision which after all that's what medical people are involved with.

Ritchie had joined the Family Planning Association in England on his return from Africa and 'they talked about certification for Irish people and rightly they said well, really, we should be doing that ourselves. So, that's one of the reasons we got started with both the clinic and advice and so on'. The clinic received initial financial support from the IFPA and the IFPRA, and started out offering consultations from 7–9 p.m. on Tuesdays, Wednesdays and Thursdays.[59]

Cathie Chappell (LFPC) moved to Limerick from England in 1976. She joined the Limerick Women's Action Group. At a group meeting Chappell expressed her frustration at being unable to get the pill she had been taking in England at the Limerick Family Planning Clinic and told the group that 'You can't have a family planning clinic without the pill or the other methods.' Chappell explained that at the time, the clinic was a 'small outfit' being run by Jim Kemmy

with a group of like-minded socialist people, mainly men, and they had a little office, they had a few condoms, they gave advice, that was it. So, the Women's Action Group *en masse* – which was about maybe ten of us women – we joined the Family Planning Clinic, we took it over. […] And one by one the guys kind of melted into the background because we said, you know, we have to do something about this.

Ferga Grant, one of the volunteers from the Women's Action Group later gave up her job as a secretary at Shannon Airport to become the first paid administrator at the clinic in 1978, at less than half of her former salary. Grant, Chappell, and Jan Tocher were crucial to the running of the clinic.

For the GFPC founders, their motivation also sprung from a combination of personal and professional experiences and indignation at the social injustice of the situation regarding contraception in Ireland. Brian Leonard, professor of pharmacology at UCG, recalled, 'There was a group of us who felt, well, look, this is completely unacceptable, it's inhuman. We got together, first of all, just a small group to discuss, "Well, what can we do?"' Leonard believed that 'I think that, as I said, a group of us just felt that, well, maybe this is something we could tackle and do something about. Have some practical value. Which it did, but it

---

[59] 'Cork family planning clinic', *Evening Echo*, 4 February 1975, p. 5.

had to be going in stages.' Pete Smith, a lecturer in biochemistry at UCG, felt that his motivation came from two areas:

One was an obvious concern for my friends and people I knew that they couldn't get access but the other came from the fact that I was teaching. And I was teaching students about medical diseases. And every year I was standing in front of them and saying, right, these are the sexually transmitted diseases, and these are the ways not to get them and it's illegal. You know? And this is sort of irritating me. So, anyhow, we sort of debated this issue with the people I was close to in the university, and it really came from those two routes. The interest in direct action and the feeling that this was an issue that had to be dealt with.

Evelyn Stevens' motivation to get involved in the GFPC came partly out of personal experience. Stevens recalled her own disappointment in relation to *Humanae Vitae*. Like many other Irish men and women she had expected that 'the Pope was going to say that people could use contraception. But he didn't. It was very disappointing. But people really were ready to change. They wanted contraception.' She further explained:

Yeah, I mean the whole thing about contraception was significant for me because of being married and because Emmet and I were both students, we didn't want to have a baby, so my first experience was going to a doctor in Galway to get the pill and I was married but he wouldn't give it to me because he said I hadn't had a child and I had to have a child first before I could get the pill. So, that was that. Then I did, I knew medical students, so I got a prescription from a medical student, so that was illegal but anyway, I managed to get the pill. And then at a later point when I wanted to come off the pill and ... I mean there was no other contraception available, but I wanted to come off the pill and then I wanted to get condoms and I became aware of Family Planning Services in Dublin and their postal service. So, I was involved with them on a very personal basis.

Mary Fahy, who had trained as a nurse in England didn't think twice about her decision to work at the clinic as their first nurse. She said: 'I didn't even think about it. My head must have been on in a different direction. I don't know, I just thought it was ... I suppose having done midwifery in England, we always had a family planning, there was a family planning section to the outpatients so it just seemed normal'. Dorothea Melvin was later taken on as an administrator for the clinic, thanks to a loan from FPS. Melvin became involved in the clinic because 'I just felt that it was wrong, that there was something wrong with a society that didn't allow couples or women, single women, I wasn't fussed about whether they were married or not to make that decision for themselves.'

Anne Connolly, who established the WWC, was inspired by 'the idea of having a centre where women could go for a whole range of contraceptive services, but more broadly, sexual health supports which didn't require a medical filter' and was coming from 'a strong campaigning point of view'.

Connolly was just 23 years old at the time, and was faced with quickly developing skills in a range of areas relating to the running of a clinic.

6.3   Challenges

The opening of the clinics was not a smooth process and founders faced a number of challenges from their local communities. The CFPC, for instance, was condemned from its opening by the bishop of Cork and Ross, Cornelius Lucey. A letter was read out at all masses in the diocese on Sunday, 9 February 1975, informing the public that the clinic had opened on Tuckey Street. The letter drew attention to the fact that there were already services available through the Catholic Marriage Advisory Service and the Ovulation Method Advisory Service which would advise on natural methods in accordance with Catholic teaching. The letter also highlighted that the founder of the clinic, Dr. Edgar Ritchie was not Catholic and that artificial methods of contraception were 'morally wrong'.[60] Indeed, Lucey's letter might have inadvertently proved a boon for the clinic in promoting its services. Writing in 1975, David Nowlan of the *Irish Times* suggested that 'the relatively high demand for services (About 50 couples have been advised in the first three weeks of the clinic's existence) may in part be the result of the fact that 97% of the population of Cork were told one Sunday morning where the clinic was and what services it provided. It may also reflect a genuine need, increasingly felt, for the means to control fertility with methods more effective than those that Dr. Lucey would endorse'.[61] Nevertheless, Lucey continued to condemn the clinic. In May 1975, speaking after the confirmation of 500 children in the south and middle parishes in Cork, Lucey again drew attention to the fact that Dr. Ritchie was not a Catholic doctor, emphasising that the contraception provided by the clinic was irreconcilable with Catholic principles.[62]

Like the Cork clinic, the LFPC faced opposition from the local church hierarchy. Bishop of Limerick, Dr. Jeremiah Newman, was interviewed on RTÉ television in summer 1975. He stated his opposition to the clinic, arguing that the demand for contraception would lead to demand for abortion and euthanasia.[63] In August 1976, Newman again spoke out against the clinic. Councillor Jim Kemmy was not afraid to challenge Church hierarchy on the issue. Speaking at a function in September

---

[60] 'Bishop's letter on family planning clinic', *Evening Echo*, 10 February 1975, p. 5.
[61] 'Business as usual', *Irish Times*, 5 March 1975, p. 10.
[62] 'Bishop opposes Cork family planning clinic', *Irish Times*, 16 May 1975, p. 4.
[63] 'Dr. Newman comments', *Limerick Leader*, 2 August 1975, p. 1.

1976, he stated, 'it is regrettable that the bishop appears to lack compassion and an understanding of the plight of countless couples suffering psychological frustrations and insecurity by trying to bring up too many children on inadequate incomes'. In Kemmy's view, the role of women had changed and women 'are no longer content to be relegated to a lesser role in marriage and in society generally, and they are increasingly regarding sexual intercourse as an expression of personality and a physical pleasure, rather than a mere means of human reproduction.'[64] Kemmy stepped down from the role of chairman of the LFPC committee before the 1977 election because of suggestions that he was using the clinic for political gain. Because the clinic only dealt in non-medical contraceptives, a doctor was not yet needed but he hoped that one would join the clinic.[65] Another limitation was that the local newspaper, the *Limerick Leader*, refused to accept advertisements from the clinic.[66] While the clinic often made front page news on the newspaper, it was often referred to as 'pill clinic' rather than given its full title.

Plans for the GFPC also faced backlash from their inception. In February 1976, the UCG Students' Union nominated the fledgling GFPA as the beneficiary of its rag week fundraising; the sum of £1,000. This proposal caused outrage; fifty local residents including then mayor Mary Byrne wrote a public letter to the UCG Students' Union, the three local newspapers editorialised against the allocation of the rag week money to the Galway Family Planning Association and the Students' Union was forced to debate the resolutions.[67] Concurrently, Galway corporation unanimously passed a motion condemning Mary Robinson's family planning bill. A member of Galway Corporation, Alderman Sheila Jordan, publicly declared her complete opposition to the plans to set up a clinic. Jordan appeared to have issue with the distribution of 'contraceptives to just anyone who asked for them. Only a doctor should judge whether a person should get them or not. A good bit of old-fashioned self-denial is the greatest thing going'.[68] In response, a spokesman for the GFPA, stressed that the main aim of the clinic was 'to advise and help in family planning. Contraceptives will, however, be available to anyone who wants them, but a doctor will be constantly available to give advice'.[69] After a heated debate, a vote was taken and 417 students voted for the rag week money to be given to the Samaritans and 379 voted for the money to be given to the GFPA.[70] The proposals to set up a family

---

[64] 'Bishop lacking family planning 'compassion', *Irish Times*, 4 September 1976, p. 11.
[65] 'Storm hits', p. 5.   [66] 'Contraception 1979', *Irish Times*, 5 January 1979, p. 8.
[67] Cunningham, 'Spreading VD all over Connacht'.
[68] 'Family plan clinic query', *Connacht Tribune*, 6 February 1976, p. 2.   [69] *Ibid*.
[70] Cunningham, 'Spreading VD'.

planning clinic were also met with passionate debate in the letters pages of the local newspapers. Writing to the *Connacht Tribune*, Michael Heneghan from Ballybane criticised 'those faceless, nameless, gutless doctors and others who belong to and are ready to promote Galway Contraceptives Centre' and argued that 'wherever contraceptives have started abortion has followed'.[71] Frank Wynne, from Wellpark, on the other hand felt that 'the decision of UCG students to withdraw their contribution from the Family Planning Association, must be a lamentable one. So much for the benefits of an academic education' and alluded to the problems brought on by unplanned pregnancies.[72] One of the few local politicians to support the GFPC was then Labour Senator and UCG lecturer, Michael D. Higgins, who had supported Mary Robinson's Family Planning Bill in the Senate in 1974, arguing that access to contraception was a civil right.[73]

In April 1976, the GFPA organised a seminar on Family Planning at the Ardilaun Hotel. The speakers included Michael Conlon, Dr. Paul Dowding from TCD, and Dr. George Henry and Máire Mullarney from the IFPA.[74] The meeting attracted about a hundred attendees as well as a small number of opponents to artificial contraception, including Deirdre Manifold.[75] As John Cunningham has noted, in addition to the opposition at the public meeting from lay Catholics, the rag week controversy 'stirred influential opponents into action', with the Catholic Marriage Advisory Council devoting more space in local newspapers to the Billings method. Deirdre Manifold set up her own Billings centre in Galway city centre in spring 1977.[76]

Public discussions of the issue of contraception could also turn heated. Frank Crummey (FPS) recalled giving a talk with Dr. Paddy Randles (who had founded the Navan Family Planning Clinic with his wife Dr. Mary Randles) at Moyle Park School Hall in Clondalkin. Crummey explained that the school principal, Brother Eamon, a Marist brother, was at the meeting but 'shall we say, wasn't friendly'. One of the attendees at the meeting was Mena Cribben, a prominent conservative campaigner, who sat in the front row. Crummey recalled the event as follows:

Anyway, I was speaking and I said something, whatever I said. Mena Cribben jumped up and said 'I have six children' and something, something, something, and started attacking me. I didn't give a shit, but Paddy mumbled to me 'they

---

[71] 'Views on family planning', *Connacht Tribune*, 20 February 1976, p. 10.   [72] *Ibid.*
[73] Family Planning Bill, 1973, Second Stage (resumed), Seanad Éireann debate, 21 February 1974, Vol. 77, No.3.
[74] 'Plans for Family Planning Clinic', *Connacht Tribune*, 9 April 1976, p. 2.
[75] 'Views on family planning', p. 10.   [76] Cunningham, 'Spreading VD'.

must have been virgin births'. [...] And she fuckin' heard him. So she threw the table on top of us. There was total bedlam. When Brother Eamon ran up, he said 'I may not approve of you, but I don't approve of violence either'.

Crummey's account here, while humorous, illustrates how divisive the contraception issue was, and as the next chapter will also show, meetings organised by women's groups on the issue were also frequently disrupted by anti-contraception campaigners.

Most of the clinics struggled with finding a premises, legal representation and a doctor. In the case of the FGC, finding a solicitor to represent the group proved challenging. Dermot Hourihane asked two school friends who were working as solicitors in Dublin but:

Neither one would touch the case. They said, 'My firm doesn't do criminal cases. This would be a crime.' I was absolutely horrified. I still am. They were very nice people to meet and I would have agreed with them and a lot of what they viewed ... They were terrified of the consequences and I didn't have the same feeling.

Solicitor Raymond Downey eventually came on board and the group set about trying to find a premises for the new clinic. Accessibility and client privacy were key concerns. Many landlords were reluctant to rent their spaces to the group when they were told about the clinic's purposes, however, a premises was eventually found at 10 Merrion Square.[77]

The GFPC experienced similar challenges in finding a premises and doctor. According to Pete Smith 'we were advised by a solicitor that the landlords of Galway would respond to money. So, if we paid over the odds, we'd get a place. And he was right'. A clinic premises was secured on Raleigh Row, a disused leather shop, but the owner had a change of heart when he received a petition from 284 local residents in the St. Ignatius parish.[78] However, the solicitor, Leonard Silke, had copper-fastened the contract and the GFPA were able to argue that the contract needed to be honoured.[79] The clinic finally opened on 21 July 1977.[80] The Raleigh Row premises was above an auto factors shop and was chosen, according to Brian Leonard, because it was 'very discreet, which of course we selected deliberately'. The next challenge was finding a doctor. According to Pete Smith 'I think doctors were nervous about being out there as the doctor who did that'. John Waldron, a GP from Tuam was recruited. Smith stated 'John was a particular person. He had very strong feelings and I say he was a particular person, so he was

[77] Solomons, *Pro-Life?* p. 28.   [78] Cunningham, 'Spreading VD'.   [79] Mary Fahy.
[80] Cunningham, 'Spreading VD'.

characteristically ... he was prepared to do it because he would be more capable of standing up to that kind of pressure'.

Ferga Grant explained how the LFPC also struggled to find a doctor: 'One of the first jobs I had, I began a kind of a ring around of doctors and I did meet some opposition there from doctors who kind of said 'Well I don't really want to get involved in family planning in Limerick". Cathie Chappell concurred: 'There was no doctor in Limerick that would touch us with a barge pole. They thought they would be ruined if they did'. The women organising the clinic got in touch with the IFPA and 'they would send down doctors to us. So, we started doing the weekly clinic and then a twice-weekly clinic and built it up that way'. The clinic eventually recruited Dr. Philip Cullen as its first Limerick-based doctor. Dr. Cullen had graduated in 1975 so was a relatively young doctor when he joined the clinic. Cullen did not have qualms about getting involved. He explained:

I didn't have any particular religious concerns about what was going on or whether it was lawful or not. I'm not from the Roman Catholic persuasion myself, I was brought up under the rules of the Church of Ireland. So, I was never particularly concerned about what they said in Rome, or they said in Dublin, or what they said anywhere else.

The WWC also had issues recruiting doctors. According to Anne Connolly, two of the originally recruited doctors were told by an eminent member of the Irish medical profession that working at the centre would be detrimental to their careers, and they pulled out. Moreover, some doctors had issues with the women-centred ethos of the clinic, which in Connolly's words 'was around empowering the woman at the centre of it'. This approach meant that women were 'handed their chart so they read it in the waiting room' and that stirrups were not used during the examination process. Attendees at the clinic were also referred to as 'clients' rather than 'patients' and were encouraged to call the doctors by their first names. Connolly explained 'that meant a number of the doctors were saying "this is not for me"'.

The clinics also faced backlash from protestors. The postal service set up in the home of Evelyn Stevens and Emmett Farrell in Galway was targeted by anti-contraception protestors, including Deirdre Manifold. Evelyn Stevens recalled the personal impact these protests had on her:

She came and said the rosary on our front garden in Ardilaun Road. It was very ... and plus, I mean even worse than that, you know, that was a bit tricky. It was terraced houses, you know, all the neighbours could see what was going on. But she said ... I mean when I met her she said, 'Your father would turn in his grave if he knew what you were doing'. It was horrible and very personal. Very difficult. That was painful.

In addition, Stevens faced pressure from family members, such as her mother who had heard that she was 'giving out condoms to 13-year-olds'. Frank Crummey also recalled personal backlash as a result of his work with FPS:

Oh, I mean it was horrendous. People shouted at me in the street at one time. The same way as they did about INFORM against corporal punishment. I was against the bishop, shouting, biting the hand that feeds you. Also, I used to visit an aunt of mine who was not married, she was a lovely aunt, one of my favourite aunts, and she could never look at me again. She would always speak directly to Evelyn [his wife] if she wanted to tell me something, because I was undermining everything she had stood for.

Conservative campaigners also organised pickets outside clinics. A group of men and women, led again by Deirdre Manifold, used to pray the rosary outside of the GFPC in its early years. Dorothea Melvin recalled:

Every time they had the clinic open, they were parading up and down outside with rosary beads and all manners of things and just saying that we were going ... telling us that we were all going to be off to hell in a handcart kind of thing. But on the other hand, I got so used to it after a while that it didn't bother me.

Similarly, Mary Fahy remembered:

... they carried a big statue of the Blessed Virgin and they carried that up and down outside and they'd stay for about an hour, hour and a half, walking up and down saying the rosary. And the women used to come in, they'd wait till they went down Palmyra Avenue and then the women would skip in and up the stairs, and then they'd have to wait until they turned back in that direction again and nip out.

Melvin was concerned about the impact that protestors would have on the clients at the clinic and that the protests might 'put people off coming to the clinic'. She felt that clients 'had to be very stiff of purpose if you were a patient coming in there' with the protestors outside. Brian Leonard faced an unpleasant personal attack when one of the leaders of the protests at the clinic found out where his teenage daughters went to school and contacted the school principal to let her know that the girls' father was 'behind the anti-Catholic family planning clinics, in Galway'. However, according to Leonard, the school principal said it had nothing to do with his daughters. In spite of the initial backlash, the GFPC soon grew and expanded its services. By the 1980s, it offered vasectomies, smear tests and sexual health screenings. It also evolved into a training clinic.

There were occasionally some quiet protests outside the LFPC. Dr. Philip Cullen recalled:

But I do know we used to get paraded outside the clinic from members of various organisations, like maybe the Legion of Mary, and things like that, they used to come and walk up Mallow Street with placards on a Saturday morning and pray for the wrath of God to fall down on us all. But apart from just waving out the window, it never bothered us, and it certainly never bothered me. [...] But I suppose we were conscious that this was out there, but it didn't really ever bother us. We never came to blows with people. They used to make their quiet protests, and that was about as far as it went.

Máire Mullarney, a founder member of the IFPA, also commented in her memoirs that 'We rather expected to be picketed by the conservative Catholic group "Maria Duce", to have bricks thrown through the window, even go to jail. Nothing of the sort happened'.[81] Interestingly, this and Cullen's testimony reflect the expectation shared by many of the family planning activists that there would be significant protests but that these did not materialise.

The WWC was picketed by anti-contraception protestors for the first two Tuesdays it was open.[82] The four picketers were from the groups Parent Concern and Mná na hÉireann and carried placards with slogans such as 'Contraception means promiscuity and abortion'.[83] This publicity, however, had a positive impact in getting the word out about the centre. Connolly stated that she had tried to encourage the press to publicise the opening of the clinic to no effect, but the picket outside the clinic 'was what saved us. So we just rang all the media, and within 10 minutes the media were outside, flashing away, and we were front page the following day. So, but we wouldn't have got that if it hadn't been for them'. Connolly's involvement in the WWC, however, had a significant personal impact. She told me, 'It was very difficult. It was very, it was very tough on, on both my parents'. She further elaborated that it was 'very, very tough on them because there was, you know, some of the profile publicly was, was pretty rough. A lot of their own peer group, you know, would have been very critical. And they were getting it, in the neck, and ... But at some level, my father in particular, who was a more rational person, would have said, you know, "It is better you, you lead ... you do what you think is right and you live by your principles". So, he would say that he admired that. Even though he found it very... He found it very tough'.

---

[81] Mullarney, *What About Me?* p. 164.
[82] 'Are you Well Woman?' *Rebel Woman*, c.1978 [Attic Press/Roisin Conroy archive BL/F/AP/1139/24], no page number.
[83] 'Family planning clinic opens to picket protest', *Evening Press*, 18 January 1978, p. 25.

6.4   Personal Risks

Founder members of the clinics took serious risks. In the early years of the FGC, clinic staff and supporters smuggled contraceptives back from England.[84] Yvonne Pim was one of the 'contraceptive couriers'. She explained:

I used to go on a regular basis over to the UK with my husband. He had a young business in air freight, and he had reason to go across to London from time to time. At that stage, Aer Lingus, because they were still in the early days, they were offering half-price spouse fares. So, if your husband's going abroad, you can go for half price. I managed to do that, and goods were delivered to my sister's house in Fetcham, in Surrey. I brought them back with my husband.

Pim believed that had she been caught, 'it would have had serious consequences' for her husband's business. She recalled business colleagues of her husband's advising him '"You're going to have to stop Yvonne being involved in this kind of thing. It's not good for business". Because our names and addresses were on the front of all the papers'. But Pim felt:

I had nothing to lose, I thought, at that stage. I was just so fired up with the enthusiasm for doing this. So, we went through with that, we brought back the goods.

Following the High Court decision after the McGee case in 1973 that the import of contraceptives was a matter of marital privacy, the IFPA had more freedom to import and distribute contraceptives and developed a growing postal service to distribute condoms to clients who were unable to travel to the clinic in person.[85] The CFPC also received supplies from contraceptive couriers. Edgar Ritchie explained 'people would bring back supplies, devices and inter-uterine devices and so on who had visited England.'

Similarly, in the early years of the contraceptive postal service in Galway, supplies of condoms were obtained from FPS in Dublin. Following the establishment of the GFPC, Brian Leonard arranged import of condoms and IUDs. Leonard had condoms posted to his daughter's address in England: 'I arranged, through some of my pharmaceutical industry contacts, because I'd been working in industry, to supply, send condoms, to her address. One way to get condoms in was going over, with a case, and pick them up, hoping that the customs wouldn't stop you over'. Leonard also had IUDs sent to his daughter

---

[84] Solomons, *Pro-Life?* p. 31.   [85] *IFPA Annual Report, 1974*, pp. 2–3.

and explained that he would 'smuggle them in, in luggage, covered up, and all the rest of it, and hopefully the customs wouldn't open the case'. Frank Crummey explained to me how the FPS system of importation operated: 'We imported from London Rubber, and they sent their shipment to Portadown, in the north of Ireland, to a house of a friend obviously, and every second Saturday it was my job to go to Portadown and to smuggle them over the border'. Crummey did not recall running into any difficulties with this, except for one occasion when he was stopped at a security checkpoint on the way back from the north and questioned about the forty thousand condoms in the boot of his car. Crummey replied, 'They are for my own personal use' and was told by the police to 'Have a nice weekend'.

All of the respondents involved in the early years of the clinic were asked about whether they had concerns about it being raided or that they might face prosecution. This question was often met with humour. For example, Dr. Edgar Ritchie (CFPC), replied, 'No, no. (laughter). We kept in touch with the appropriate Minister for Health who was called Charlie Haughey at that stage [July 1977–December 1979] and his staff. So, there was goodwill there'. The LFPC activists were anxious about the threat of raids in the early years of the clinic. According to Cathie Chappell:

so we would bring things back to our houses and we would stock the medical supplies, the condoms, all that stuff would be in our houses in case we got raided. We never did get raided but there was that threat hanging over us at one time until we began to realise, you know, nobody's ever going to shut us down. So, we kind of relaxed a bit then. But in the early days it was a bit fraught, it was.

However, Chappell admitted that, like other family planning activists, 'I don't think we really thought seriously about the consequences of what could be. We just did it because it had to be done. It was no big deal kind of thing and yet at the same time we did know that we were providing a really essential service.' In May 1979, seven members of the LFPC group set up a stall in Shannon town centre where they sold non-medical contraceptives. After almost two hours, the Gardaí arrived and confiscated £86 worth of goods. When the group asked the Gardaí what law entitled them to confiscate the contraceptives, they were told 'ye know that better than we do'.[86] Chappell recalled the incident:

We went out to Shannon for some reason and we set up a stall. We were doing this deliberately and we were selling – well, donating with contributions – very openly in the street, in the shopping centre there and the Guards came and they

---

[86] 'Around the country; Limerick'.

took all our stuff. And we thought oh, God, we're going to go to jail. We didn't really think very seriously that it was going to be actual jail. But there was a time when we thought, you know, maybe we could actually go to jail.

Respondents felt that Gardaí turned a blind eye to the clinics. Mary Fahy (GFPC) explained to me 'It was a nod and a wink. Like the law said you shouldn't be operating but highly unlikely that anybody would ever raid us or stop us'. Similarly, Pete Smith (GFPC) recalled, 'I mean we moved from there to another premises and I remember being in those premises minding the shop more or less when the Guards raided us. Nothing happened. A couple of Guards went around, saw everything we'd got, we had shelves full of, you know, a full range. And they did nothing'.

Some of the activists would have welcomed prosecution. Ferga Grant (LFPC) felt 'we would have gladly, you know, gladly have been arrested, as we always said. But we kind of, we felt I think that the authorities were a bit clever I think they knew that if they did this, they would give us, you know, publicity which they felt, probably, that we didn't deserve or need'. Similarly, Anne Connolly (WWC) felt that the police did not prosecute because 'on some level, somewhere, people were being sensible, and realised that we would have relished the day in court and it would have given the profile we wanted to increase awareness and that it would do more harm than good to prosecute'. Because the other clinics had already demonstrated that the law on contraception could be flouted, Connolly had no concerns about prosecution. However, she felt that the WWC was more radical and that it made some of the other clinics uneasy because 'we were very explicit about the fact that you did not have to be married [...] we went in there, you know, very clearly communicating 'This is contraception for everybody'''. Connolly also felt that 'we were fairly confident we were okay referring people for abortion because this was before '83'. In fact, Connolly's interactions with the police were largely positive and described with humour. She explained:

So, we had a very large mail-order service and, the guards, every so often, would come down. There was a guy in the vice squad in Dublin Castle. He used to come and visit every so often, and he was just so nice. And he, he'd sit down in front of me, he'd raise his eyebrows to heaven, he'd say, 'I have another complaint here'. And he'd laugh, and I'd laugh.

6.5   Clients and Medical Authority

The history of the early family planning clinics also highlights interesting tensions around medical authority. Lay volunteers played an important role in the early years of all of the clinics. In relation to the FGC, four doctors, Michael Solomons, Jim Loughran, Joan Wilson and Anne Legge, took it in turns to attend the one hour sessions on Tuesday and Friday evenings, accompanied by Máire Mullarney, Yvonne Pim and two lay workers, Nora O'Laoghaire and Betty Young.[87] Cecelia Homan, who volunteered as a lay worker at the clinic in its early years, joined the IFPA because she felt 'that it was important that women should have the means and the right to decide on the number of children they have'.[88] The lay workers had an important role in reassuring and meeting new clients to the clinic and also noted their addresses and family sizes.[89] Recalling her work at the clinic, Yvonne Pim (IFPA) stated:

That was great fun because we worked obviously with the patients coming in, and of course some of them coming in may be coming in with a sister or somebody, not knowing what was going to happen. It certainly was quite extraordinary. They didn't have to pay then for their contraceptives, so they just paid for their consultation. They were all delighted. There were well-known people crossing our doors as well. Took a while for them obviously, because of where we were situated, which was Dublin 2.

Both the Galway mail order service and FPS relied on posting condoms to individuals around the country. By 1974, FPS volunteers realised that they had to take on medical staff in order to develop their services. In 1975, the services of FPS were expanded to include medical contraception, and a clinic was opened in April of that year to offer a complete family planning service.[90] The postal service in Galway also operated for a few months before the group realised that there was a need for a clinic service or involvement from a medical professional. According to Pete Smith:

And then we started to get into what we thought was a problem. Partly it was obvious that we were only dealing with condoms. We couldn't deal with the coil, we couldn't do diaphragms, we couldn't do the pill. That was one thing. But the other was that we were getting worried about some of the letters. We got not just applications for supplies, but those frequently had letters associated with that. And you started to read some of those letters and you thought I'm not certain just sending something back in the post is the correct response. There was a greater need there. So, we said, right, we've got to move from this postal service – which at that stage was working quite well, it had good turnover, you know – so we recontacted the other group in Galway.

[87] Solomons, *Pro-Life?* p. 28.
[88] 'Dedicated to a cause', *Woman's Way*, 10 November 1978, p. 11.
[89] Mullarney, *What About Me?* p. 164.   [90] Bolt, 'Who's who', p. 7.

In the early years of the GFPC, clients were counselled by lay volunteers about their options. Pete Smith explained the rewarding nature of this work:

And that's probably the best teaching I did in my life was sitting down with these women explaining to them what options they had and this was exactly the information they wanted. We used to do this talk before they saw the doctor and said this is the pros and cons, disadvantages and advantages of each of the methods available. I enjoyed it tremendously, you know?

However, the clinic soon transitioned to what Brian Leonard described as 'much more of a sort of professional thing, rather than a very amateur volunteer-type organisation'. The movement to a more professional, medical model helped to further legitimise the clinic but was a source of disagreement among the original founders. Evelyn Stevens stated, 'we were very keen to have as many laypeople as possible involved. It was a kind of an almost peer support so there were quite a lot of volunteers. [...] And the volunteers used to come in and do sessions where they'd talk to people that came in and provide the information that they needed and then if they needed to see the doctor, they'd get an appointment'. This contrasted with doctor John Waldron's view, with Stevens stating that he 'was of the opinion that this needed to be a doctor-led service, that it should be a professional service'. According to Pete Smith, 'We ... I think I had anyhow, a very strong feeling that the clinic should be client rather than medical driven. I didn't want it to be another place where women were told what they could do. I wanted a place where women could come and get what they decided they needed. That didn't survive. I lost that'. Smith left the clinic after two years. Likewise, Evelyn Stevens, who was also dissatisfied with the clinic 'squeezing out the volunteers' left in 1980.

The hard cases of women with low incomes who were unable to afford their children, were often put forward as an important reason for the clinics' existence. However, in reality, some of the clinics were not reaching women from lower income groups that they had originally envisaged would be the most significant clients. A report on the IFPA clinic in *Woman's Choice* magazine in 1970 explained it was not attracting individuals most in need of contraceptive advice. The magazine asked 'Where are the mothers-of-ten? The women whose large families tax their resources physically, mentally and financially: the women who have no particular religious convictions; who don't think about not having babies because having them is part of married life; because no one has ever said anything to them personally about contraception?'[91]

---

[91] 'Ireland's only family planning clinic', p. 55.

Similarly, anti-contraception group the Irish Family League critiqued the family planning clinics in 1973, arguing that they did not 'cater mainly for the poor and for women with 16 children. They cater for people with better means than most.'[92] Indeed, reflecting on this issue in his memoirs, Michael Solomons wrote that he 'regretted that the so-called 'blue card' holders, the majority of whom were working-class, were not turning up to any great extent'. He believed this was due to problems with the clinic's information networks but also 'revealed the extent to which conservative teaching continued to dominate people's lives'.[93]

The IFPA also arranged a mail order service through the IPPF for condoms, spermicides and diaphragms. According to Solomons, small packages with hand-written addresses usually got past the customs officials, but larger packages containing spermicide were sometimes intercepted.[94] For patients who wished to use the diaphragm or cap with spermicidal jelly, these cost 8s plus 3s 6d for two tubes of jelly, and these were posted to the client's address.[95] In addition, doctors who were based in Northern Ireland and sympathetic to the aims of the clinic would drive to Donegal and post supplies such as spermicidal jelly from there to Dublin.[96] Women who required IUDs in the early years of the clinic were sent to the Royal Victoria Hospital in Belfast to have this fitted free of charge but were asked to make a donation to the Northern Ireland Family Planning Association. A check-up was provided in Dublin a month after insertion and another year later.[97] By September 1970, following training provided by Joyce Neill from the Northern Ireland Family Planning Association, the clinics began providing IUDs.[98]

A fear of being seen going into the clinic was a real concern for clients. Cathy (b.1949) for instance, explained:

I went on the pill a couple of months before I got married, and I used to go to the family planning clinic in Mountjoy Square. That's where they were. But I remember, I'd go to the door and I'd be looking over my shoulder before I'd go in, making sure nobody saw me. Because I told nobody I was on it.

Cathy's account is not unusual. However, the bravery of women like her in taking control of their fertility, helped, in Yvonne Pim's view, to push the movement forward:

[92] Irish Family League, *Is Contraception the Answer?* p. 15.   [93] Solomons, *Pro-Life?* p. 30
[94] *Ibid.*, p. 31.   [95] 'Ireland's only family planning clinic', p. 55.
[96] Solomons, *Pro-Life?* p. 31.   [97] 'Ireland's only family planning clinic', p. 55.
[98] Solomons, *Pro-Life?* p. 33.

They felt the conscience was certainly pricking them if they had any thoughts at all about controlling their fertility. They struggled with their consciences to get involved, but through the family planning clinic, people did bit by bit.

While some anti-contraception groups claimed that family planning clinics such as the IFPA were money-making ventures, it is clear from their accounts in the early years that their profits were marginal. Indeed, the clinics would not have survived without the financial support of the IPPF.[99] For instance, in the period from February to December 1970, the FGC made a total of £10,772 in income, with £7,389 of this comprising patients' contributions and £3,000 comprising a grant from the IPPF. Their expenditure came to £11,040, which in addition to £256 depreciation meant that they had a profit of just £534 for that year.[100] Indeed, in 1974, the IFPA reported that in the spring of that year, they had been unable to meet the salaries bill and without the grant of £3,000 from the IPFF, the organisation 'would have been bankrupt'. This financial situation was attributed to escalating costs of post, heating and lighting as well as clinic supplies and printing.[101]

The clinic could not advertise its services, however, a large number of clients found out about its existence through word of mouth, mention in the press, and from GP referrals.[102] In 1971, a total of 4,912 patients were seen at the Merrion Square Clinic, with 1,907 seen at Mountjoy Square. 2,182 of these were new patients. The majority of patients came from Dublin city (1,371) and Co. Dublin (377), however, there were patients from all of the 26 counties of the Republic, as well as 1 person travelling from Co. Fermanagh and one from Co. Tyrone. 80.9% of new patients at the Merrion Square clinic were married and 19.1% were single while at the Mountjoy Square Clinic, 90.1% were married and 9.9% single.[103] Of new patients at Merrion Square, 33% were in the 20–24 age range and 31.2% in the 25–29 age range, while at Mountjoy Square, 30% were in the 20–24 age range and 31.6% in the 25–29 range. At both clinics, the largest percentage of new clients had no children (28.8% at Merrion Square and 21% at Mountjoy Square), with 15.8% of new clients at Merrion Square and 12.9% of clients at Mountjoy Square having 1 child at the time of their first visit. The statistics relating to the

[99] For example, the IFL claimed that the family planning movement was 'a sordid business, involving money, big business, and new vistas for medical careers.' 'Breaking the law', *Irish Press*, 25 July 1973, p. 8.
[100] Fertility Guidance Company, *Annual Report for 1971* [IFPA Archives].
[101] *IFPA Annual Report, 1974.*
[102] 'The Dublin clinic that defies convention', *This Week in Ireland*, 7 November 1969, p. 23. Courtesy of Susan Solomons
[103] Fertility Guidance Company, *Annual Report for 1971* [IFPA Archives], p. 3.

clinic clearly illustrate the urban-rural divide and that the most clients were young, urban-based women, the majority of whom had no children.

Irene (b.1942) from the rural south-east, recalled women she knew travelling to the family planning clinics in Dublin for contraception because access was limited in her area, but also for purposes of anonymity:

When I was living here then, I knew after a few years, people going up to ... because there was nobody in town. So women were going up to Dublin for the coil and stuff. Do you know what I mean? Some people went up because the husbands wouldn't know anything about it. Honestly.

The existence of the family planning clinics also meant that women did not have to ask their GPs for contraception and face the possibility of refusal. Judith (b.1950) told me 'They didn't want to go to the doctor and ask. In case the doctor said no'. Judith went to an IFPA clinic to obtain the pill instead because 'You knew you were getting it in there'. While she felt there was a possibility that she could have obtained contraception from her GP, she said, 'I didn't know to go in and ask'.

By 1975, 30.0% of patients at Mountjoy Square were single, and 48.14% of patients at Synge Street (formerly Merrion Square) were single.[104] In her report on the Synge Street clinic in 1975, Nora Harkin suggested that this was due to the fact that 'today women in Ireland, as elsewhere, find it necessary to continue working after their marriage and therefore seek advice on family planning beforehand'.[105] By 1981, 48% of visitors to the Cathal Brugha Street clinic were single and 43% married while 46% of visitors to the Synge Street clinic were single and 54% were married.[106] The 1980 annual report stressed however, that the 'single' statistic was misleading because 'many first attendees will have married by their second visit'.[107] However, what is clear is that by the mid-1970s, it was becoming more acceptable for clients to visit the clinic prior to marriage and by the late 1970s, numbers of married clients were almost equal to numbers of single clients.

A significant percentage of first-time clients at the IFPA were individuals wishing to plan their first pregnancy, rather than women who had experienced multiple pregnancies.[108] While discussions of 'hard cases' such as of women who had experienced multiple pregnancies were clearly at the heart of public discussions around family planning in the 1970s in Ireland, the evidence from the IFPA suggests that these were not the women who were being served by the clinics; a pattern also

---

[104] *IFPA Annual Report 1975*, p. 9.   [105] *Ibid.*, p. 7.
[106] *IFPA Annual Report 1981*. No page number.   [107] *IFPA Annual Report 1980*, p. 12.
[108] See Appendix: Table 2.

borne out in some of the other clinics. For instance, in the case of the Navan clinic, the majority of clients were women in their early twenties who were about to marry, just married or married a short time with one or two children.[109] Oral history evidence from staff at the other clinics suggests similar patterns in relation to clients.

The majority of new clients at both IFPA clinics came on the recommendation of a friend, with the second largest number of clients finding out about the clinic from women's magazines, newspapers and the media. Smaller numbers were referred to the clinic by hospitals and family doctors.[110] Female-centred forms of contraception were the most popular methods, particularly the pill. Male-centred forms of contraception such as condoms were less popular at the Irish clinics. Similar patterns occurred at the other family planning clinics established later in the 1970s. In 1971, 47.1% of first-time visitors to the Merrion Square clinic and 48.0% of first-time visitors at Mountjoy Square were prescribed the pill. The cap was the next most popular (23.5% at Merrion Square and 20.2% at Mountjoy Square), followed by the IUD (15.2% at Merrion Square and 14.9% at Mountjoy Square), condoms (2.1% at Merrion Square and 6.4% at Mountjoy Square), the temperature method (3.5% at Merrion Square and 2.0% at Mountjoy Square). 8.6% of clients at Merrion Square and 8.5% of clients at Mountjoy Square were described as looking for 'advice'.[111]

In 1972, there was a significant increase in clients choosing the IUD, (10% at Merrion Square and 25.1% at Mountjoy Square), with a decrease in clients selecting the cap. This increase in IUD usage was said to reflect 'the particular suitability of this method in the Irish situation'.[112] Over the next eight years, there was some fluctuation in the popularity of the IUD, but evidently, at the Mountjoy Square (and later Cathal Brugha clinic) which served a higher percentage of clients from lower socio-economic groups, the IUD continued to be popular.[113]

---

[109] 'Navan family planning clinic', *Family Planning News*, 1:1, (August 1975), p. 2.

[110] 434 clients at Mountjoy Square and 524 at Merrion Square came to the clinic on recommendation of a friend, 128 at Mountjoy Square found out about the clinic through newspapers and women's magazines and 52 from radio and TV (no figure given for Merrion Square). 90 new clients at Mountjoy Square and 89 at Merrion Square were referred by hospitals, and 104 at Mountjoy Square and 137 at Merrion Square were referred by family doctors. *Fertility Guidance Company Annual Report for 1971* [IFPA Archives], pp. 5–7.

[111] Fertility Guidance Company, *Annual Report for 1971* [IFPA Archives], p. 4.

[112] *F.G.C. Annual Report 1972*, p. 4

[113] As Necochea López has suggested, the IUD gave more control to the medical profession over women's reproductive choices, reinforced medical authority, and 'converged with the goal of international birth control organisations of arresting rapid

A study by Dr. Helena Watson looked at the medical and socio-economic characteristics of women who used the IUD, based on research on 130 first-time visitors to the IFPA Mountjoy Square clinic in 1977 who decided to be fitted with an IUD. Watson also acknowledged that 'the distance many are prepared to come for advice, or to be fitted with an IUD, also indicate high motivation', with 8.5% of IUD users travelling from Donegal, Mayo, Clare, Limerick, Cork and Kerry. She found that the majority of women being fitted with IUDs came from lower socio-economic groups: 35.4% of the IUD users had a medical card in contrast with only 8.9% of women given 'other methods'. Watson believed the IUD's popularity was because of the fact that 'once in place, it requires little further effort and expense on the user's part' and for women who were less mobile, the necessity of regularly renewing a prescription for the pill may have been a deterrent.[114] As Chikako Takeshita has shown, the IUD had been developed by population control advocates in the 1960s with the discourse around the IUD positioning it as a contraceptive for the masses, while user-controlled contraceptive methods such as the pill or the condom 'were characterised as appropriate only for educated upper- and middle-class Western individuals'.[115]

The services of the IFPA expanded over time. By September 1970, women were no longer being sent to Belfast for IUDs and these were being fitted initially at the clinic in Mountjoy Square.[116] The first vasectomies were conducted at the IFPA Mountjoy Square premises in the summer of 1974 by a female ophthalmic surgeon who had been flown into Ireland to carry out the procedure. Dr. Andrew Rynne also attended this as he had conducted vasectomies in Canada. Following this, Rynne was taken on by the IFPA to do three or four vasectomies per week.[117]

The other clinics also expanded quickly. For instance, in spite of the condemnation from the Church hierarchy, the CFPC also proved popular. In its first year, 800 first visits were paid by individuals from all over Munster and other parts of the country, an average of 60 people attending for the first time each month.[118] By 1977, it was necessary for the clinic to move to a larger premises.[119] The clinic also, in Ritchie's words, engaged in 'a good deal of sensible collaboration and that clinic

population growth in parts of the developing world'. Necochea López, *A History of Family Planning in Twentieth-Century Peru*, p. 91.

[114] 'The case for IUDs', *Irish Times*, 3 September 1982, p. 10.

[115] Chikako Takeshita, *The Global Biopolitics of the IUD: How Science Constructs Contraceptive Users and Women's Bodies* (MIT Press, 2011), p. 71.

[116] Solomons, *Pro-Life?* p. 33.   [117] Rynne, *The Vasectomy Doctor*, pp. 120–1.

[118] '800 first visits to Cork Family Planning Clinic', *Evening Echo*, 6 April 1976, p. 7.

[119] 'Family planning clinic is run by company', *Evening Echo*, 24 February 1977, p. 4.

provided what were called temperature methods, advice and so on. And we would have had one or two people come in to provide that advice who would be working in perhaps a Catholic clinic'. According to an early report on the clinic, men and women from surrounding counties such as Limerick, Tipperary, Kerry and Waterford, travelled to the Cork clinic and a large amount of correspondence from these areas was also noted. For clients who were unable to travel to the clinic, a postal service for non-medical supplies was available. Clients were primarily women in their early twenties, 'about to marry, recently married, or married a short time with a couple of children'. The report expressed concern that, as was the case with other family planning clinics, that there was a relatively small attendance from women who already had large families and women from lower socio-economic groups, or medical card holders.[120] By 1978, total patient attendances reached 3,772 for the year from February 1977 to February 1978 and medical card holders comprised 43% of new patients. From December 1977, the clinic was able to remain open five days a week.[121] As with the other family planning clinics, the Cork clinic provided contraceptives to unmarried as well as married individuals, leading one writer to the *Evening Echo* in 1979 to query 'the number of young teenagers into whose hands these [artificial contraceptives] fall into'.[122]

Again, and similar to the case of the Cork clinic, the LFPC quickly became popular in spite of Church condemnation. By October 1976, Jim Kemmy claimed that they had 150 enquiries per week, with about 50 coming from Co. Limerick and the remaining 100 coming from Limerick city as well as a few from Kerry, Clare and sometimes Galway. The clinic moved to a new premises on Myles Street that month as a result of an expanding service. Kemmy stated that the majority of the people visiting the clinic were 'in their thirties and married with families already'. At this point, the clinic still did not have the services of a doctor and about a third of their business was through the post.[123] The Limerick clinic, in contrast to the other clinics in Ireland, with the exception of the WWC established later, took a more feminist approach. Chappell recalled that the women involved in the clinic became known as 'Kemmy's Femmes', which perhaps highlights the continued association of Kemmy with the clinic and perceived hierarchies. In addition to becoming involved in the LFPC, members of the Limerick Women's Action Group were also involved in setting up the Limerick Rape Crisis Centre. Information on

[120] 'Cork Clinic', *Family Planning News*, 1:1, (August 1975), p. 2.
[121] 'More attend clinic', *Evening Echo*, 4 April 1978, p. 7.
[122] 'Contraception: Agrees with Mr. O'Connor', *Evening Echo*, 5 February 1979, p. 5.
[123] 'Contraceptives clinic moves', *Limerick Leader*, 16 October 1976, p. 1.

the clinic's activities was largely spread by word of mouth. The clinic initially started solely providing contraception but soon began offering other services such as smear testing.

The majority of clients at the clinic were women and they came from a range of social backgrounds. According to Ferga Grant:

There was a lot of rural people I remember, sad stories, people who had, you know, large families, didn't want any more children. [...] actually some women I remember telling me at the time, they had more opposition from their doctors than they had from their priests about using contraception, which surprised me.

Grant's testimony here is revealing in it further highlights the power and authority that the medical profession held over individuals' access to contraception at the time. Grant stated that as feminists clinic workers 'we would be saying, "Look, this is your body, you have a right to want to do this, you know."'

The LFPC did not just serve the Limerick city area but according to Cathie Chappell, word spread, and the clinics also served women from surrounding counties, including Clare, Kerry and Tipperary, who struggled to get contraception from their local GP.[124] Moreover, the clinic provided contraception to both married and single women and women were not asked about their marital status when visiting.[125] According to Dr. Philip Cullen, the pill, over the counter sales of condoms, and IUDs were the most popular forms of contraception. The clinic moved premises again in 1978 to Mallow Street and extended its hours to 16 hours six days a week as a result of increased demand. By this stage, the clinic was offering medical and non-medical contraceptives. From 1982, Dr. Cullen began providing a vasectomy service.

The GFPC also had a range of clients who travelled in from other parts of the west of Ireland. Evening sessions also facilitated some level of secrecy for individuals who had a fear of being seen going into the clinic. Melvin explained that 'the evening times were the times when local people came in. Under cover of darkness'. As with the other clinics, there was a real fear from clients about being seen. Richard (b.1954) who attended the clinic for contraception before he and his wife got married recalled his visit vividly and with humour:

It's strange but I can still remember going down to the family planning office. Kind of six months before we got married. You know, one of these kind of mile stones that stick out. You know. I mentioned it earlier. But, like, looking behind your back to see your, do I know anyone. (laughs).

---

[124] Cathie Chappell.   [125] *Ibid.*.

Richard had a positive experience at the GFPC, explaining, 'It was very kind of open. And we were surprised. We thought that it would be much, much more, that they'd be much... but they were very, very open. Very informative. And provided lots of details on the options and all of that. And the implications'.

Word about the clinic soon spread. Mary Fahy recalled the Thursday evening sessions as follows: 'And you could hardly walk up the stairs to the clinic rooms because people would be ... girls, women everywhere. Very few men attending. But just so busy. People coming from all over the place in spite of Church teaching and stuff'. According to Stevens, Melvin and Fahy, the contraceptive pill and the coil (IUD) were the most popular forms of contraception in the early years of the clinic, although they also supplied diaphragms and condoms. In the early years of the GFPC, women who required sterilisations were sent to Dr. Edgar Ritchie in Cork, and later a vasectomy service was provided by Dr. John Waldron.[126] Smith recalled being surprised that few university students attended the clinic and that the majority of clients were married women who had children already, 'the typical person we saw were 30-year-old women with two children who didn't want any more'. Clinic workers often had to deal with difficult cases. Melvin recalled, 'it was shocking some of the stuff that came in the door. It took a while, not being social workers, not having the kind of training of a social worker, it could affect you quite profoundly'.

It is evident from the oral history interviews, that activists from all of the clinics viewed Irish women as being important drivers of change. These women were beginning to reject Church teachings and exercise their own agency over their reproductive choices. Evelyn Stevens told me:

and I think that was *the* most noticeable thing or most notable thing that most of the people that came in would have been from Galway and County Galway, specifically the west of Ireland and more than likely would have been raised as Catholics, but they just did not want to have more children or children for a certain period of time, so they were going to avail of contraception no matter what.

Similarly, Mary Fahy (GFPC) recalled a group of women from Connemara who had lived in England:

they all had their coils fitted and stuff like that when they came home and no place to have them changed or do anything about them. So, they used to come in, a carload of them would come in on the Thursday night or a Wednesday night and they were great, you know, they just didn't pass any remarks, they just thought it should be ... that's how it should be, that they were entitled to the service.

[126] Dorothea Melvin, Mary Fahy.

Yet, in her view 'for a lot of women, there was a huge anxiety about it being against the teaching of the Catholic Church. And that was the ... we weren't in a position to make those kinds of decisions for people. It was something they had to come to grasp or to terms with themselves'. Edgar Ritchie (CFPC) believed 'in practice the tide was flowing in the direction of taking responsibility, looking for ways of limiting their family and of course, in fact of ability to conceive and so on'. These testimonies suggest that many women were beginning to reject Catholic teachings on birth control and come to their own decisions on the matter.

Like feminist health centres in the United States, the WWC encouraged women to take ownership of their health and tried to empower women through the provision of information such as on, for example, self-examination of the cervix and breast examinations. An emphasis was placed on making the WWC a friendly and comfortable environment with Connolly recognising that, 'Many women are reluctant to attend GPs about these kind of matters and feel more confident coming to a centre where there is a confidential and specialised service'.[127] The waiting room of the WWC was designed to be welcoming, with one article describing 'its brown and cream décor, chrome easy chairs with brown corduroy upholstery, chrome and glass coffee tables, green plants and soft white net at the window' as well as a box of children's books, toys and games. Tea and coffee making facilities were also provided with Connolly noting that 'People tend to be nervous when they come to a place like this, and a hot drink sometimes helps'.[128] Indeed, Connolly found that large numbers of women came from other parts of the country to the Well Woman because they found it difficult to talk about women's health issues with their local GP[129]

As with the other family planning clinics, WWC clients tended to come from the middle-classes; the fees were relatively expensive at £5 for a first visit and £3.50 for every other visit. The centre did not accept medical cards.[130] A critical view of the clinic was published in *Rebel Woman* magazine which stated that the WWC 'is more 'sophisticated' and indeed ruthless than the 'traditional' ones: it uses a 'hardsell' approach. No white coats here...but plush carpets and first names for doctors and patients.' The magazine also raised concerns that, in its view, 'it advocates strongly male and female sterilisation as a form of birth control – an attitude common to population control clinics in Asia and Latin

---

[127] 'Well Woman Centre opens in Dublin', *Irish Independent*, 16 January 1978, p. 8.
[128] 'Dedicated to a cause', *Woman's Way*, 10 November 1978, p. 12.
[129] 'Can you talk to you doctor?', *Irish Independent*, 26 April 1978, p. 6.
[130] 'Are you Well Woman?'

America'.[131] In Anne Connolly's view, as with the other clinics, there was evidently a demand for the WWC's services. She told me, 'You know, women voted with their feet, they wanted to be able to access the service which was very pro-woman, which put as much of the decision-making as possible in the woman's hand'. Oral history testimonies suggest that women who attended the clinic viewed it in a positive light. Ger Moane (IWU), visited the WWC in her final year of university in Dublin. She explained, 'It was a positive experience, is all I can say. It felt bold, and it felt like a right in the one way that I was doing something for myself, and for us. All this liberation had obviously gone to my head. Yeah. I went to the Well Woman Centre, and got the pill. Went on the pill, did the whole thing. Had sexual intercourse, felt great about it. I remember leaving the Well Woman Centre feeling like, "Wow! I've grown up!" You know? That this is kind of a strong thing to do'. Similarly, Mairead (b.1953) stated, 'I remember the Well Woman Centre was great like, you would have all the information and stuff. And they would be very sort of, caring and things and supportive exactly, yeah'.

In addition to providing family planning services including vasectomies, the clinic also provided mail order contraceptives, information on STDs, pregnancy testing, advice and referrals for female sterilisation, smear tests, pregnancy counselling, and advice on the menopause and pre-menstrual tension.[132] The centre referred women to BPAS clinics in the UK for abortions and also conducted pre- and post-abortion counselling.[133]

Counselling in relation to unplanned pregnancy was also provided at other clinics in the era before the introduction of the eighth amendment in 1983. Dr. Philip Cullen (LFPC) recalled:

We would have said to people, okay, we'll arrange for you to have a termination in London, and in the clinic, we would have quietly made the necessary arrangements. But then of course, when the Eighth Amendment came along, you really couldn't do that, because you would have taken the risk of really being locked away if you did it.

Similarly, Evelyn Stevens (GFPC) also recalled counselling women in the late 1970s who were experiencing unplanned pregnancies:

that was a very tricky area, but there would have been people who came in who were pregnant and didn't want to be pregnant. And I would step outside the

---

[131] 'The Battle of the Clinics', *Rebel Woman*, c.1978 [RCAPA, UCC, BL/F/AP/1139/24], no page number.
[132] The Dublin Well Woman Centre leaflet, [RCAPA, UCC, BL/F/A[/1221/2].
[133] Anne Connolly, 9 December 2019.

clinic sort of thing and just on a one-to-one basis I'd just give them a phone number in England, because I couldn't do it really as per the clinic work and these people were desperate and I just had that bit of information so I passed that on to people. That was very difficult.

Stevens felt that 'I suppose, the advantage of getting it from somebody like me was that I ... I'd had contact with places, I knew that they were trustworthy and people had come back and said that they were trustworthy'.

The clinics were also involved in education around family planning. As mentioned in Chapter 3, the FGC published an educational booklet, *Family Planning*, written by Jim Loughran and Robert Towers in 1971. In addition, members of the organisation were involved in outreach activities. In 1972, Loughran gave lectures on family planning to the Dublin and North Wicklow branch of the Irish Medical Association, to senior midwives from the midwifery training hospitals and to final year students at the Royal College of Surgeons. Máire Mullarney presented lectures on family planning to more than twenty Ladies' Clubs in the Dublin region.[134] Frank Crummey and Pat O'Donovan (FPS) also gave regular talks to ladies' clubs.[135] In Frank Crummey's words, 'messengers were sent out on educational missions all over the country, to talk about contraceptive methods and choices'.[136] Moreover, an important element of the clinics' work was the provision of training in family planning. Edgar Ritchie (CFPC) felt:

really the important thing was training doctors out in the provinces and so on. How to advise people and that was I think the most important thing we did. In a sense that it was no longer something that was restricted to a few people in gynaecology or in family planning clinics, but right across the country. It could be taken up as a proper service both in method and advice by family doctors across the country.

6.6   Conclusion

The history of the Irish family planning clinics provides a number of important insights into the history of contraception. As scholars such as Cloatre and Enright have already shown, the clinics played an important part in challenging the law on contraception in Ireland. While oral history respondents felt that the risks of arrest or raids were minimal, or as Dorothea Melvin (GFPC) described it, 'We were a little bit afraid but not too afraid', it is still clear that they were taking significant risks through their involvement with the clinics, and in some cases this could have

---

[134] F.G.C. *Annual Report 1972*, p. 8.   [135] *Crummey v Ireland*, p. 100.
[136] *Ibid.*, p. 99.

substantial personal impact. It is evident that activists had a range of reasons for becoming involved in family planning activism, but often this motivation stemmed from personal experience. Many had a firm belief in responsible parenthood and contraception as a human right and as such positioned themselves within the wider international family planning movement. Networks were crucial to the development of the Irish family planning clinics. In particular, the IPPF was an important transnational network without which, the Fertility Guidance Company/IFPA would not have survived, while the Marie Stopes foundation in the UK was integral to the setting up of the WWC. Regular international meetings and financial support from the IPPF enabled the development of the IFPA clinics but arguably impacted on the direction of the services provided. National networks were integral in providing a sense of community and in exchanging support and advice among workers involved in the clinics across the country. While it was often not possible for clinics to publicly advertise their services, information on them was spread by word of mouth and protests by conservative campaigners arguably helped to publicise them.

It is evident, from oral history interviews and archival evidence, that women were predominantly the main clients of the family planning clinics. While all of the clinics eventually began to expand their services, female-centred forms of contraception such as the pill, IUD and the diaphragm, remained the most popular methods, in line with those being promoted by international family planning organisations such as IPPF. While the majority of clients were young, middle-class and urban-based, the clinics provided an important service, and travel from rural areas to the urban clinics for family planning advice was a common practice. Moreover, discussions about the clinics in the press helped to spark debate around the issue more broadly. The clinics were not just providing advice on family planning, and over time their services expanded widely. Additionally, several of the clinics also provided advice on unplanned pregnancy to women. It is clear also that the clinics became an important setting for the medicalisation of family planning in Ireland. Medical authority was essential in the cases of all of the clinics so that a full spectrum of contraceptive options could be provided, although the WWC attempted to negate this with a feminist health approach. Organisations such as FPS and the Galway mail order service which initially began providing non-medical contraceptives, soon realised the necessity of providing a full service. The cases of the Limerick and Galway clinics also reveal the tensions between grassroots activism and a more medical, professional model. Indeed, arguably, the involvement of medical professionals helped to give clinics more legitimacy and a more professional identity and meant that training could be provided.

7 Feminist Campaigns for Free, Safe and Legal Contraception in the 1970s

On 23 May 1971 at mass at Knock Shrine, in Co. Mayo, the Bishop of Clonfert, Rev. Thomas Ryan declared that 'probably never before, certainly not since the penal days, had the Catholic heritage of our country been subjected to so many insidious onslaughts on the pretext of conscience, civil rights and women's liberation'. In Ryan's view, 'It was no exaggeration to say that the mass media of communication in Ireland were being misused and were providing too easy a platform for those who seemed intent on attacking the Church and destroying our Catholic heritage'.[1] The subjects of Ryan's attack were members of the Irish Women's Liberation Movement (IWLM), who, one day earlier, had embarked on a trip by train from Dublin to Belfast to purchase contraceptives in order to highlight the hypocrisy of the Irish ban on contraception.

As Raewyn Connell has shown, women's liberation and gay liberation movements 'reflect crisis tendencies of a general kind, and are historically novel in the depth of their critique of the gender order and the scope of the transformation they propose'.[2] In addition to the ban on contraception, women living in 1970s Ireland suffered from a range of inequalities that had been in existence since the early twentieth century, including lack of equal pay for equal work and the marriage bar.[3] This chapter therefore explores the activism of feminist groups who critiqued these conditions, and particularly focuses on their campaigns for the legalisation of contraception in the 1970s. As well as examining the contraception campaign of the IWLM, I will also explore the work of two groups that have received much less historical attention, Irishwomen United (IWU) and their offshoot, the Contraception Action Programme (CAP). This chapter will illuminate the personal experiences of Irish

---

[1] 'Onslaughts on faith deplored', *Irish Press*, May 24, 1971, p.4.
[2] R. W. Connell, *Gender and power: society, the person and sexual politics* (London, 1987), p. 279.
[3] Hug, *The politics of sexual morality*, pp 79–82.

feminist activists and illustrate the nuances of feminist demands for reproductive rights within the Irish case study. Moreover, as well as service provision, later groups such as IWU and CAP drew attention to the important class and geographic inequalities with regard to access to contraception in Ireland.

7.1   The Irish Women's Liberation Movement

The IWLM was the first Irish women's group to take a stand on the Irish government's laws on contraception, and in doing so; they not only took on the state but also the Catholic hierarchy. A largely middle-class group of Irish women including left-wing activists, trade unionists, journalists, and stay-at-home-mothers had formed the IWLM in 1970. The idea for the group started with five women: Margaret Gaj, the owner of a Dublin restaurant that often housed meetings of left-wing groups, Mary Maher, journalist for the *Irish Times*, Moira Woods, a doctor, Máirín de Burca, a left-wing activist who had been involved in Sinn Féin and the Dublin Housing Action Committee, and Máirín Johnston, a left-wing activist who had also been involved in the Dublin Housing Action Committee.[4] The IWLM soon expanded to include Mary Kenny, Nell McCafferty, June Levine as well as Nuala Fennell, Mary Anderson, Mary McCutcheon, Marie McMahon, Nuala Monaghan, and Dr. Eimer Philbin Bowman. The first meeting of the IWLM took place at Mary Maher's home in Fairview, Dublin, in October 1970, with another scheduled soon after at Mary Kenny's flat. Subsequent meetings were usually held on Mondays upstairs at Gaj's restaurant on Baggott Street.[5] Several of the founder members of the IWLM held prominent positions as journalists, while others had backgrounds in left-wing and republican politics. Dr. Eimer Philbin Bowman explained, 'They were a very exciting group of people because they were at the forefront of the ... the editors of the women's pages in the three newspapers, Mary Maher and Mary Kenny and ... Mary Maher was in the Irish Times, Mary Kenny was at the Irish Press and Mary McCutcheon who's sadly died, was in the Independent. They were an exciting group of people to be in touch with'. Their links with the major Irish newspapers meant that 'the small group had a considerable reservoir to draw on when seeking to disseminate feminist ideas and information in a country still quite insular in its social perspectives'.[6]

[4] Stopper, p.23 and p.49.
[5] 'List of activists in the IWLM', [RCAPA, UCC, BL/F/AP/1110/2] Stopper, p.41.
[6] Galligan, *Women and Politics*, p.52

In their first publication, *Irishwomen Chains or Change*, published in early 1971, the group set out the key problems facing Irish women in the early 1970s. These included the legal inequities such as the fact that women could not be called upon for jury service. Additionally, under Irish law, a married woman was 'still regarded as the chattel of her husband'. Moreover, a husband could desert his wife for as long as he chose, but if a wife were to do this, she would forfeit all of her rights, including access to the marital home and to her children.[7] The document also drew attention to the inequalities faced by Irish women in the workplace. They were not paid equally for equal work and the Irish marriage bar meant that women working in the civil service, state bodies and much of private industry were forced to leave their jobs upon marriage.[8] Importantly, *Irishwomen Chains or Change* also drew attention to the plight of widows, deserted wives, unmarried mothers and single women, whom they labelled 'Women in distress'. In a deliberately provocative move, the pamphlet concluded with five reasons why it was better for Irish women to 'live in sin' than get married.[9]

Contraception became a 'unifying question' for the IWLM.[10] On this issue, Nell McCafferty explained in an oral history interview: 'Which would be fun since I was born gay but I knew enough to know the despair that women felt when they're pregnant'. McCafferty was also angered by the hypocrisy around the law on contraception in Ireland. She stated:

And there's always an underground doctor to say he would give you the pill for what's it called to regulate your menstrual flow and we had, and this is a fact, the highest rate in the world of irregular menstrual flow. But you had to be a certain type of person, educated or middle–class, the working class wouldn't have known those things. And probably couldn't have afforded a doctor.

The Irish laws against family planning were critiqued in a section of *Irishwomen Chains or Change* entitled 'Incidental facts' which also noted the lack of childcare facilities, playgrounds and creches, baby-minding regulations, the option to divorce, and re-training facilities for women. The section on the family planning laws drew attention to the hypocrisy of the law in that it was possible for Irish women to get access to the contraceptive pill as a 'cycle regulator' and reported that '25,000

---

[7] *Irishwomen Chains or Change*, (Dublin: Irish Women's Liberation Movement, 1971), pp.1–4. [RCAPA, BL/F/AP/1139/15].

[8] *Irishwomen Chains or Change*, pp.5–9. On the marriage bar, see Hartford and Redmond, "I am amazed at how easily we accepted it'.

[9] *Irishwomen Chains or Change*, pp.30–1.

[10] See: Connolly, *The Irish Women's Movement*, Ailbhe Smyth, 'The Women's Movement in the Republic of Ireland, 1970–1990', in: Ailbhe Smyth (ed.). *Irish Women's Studies Reader*, (Dublin: Attic Press, 1993), pp.245–69.

Irishwomen use it, ostensibly under the guise of a medicine to regularise the menstrual cycle'. According to the authors, 'The moral question is not here under discussion: the fact remains that Irishwomen who do not adhere to orthodox Roman Catholic dogma are technically criminals, and when caught, are punished by deprivation of their right to plan their families as they wish.'[11]

Following the publication of *Irishwomen Chains or Change*, the IWLM began to receive more attention from the public. A dramatic appearance on the popular television programme The Late Late Show, hosted by Gay Byrne, in March 1971, where members of the IWLM became embroiled in an argument with politician Garret FitzGerald, resulted in increased media attention. In an article published in the *Irish Times* shortly after, founder member Mary Maher, stated 'We're not asking anyone to join us; we are just hoping that Irishwomen will start to join each other, to form groups in whatever situation they find themselves in – offices, factories, housing estates, high-rise flats – to discuss the concept of liberation and how it applies to them immediately'. Maher went on to express her hopes that the women's movement would take off in Ireland as it had done in other countries.[12] On 14 April 1971, the first major public meeting of the IWLM was held in the Mansion House, Dublin, with over 1,000 people, mostly women, attending.[13] According to founder member Máirín Johnston:

We couldn't believe that the women of Ireland were… each individual was so aware of what was happening and what had happened to them and the situation, in the country, as regards women. Nobody ever spoke about it. This was a big, big open meeting and it was very, very good.

Women aired their grievances at this meeting and the movement grew into twenty-eight groups, largely based on geographical location.[14] Contraception was an important mobilising issue for the newly expanded IWLM. According to June Levine, one of the founding members, 'We certainly all agreed on contraception being a basic issue of women's liberation, most claiming it as the central issue. Out of that first meeting of delegates came the decision to do something "worthwhile" about it'.[15]

Archbishop John Charles McQuaid faced particular criticism from the IWLM after the publication of his pastoral on contraception in March 1971. As a dramatic act of defiance, the IWLM organised walk-outs of

---

[11] *Irishwomen Chains or Change*, p. 25.
[12] 'Women first', *Irish Times*, 9 March 1971, p. 6.
[13] Galligan, *Women and Politics*, p. 53.   [14] *Ibid.*.
[15] June Levine, *Sisters: The Personal Story of an Irish Feminist* (Cork: Attic Press, new edition, 2009), p. 138.

Dublin churches after the reading of the pastoral. Eight women and one man left the Pro-Cathedral in Dublin after the pastoral was read, 'in protest at what they described as blatant interference of the Church in State affairs and an attempt to deny civil rights to those whose consciences permitted the use of contraceptives'.[16] June Levine, who was Jewish, described how her anxiety the night before the walk-out manifested itself in a nightmare about the Archbishop.[17] She wrote that as she left the cathedral in protest she felt 'Eyes' on her back.[18] Mary Kenny and Máirín Johnston walked out of mass at Haddington Road Church. When the priest read the line 'any contraceptive act is wrong in itself' from the pastoral, Kenny stood up and said: "This is a wicked pastoral. It is disgraceful and contrary to *Humanae Vitae*. This is Church dictatorship." Máirín Johnston also rose and said "This is a matter that should be decided by women alone. Why should men dictate to us how many children we should have? We are leaving this church in protest".[19]

Not all mass-goers that day felt the same as Kenny and Johnston. Numerous letters sent to Archbishop McQuaid illustrate the polarised opinions of Dublin residents on the matter. One male parishioner, who had been present at Haddington Road mass wrote to Archbishop McQuaid to say 'I listened with admiration and gratitude to your pastoral letter this morning in St. Mary's, Haddington Road. My simple reaction was, thank God for a bishop who accepts and discharges his apostolic obligation to teach his people God's law'.[20] Another Dublin man wrote 'I have just heard on the 10 p.m. news of the protests made about your letter on "contraception", which was read at all masses today. I have no doubt that these protests will cause you great pain, because of your obvious concern for all of us, both spiritually and temporally. May I as a Dublin Catholic apologise for the activities of my fellow citizens and co-religionists. I ask you to adopt the patience of Christ who prayed for His enemies, "Father, forgive them, for they know not what they do."'[21]

A demonstration outside the Archbishop's house was organised by the IWLM for the evening after the walk-out. According to the *Irish Examiner*, thirty 'picketers formed a 40-foot chain across the entrance to the Archbishop's House at Drumcondra, Dublin. They carried placards

[16] 'Women protest in pro-Cathedral: archbishop denounces contraception', *Irish Times*, 29 March 1971, p. 1.
[17] Levine, *Sisters*, p. 136.   [18] *Ibid.*, p. 137.
[19] 'Women protest in pro-Cathedral', *Irish Times*, 29 March 1971, p. 1.
[20] Letter to Archbishop John Charles McQuaid, 28 March 1971. [DDA: McQuaid Papers, XX/82/4].
[21] Letter to Archbishop McQuaid, dated 28 March 1971 [DDA: McQuaid Papers, XX/82/10(1)-(2)].

saying that the Archbishop's letter was dictatorial.'[22] The divisiveness of the contraception issue is evident by the reaction that one of the protestors, a woman from the north of Ireland, received from passers-by. She was allegedly told to 'get back to where you came from' and after revealing that she was a Catholic, was told 'Go back up there and shoot yourselves'.[23]

The IWLM later released a statement on McQuaid's pastoral arguing that he 'had gone outside his brief in making this statement. It is clearly an intolerable interference with the role of the State in the framing of civil laws. Furthermore, it denies the existence of the civil law'. The IWLM also drew attention to previous interference by the Church in the country's legislative and democratic processes, citing in particular, the Mother and Child scheme of 1951.[24] Notably, they highlighted that fifty-one Irish women had died as a result of pregnancy according to the 1968–9 Maternal Mortality report, arguing that most of these women were 'dependent on State medicine. For most of them pregnancy was already a serious medical hazard because they suffered from heart conditions, strain from too much childbearing, etc. These women, mainly working class, were in effect killed by lack of contraceptive aid. Many of them left large families motherless'. In their view, the pastoral letter was 'an attack on the integrity of the people of Ireland, North and South, firstly in its implication that the legislation of contraception would bring about widespread moral degradation, and, secondly, in that it tries to use its moral authority to prevent civil law being enacted'.[25]

The walk-out of mass at the end of March 1971 and the subsequent picket marked a new phase of direct action for the IWLM. On April 1, 1971, fifteen members of the group, along with a dozen children, marched outside Leinster House, the home of the Irish parliament, before bursting through the entrance, to the surprise of army and police security, who refused to allow them entry to the building. The women began singing 'We shall not be moved', later changing the lyrics to 'We shall not conceive'. The singing attracted the attention of curious members of parliament and senators. Three of the women, Máirín de Burca, Hilary Orpen, and Fionnuala O'Connor then entered Leinster House through a lavatory window and asked to meet with three senators. They were told that the senators were 'unavailable' but were met by one, Bernard McGlinchy of the Fianna Fáil party. Upon being escorted outside, the

---

[22] *Irish Examiner,* 29 March 1971, p. 7.   [23] 'Women protest in pro-Cathedral', p. 1.
[24] For a detailed discussion of the Mother and Child scheme, see Earner-Byrne, *Mother and Child.*
[25] 'Archbishop criticised by women', *Irish Times,* 31 March 1971, p. 13.

women met with the other members of the group. Hilary Orpen claimed she had been struck by a garda officer and the group went to Pearse Street Station to register a complaint.[26] Two days later, members of the IWLM picketed the Eurovision Song Contest which was taking place in Dublin that year. Leaflets were distributed to European personalities which informed them that contraception was illegal in Ireland, a fact that 'seems especially repugnant in view of the fact that Ireland as a member of the United Nations is not bound by this organisation's universal declaration of human rights'.[27] The following month, international members of the medical profession were also targeted. On 19 May 1971, twelve members of the IWLM picketed the Nineteenth British Congress of Obstetrics and Gynaecology in Dublin. With placards that had slogans such as 'Gynaes – be logical' and 'Ceart an duine is ea frithghinnuint' (the Irish for 'Contraception is a human right'), protestors confronted delegates at the conference and handed out leaflets.[28]

The most significant protest organised by the IWLM, however, was to occur later that month. On 22 May 1971, forty-seven members of the IWLM boarded the 8 a.m. train from Dublin to Belfast with the aim of purchasing contraceptives in the north and travelling back with them. According to Mary Kenny, reflecting on what became known as the 'Contraceptive Train':

A stunt is often a good way to move political ideas forward: the Suffragettes had done it with their demonstrations – some of which were hair-raisingly violent, and environmental organisations like Friends of the Earth and Greenpeace have been imaginative in their various forms of direct action.[29]

For Nell McCafferty, the Contraceptive Train represented

a chance to draw the eyes of the world to Ireland and its punitive laws against the use of birth control: we would go to Belfast, purchase contraceptives, show them to the customs officers in Dublin and challenge them to arrest and charge us, or let us pass, thereby proving the law both hypocritical and obsolete.[30]

Members of the IWLM were concerned by the fact that the contraceptive pill was often prescribed as a cycle regulator to Irish women, despite the fact that this may not have been the most suitable contraceptive for them, and sometimes produced side effects. Other contraceptives, such as the diaphragm, condoms and the coil were available to middle-class women

---

[26] 'Protest at Leinster House by 15 women', *Irish Times*, 1 April 1971, p. 1.
[27] *Succubus*, May 1971, (RCAPA).
[28] 'Gynaes – be logical' urge feminists', *Irish Times*, 20 May 1971, p. 13.
[29] Kenny, *Something of Myself and Others*, p. 152.
[30] Nell McCafferty, *Nell*, (Dublin: Penguin Ireland, 2004), p. 222.

through family planning clinics or to women who were able to travel to the UK to obtain them. Writing in her memoirs, June Levine explained:

The point was that the Contraceptive Law affected those who most needed contraceptives, the poor and women who could not take or get the pill. Anyone who could take the train to Belfast could have all the contraceptives they wanted. The customs people never bothered about them when they came back to Ireland. The idea of Women's Liberation was to show up the hypocrisy...[31]

The stunt was controversial among members of the IWLM and some, such as Nuala Fennell, did not go on the train. Being seen on the train could potentially have professional consequences. Dr. Eimer Philbin Bowman, for example, explained, 'The reason I knew I couldn't go on it was because I knew that any hope I had of getting a job, and I still was hoping to go back to medicine, would have been put at risk if I had been photographed coming back on the train'.

After arriving in Belfast, the group of women, followed by the reporters and cameras from the international press, went into a chemist shop. According to several newspaper articles, and IWLM members' memoirs, for many of the women it was their first time ever seeing contraception. Some women were reported to have had difficulty in choosing an appropriate contraceptive.[32] The lack of knowledge that many women on the train had about contraceptives was apparent. The chemist remarked, 'They certainly could do with a bit of education. You have to know something about the subject before you can buy contraceptives – it's usually the men who buy the kind these women bought. It's surprising how little they know'.[33] Many of the women did not realise that most forms of contraception required a prescription. Nell McCafferty recalled:

And we got to Belfast and I lead them across the street there at the train station across the street to the pharmacy and went into the pharmacy and I was the spokesperson. And I walked up and I said 'Have you any contraceptive pills?' and he went 'certainly where's your prescription?' I went 'What do you mean prescription?' he says 'Give me your prescription' I says 'Well then I'll have the coil please' 'where's your prescription?' and I said 'I'll have to look' he says 'Where's your prescription?' and I thought Christ, if we go down South with condoms, there's two things wrong with it. One it's going to draw attention to the penis and two its giving men control over fertility. We are going to be wrecked.

Fearful of the stunt collapsing, McCafferty, had a brainwave: 'Uninformed I was, but stupid I was not. I did not fancy us returning to Dublin armed

---

[31] Levine, *Sisters*, p. 139.
[32] 'Women's Lib shopping trip tests law', *Irish Examiner*, 24 May 1971, p. 20.
[33] 'Innocents, too, on Pill train!', *Sunday Independent*, 23 May 1971, p. 1.

only with condoms, which would have concentrated the mind of the nation on male nether regions; on sex; on anything but birth control. Unthinkable. So I bought hundreds of packets of aspirin'.[34] McCafferty dispersed these among the group, with women instructed to pretend they were birth control pills and to swallow them in front of the customs officials in Dublin. Other women purchased condoms and jars of spermicidal jelly. Máirín Johnston, for instance, who went on the train with her son and partner commented:

The chemist was highly amused at the whole thing and he was putting all the goods out on the thing. I didn't want to be burdened with too much, so I just said I'll buy jelly. Spermicidal jelly. That's what I got.

As the return train approached Dublin, the women grew more worried. Several of the women reflected on their anxiety. Mary Kenny, in her memoirs, wrote 'I knew that this was something which had to be done, because it would make a point dramatically, sensationally, even historically. But I was also wretched about doing it. I knew how upset my mother would be – how mortified to see her daughter in the headlines, even identified as a ringleader, in a stunt which involved buying French letters in Belfast'.[35] Similarly, McCafferty wondered "What would our mothers say? What would our editors say? Would we still have jobs?"[36] In an oral history interview I asked Máirín Johnston if she was worried she would be arrested. She replied:

I was, yeah. Oh yeah, I was very worried about it because I was involved in a lot of things. I was involved in the Housing Action Committee, and we were beaten off the streets. I knew what it was to get the blow of a baton and I didn't want … Since I was pregnant, I didn't want to be dragged around by any policeman because they had a special branch, there was the heavy gang, the heavy gang they called them. They were vicious, absolutely vicious. I didn't like that. Still, I mean, I was willing to. Somebody has to do it. If you don't, if you're afraid all the time, you'll just …

However, as the train drew closer to the station, the women on the train became reassured after hearing a huge number of voices singing 'We Shall Overcome'. Levine wrote: 'I gave up the fear of spending even five minutes in a cell. We'd been scared, but now we'd see it through. The station was a teeming mass of people with banners, cheering. We unfurled our banner, with the Sutton group carrying it, and Colette O'Neill marching in front of it, mother of four, singing at the top of her lungs'.[37] Similarly, Mary Kenny remarked that there was 'an atmosphere of

---

[34] Nell McCafferty, *Nell*, p. 223.   [35] Kenny, *Something of Myself and Others*, p. 153.
[36] McCafferty, *Nell*, p. 227.   [37] Levine, *Sisters*, p. 144.

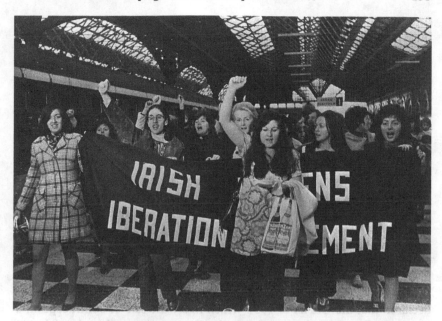

Figure 7.1 Irish Women's Liberation Movement Contraceptive Train protest, 22 May 1971.
Photograph by Eddie Kelly. Courtesy of the *Irish Times*.

carnival at the Dublin railway station and that some of the activists began to blow condoms up like balloons.[38] The scenes at Connolly Station were ones of jubilance (Figure 7.1). The members of the IWLM were met by a 200-strong crowd of supporters, which had been organised by founder member Máirín de Burca. Men and women carried placards with slogans such as 'Men care too', 'Women are only baby machines' and 'Welcome home, criminals'.[39]

On approaching the customs officials, a woman was asked if she had 'any of those things with you?' She replied that she had and that she was wearing it. The customs official appeared not to hear her and told her to 'Go ahead'. The next two women to approach the customs officers declared their purchases but refused to hand them over. The third told the official she had twelve packets of contraceptives in her handbag and that she would not be handing them over. The customs officer declared 'I'm not interested' and the three women marched past the barrier.[40]

[38] Kenny, *Something of Myself and Others*, p. 154.
[39] 'Victory for women's Lib.!', *Sunday Independent*, 23 May 1971, p. 4.
[40] 'Victory for women's Lib.!', p. 4.

Another woman declared her 'contraceptive pills' before swallowing them and stating, 'I have just asserted my constitutional rights. What are you going to do about it?'[41] According to a report in the *Sunday Independent*, a scuffle broke out between station officials, the Gardaí and a section of the crowd when a woman tried to push through on to the platform. No searches were made of any of the women.[42] As women marched through the barrier they chanted, 'The law is obsolete; we have enforced the Constitution'.[43] In Nell McCafferty's words: 'A woman shouted 'Loose your contraceptives', and 'packets of condoms flew through the air. As did packets of aspirin. And containers of spermicidal jelly. They landed beyond the barrier. The noise from there grew, and it sounded like a victory'.[44] The crowd then marched to Store Street Garda Station where they stood outside waving contraceptives and chanting, 'The law is obsolete'. No arrests were made.

Nell McCafferty read a statement to the crowd which outlined the views of the IWLM and the reasons for their protest. She explained that through their actions on the Contraceptive Train, the IWLM had enforced the Constitution and challenged the criminal law.[45] She further declared that the CLAA of 1935 which made the sale of contraception a criminal offence was 'repugnant to the Constitution and to the rights of man and woman, as guaranteed by the U.N. Declaration of Family Planning, which was signed by Ireland as a member nation'. Boldly, the IWLM accused the State of 'political timidity' in refusing to discuss or debate the matter in parliament and for being 'manipulated by forces outside of the electorate'. The Irish government was also accused of 'criminal irresponsibility' in permitting 26,000 women to use only the contraceptive pill because that was the only contraceptive available to them, despite the fact that the pill was in many cases 'medically unsuited and damaging to the woman who might otherwise, in all conscience, choose other methods at present illegal'.[46]

Moreover, the significant publicity that the Contraceptive Train raised meant that it stood out in the memories of individuals who were young men and women at the time. Many oral history respondents mentioned it in their interviews. Mark (b.1952) recalled: 'There was a train that came down from Belfast at some stage and a bunch of liberal women from the liberal women's movement back in the early 70s, people like Nell McCafferty, and people like that. Journalists, Mary Kenny and people

[41] 'Women's Lib. in station scenes', *Sunday Independent*, 23 May 1971, p. 1.
[42] 'Women's Lib. in station scenes', p. 1.   [43] 'Victory for women's Lib.!', p. 4.
[44] McCafferty, *Nell*, p. 225.   [45] 'Victory for women's Lib.!', p. 4.
[46] 'Women's Lib defy law on contraceptives', *Evening Herald*, 22 May 1971, p. 1.

like that. They came down distributing contraception, contraceptives all around Dublin at the train station. I think they were all arrested and charged'. Evelyn (b.1940) stated, 'I think people thought it was great. It was a gas thing to do type of thing'. Some oral history respondents also misremembered Mary Robinson being on the train, likely because she was campaigning to have a bill passed on the issue around the same time. For example, Brigid (b.1945) referred to the contraceptive train as 'that famous train journey up to the north, Nell McCafferty and all of those people. Mary Robinson, and I can't remember who else was there'.

Others were less positive about the stunt. Nuala Fennell, one of the IWLM founder members, believed that the Contraceptive Train had been too sensationalist and she resigned soon after. Winnie (b.1938) recalled, 'I remember reading about these two women, Mary Kenny and the other woman from Derry. Uh, you wouldn't pay much heed to it now. But we just thought they were...Weird. You know? Women's libbers and makin' a fuss'. She added, 'I don't know what the whole thing was about. Just a bit of publicity'. Some citizens wrote to the Taoiseach to express their outrage. 'Three elderly Irish-born Sisters of Mercy who love Ireland dearly' wrote to Jack Lynch in May 1971 in relation to the Contraceptive Train 'to assure your government of the fact that thousands and thousands of Irish exiles throughout the world are praying every day that Ireland will be spared the unspeakable tragedy of contraception and abortion'.[47]

On the evening of the Contraceptive Train, Mary Kenny and Colette O'Neill appeared on The Late Late Show. The Late Late Show appearance clearly helped to further publicise the stunt. Mary Kenny held up some of the condoms bought in Belfast and showed them to the TV camera in order to make the point that 'the law had been successfully challenged, and no one arrested'.[48] The government, in particular, George Colley, who was then Minister for Finance, claimed that the contraceptives had been seized by customs officials on the day. However, in a reply published in the Irish Times, the IWLM claimed that contraceptives were still in the possession of its members and that their names were available to the Minister, writing: 'We have broken the law. We will continue to break the law'.[49] In Mary Kenny's view, the Contraceptive Train had been a successful stunt 'because it did help to lead, eventually, to an outdated law being rescinded, through the proper

---

[47] Letter from Sister M. Fidelis, Convent of Mercy, Greymouth, New Zealand, 31 May 1971. [NAI, 2002/8/459].

[48] Kenny, Something of Myself and Others, p. 155.

[49] 'Reply to Colley by Women's Liberation', Irish Times, 3 June 1971, p. 13.

legislative challenges'.[50] Although the IWLM disbanded soon after, their contraception campaign had an important influence on feminist groups which followed them.

7.2   Irishwomen United

Following the disbandment of the IWLM in 1971, a new group calling themselves the Women's Liberation Movement, Ireland, emerged, which lasted for about two years. The Women's Liberation Movement, also called the Fownes Street Group, put forward a non-violent approach to activism, including methods such as boycotting, picketing, strikes, fasts, and civil disobedience, arguing that non-violence was 'the only method possible for women who hope to create a new society'.[51] The group published a monthly publication called the *Fownes Street Journal*. The Women's Liberation Movement held workshops on the theme of contraception monthly, with the first of these beginning in May 1972. These workshops included an educational talk on family planning and contraceptive methods as well as informal discussion, with meetings being open to anyone who wished to attend.[52] However, it was not until the formation of Irishwomen United (IWU) in 1975 that there was 'a women's liberation group of any comparable scale to the IWLM'.[53]

Although they used similar tactics to the IWLM, such as direct action and consciousness raising, IWU was arguably more politicised.[54] Looking back on the period of IWU's existence, former members of the group recalled the sense of optimism they felt in contrast with the disenchantment of the period from 1983 to 1990 which was characterised by 'severe repression, socially and economically'.[55] As Betty Purcell (IWU/CAP) explained:

I remember the atmosphere of it very strongly, in that it was a very optimistic time and it was a very brave time. There was a lot of, 'We're going to do this'. You know? 'There might be only 40 of us in the room but we'll change that, let's just take that and change it'. There was a great can–do thing.

IWU had been founded in 1975 by activists who had been involved in socialist and radical politics, encompassing 'a diverse grouping of left-

---

[50] Kenny, *Something of Myself and Others*, pp. 155–6.
[51] 'Women and nonviolence', *Fownes Street Journal*, Vol.1, No. 2, June 1972, no page number.
[52] 'Women's Liberation Contraception Advisory Service', *Fownes Street Journal*, 1:1, (May 1972), no page number.
[53] Connolly, *The Irish Women's Movement*, p. 129.
[54] Connolly, *The Irish Women's Movement*, pp. 130–1.   [55] *Ibid.*

wing philosophies'.[56] This differentiated them from the IWLM and interviewees viewed IWU as being more radical and interested in theoretical socialist approaches. According to Ger Moane (IWU):

They [IWU] came from political backgrounds like republicanism, trade union movement, civil rights. Whereas, IWLM were more from paternalistic ... Women's rights without political analysis of patriarchy and systems, and wouldn't touch capitalism. You know? That system thing, it makes you more radical.

Anne Speed (IWU/CAP) acknowledged the importance of the introduction of free secondary school education in 1967 for this generation of activists. The 1960s was a period of significance and opportunity for many young people and, as Carole Holohan has shown, 'those with a secondary school or third-level education, benefited from a more diverse employment market often in Irish cities'.[57] For Speed, the civil rights movement and the American women's movement also had an important influence:

The women who came to Irishwomen United came from the left and feminism, and we were all kind of, inspired by the Vietnam war, by the resistance to the Vietnam war. By the rise of the civil rights movement in the north. By the rise of the women's movement internationally, in the US in particular. A lot of young feminists who came through free education, which had been developed in the late 60s, 1967 I think it was introduced. So they got a chance to go to university, to reach beyond what might have been expected. These would have been women say of skilled working-class families or lower middle-class. But by the time they came out of university, they realised that the kind of Ireland they were entering to wasn't giving them any opportunity really. There wasn't equal pay and women were still very much discriminated against. They were radicalised by that.

Moreover, interviewees emphasised that their youth and experiences differentiated them from earlier women's groups. In 1970 the Irish government established the Commission for the Status of Women to report on the injustices facing Irish women. As Chrystel Hug as argued, however, 'there is little doubt that it viewed it with ambivalence and paternalism'.[58] The commission was viewed with scepticism by some IWU members. Taragh O'Kelly (IWU/CAP), for instance, explained:

I knew we had a battle on our hands, I knew that it was up to young women. I felt like there was a great divide between the likes of the Irish ... Most were professional university educated, doctors, whatever, or married to quite well to do men. They really had no ... conception of what reality was, for the majority of

---

[56] *Ibid.*, p. 131.   [57] *Ibid.*, p. 97.
[58] Hug, *The Politics of Sexual Morality in Ireland*, p. 89.

women. The majority of young working–class women, who left school at 16 or 17, went to work in factories and got married and had far too many children.

Following their first public conference, in Dublin in June 1975, the IWU group agreed on a charter of demands and began to mobilise. Surviving minutes from meetings in 1975 show that attendance varied from nine-teen women at a meeting in August 1975 to thirty seven at a meeting in October of the same year.[59] The IWU charter demanded the removal of all legal and bureaucratic obstacles to equality, the right to divorce, free, legal contraception, the provision of twenty-four-hour nurseries, free of charge, as well as equal pay for equal work, and equality in education.[60] Like feminist groups around the world, IWU activities included weekly meetings (in Dublin), joint action through pickets, public meetings, workshops (on issues such as women in trade unions, contraception, social welfare and political theory), and consciousness-raising groups.[61] IWU also produced their own magazine called *Banshee*, which had a rotating editorial board. Contraception was a 'pivotal mobilising issue' for IWU from its foundation.[62] Members wanted free legal contraception to be provided through state-financed birth control clinics, as well as sex education programmes and the right to publish literature on sex education.[63]

IWU differed from IWLM, in that lesbian women represented a signifi-cant voice in the former group and issues around lesbian sexuality were discussed. Although IWU used similar tactics to the IWLM, such as direct action and consciousness raising, it was arguably more politicised.[64] During its eighteen-month existence, IWU engaged in regular protests such as at traditionally male-only spaces including the Fitzwilliam Lawn Tennis Club and the 'men only' Forty Foot bathing area in Sandycove, Dublin. In October 1975, almost one hundred members and supporters of IWU held an hour-long, torch-lit picket outside the house of the Catholic Archbishop of Dublin in Drumcondra, demanding that there should be an immediate change in the laws relating to contraception in Ireland. The group chanted, 'Not the Church, not the State, women must decide their fate' and 'We demand the right to choose', while marching outside the main gates to the grounds and holding placards. In a statement

---

[59] Minutes of a meeting of IWU, 2 August 1975 [RCAPA, BL/F/AP/1175/1]; minutes of a meeting of IWU, 12 October 1975 [RCAPA, BL/F/AP/1175/15].

[60] IWU 'Women's Charter' [RCAPA, BL/F/AP/1111/1].

[61] 'Editorial' in *Banshee: Journal of Irishwomen United*, 1:1 (1976?), p. 2.

[62] Connolly, The Irish Women's Movement, p. 131.

[63] 'Contraception: the slot machine government' in *Banshee: Journal of Irishwomen United*, 1:1 (1976?), p. 5.

[64] Connolly, *The Irish Women's Movement*, pp 130–1.

released by IWU following the picket, they argued 'Historically the interference by the Catholic Church in the legislative affairs of this State has been effective in blocking social and political change'.[65] The cheery atmosphere of the picket is immortalised in IWU member Evelyn Conlon's short story, 'The Last Confession' where a man recalls the atmosphere at the protest when he arrived to collect his sister, an IWU member:

When I arrived more snow had fallen, it vainly tried to look white. It was so cold I could have cried. But the women were cheerful; they were up against such odds they laughed a lot.[66]

Betty Purcell (IWU/CAP) recalled of the demonstration:

That was great, very exciting. Great shouting, great slogans, big megaphones and, of course, the gates and the walls of the Archbishop's palace are so daunting ... An awful lot of it was in the best of spirits and good fun. To be honest, we kind of didn't really think about getting arrested. For those ones where we were out of doors, the guards never moved to arrest us.

Regular public meetings were held, including a meeting on 'Women in Trade Unions' in September 1975, and a contraception rally held in Liberty Hall in November 1975. In January 1976, IWU picketed and occupied the offices of the Federation Union of Employers and, in April, members protested at Irish government buildings over the contraception debate.[67] IWU members also challenged politicians who were publicly anti-contraception.[68] The group attracted media attention and their activities were regularly reported in Irish newspapers, however, interviewees reflected on their lack of experience. Considering the IWU charter of demands, Anne Speed (IWU/CAP) recalled:

It was so ultimatistic [sic] in its aspirations and sure why not? We were young, we wanted to change the world. We didn't really have any sense or experience of how to build a broad front and you know, finding points of contact with groups of women that you wouldn't have that much politically in common with. But anyway, we took this charter and we started to organise a number of meetings.

---

[65] 'Archbishop's house picket by women', *Irish Press*, 30 October 1975, p. 2.
[66] Evelyn Conlon, "The Last Confession", in: *Telling: new and selected stories*, (Blackstaff Press, 2000), pp. 202–211, on p. 207.
[67] 'Activities of Irishwomen United – May 1975–May 1976' in *Banshee: Journal of Irishwomen United*, 1:3, (1976), no page number.
[68] Mary McAuliffe, '"To change society": Irishwomen United and political activism, 1975-1979' in Mary McAuliffe and Clara Fischer (eds.). *Irish Feminisms; Past, Present and Future* (Dublin: Arlen House, 2014), p. 97.

However, in Joanne O'Brien's (IWU/CAP) words, 'despite the fact that we didn't necessarily handle the media in a sort of professional way, if you like, we kept them guessing. They didn't know what we were going to do next. We were a perennial source of fascination'.

While IWU also addressed a number of important women's issues in their campaigns and charter, the contraception issue represented, in the group's words, their 'most sustained public campaign', and positioned them in opposition to the Catholic Church, the government, employers and political parties.[69] IWU believed that their perspective was different from other groups campaigning for change because their demands were 'based on the fundamental right of all women to control their bodies'. The link between contraception and economic independence was stressed, while the group also argued for women's right to a self-determined sexuality.[70] According to O'Brien (IWU/CAP): 'We were challenging the idea of the downtrodden woman with children hanging out of her and so on, that there was some inevitability about that, we challenged that completely'. Feminist campaigners compared the plight of Irish women in relation to birth control with the rights of women in other EEC member states. In 1974, Betty Purcell, IWU member and founder of the Women's Group at UCD, wrote 'The fact that Ireland is one of the last European countries to keep contraception illegal has a lot of significance for Irishwomen today. Without the fundamental right of a woman to control her own fertility being recognised, all other rights give only a sham equality.'[71]

At an IWU Contraception Workshop in 1975, participants agreed that if women were given control of their bodies through access to contraception, it would be possible for them to gain more freedom in relation to employment opportunities.[72] In August 1975, a panel was established by IWU to devise a strategy for their contraception campaign. This initial panel consisted of five volunteers: Anne Speed, who would go on to be a key figure in the CAP campaign, Karen Snider, Patricia Kelleher, Patricia Cobey and Pat Farrell.[73] Over the following months, this group of women, which occasionally included others, met to discuss the campaign. The

---

69 'Irishwomen United and birth control', undated statement [RCAPA, BL/F/AP/1177/13].
70 'Irishwomen United Contraception Workshop', 9–10 May 1975 [RCAPA, BL/F/AP/1177/24].
71 Betty Purcell, 'Contraception – a woman's right to choose' in Bread and Roses (c.1974) [RCAPA, BL/F/AP/1517/3].
72 'Irishwomen United Contraception Workshop', 9–10 May 1975 [RCAPA, BL/F/AP/1177/24].
73 Minutes of a meeting of Irishwomen United, 2 August 1975 [RCAPA, BL/F/AP/1197/42].

class issue was vital to the IWU contraception campaign from the beginning. At a panel meeting in September 1975 to devise a leaflet outlining their aims, they agreed that it ought to 'specifically focus on the fact that the advertising of contraceptives is not permitted and that therefore the availability of contraceptives is confined to specific classes and geographical areas'.[74] The IWU campaign focused on reaching women from working-class backgrounds. In October, a leafleting campaign was devised which specifically targeted more disadvantaged, working-class areas in Dublin, such as Crumlin, Ballymun and Tallaght.[75]

IWU was also a source of knowledge about contraception for women. Meetings provided members with practical information about contraceptive options and advice on sympathetic doctors who would prescribe the pill as a cycle regulator. According to Joanne O'Brien (IWU/CAP), 'Information was exchanged as to who were friendly doctors because I think you could get the pill on prescription supposedly to regulate your periods'. Taragh O'Kelly (IWU/CAP) remarked that in Dublin 'you just went to a Jewish doctor and he/she gave you a prescription with no questions asked and you went to a Jewish chemist or Protestant chemist, no questions asked'. Women who were anxious to obtain contraception also attended meetings. According to Betty Purcell (IWU/CAP):

I remember myself counselling women who would come along to our meetings and were talking about things like their doctor had said, 'If you have another pregnancy, you'll die'. This was what was driving them to come to our meetings. You had women in those kind of situations saying, 'I've just got to get my hands on contraceptives'. They were the real cases in point, if you like, that ... then there were other women who wanted to have careers and wanted to establish their families in an ordered way.

In this way, IWU became a women's network for information about contraception.[76] IWU also stressed the problems created by the increased medicalisation of women's bodies, in a similar manner to members of the American feminist movement in the early 1970s.[77] This was in contrast to Spain, where as Agata Ignaciuk and Teresa

---

[74] Minutes of the meeting of the panel for the 'Contraception Campaign', 2 September 1975 [RCAPA,BL/F/AP/1177/16].

[75] Minutes of a meeting of the 'Contraception Group', 7 October 1975 [RCAPA,BL/F/AP/1177/20].

[76] Leanne McCormick has similarly shown, for an earlier period in Belfast, how women's networks were integral to the dissemination of information around abortion, particularly in Protestant neighbourhoods (McCormick, 'No sense of wrongdoing', pp. 125–48).

[77] See Watkins, On the Pill, p.3. See also: Wendy Kline, Bodies of Knowledge: Sexuality, Reproduction, and Women's Health in the Second Wave (University of Chicago Press, 2010).

Ortiz Gómez have shown 'family planning activism was initiated in medical circles during the late 1960s before it exploded in the following decade thanks to the commitment of radical women's organizations and their cooperation with liberal medical professionals', with similar patterns in France and Italy.[78]

In 1976, IWU stated: 'We demand the BEST and SAFEST forms of contraceptives FREE. Women are not guinea-pigs. We don't want to have to put up with expensive contraceptives that either don't work or make us feel ill or depressed.'[79] Similar statements were also circulated within the American and British women's movements. In the United States, in the late 1960s and early 1970s, the perceived over-prescription of the contraceptive pill was critiqued by feminist activists who believed that women's reproductive healthcare had become over-medicalised and were concerned with the side effects.[80] With the publication of Barbara Seaman's *The Doctor's Case Against the Pill* (1969), American feminist activists were inspired to 'vocalise the shared perception that the medical profession was "condescending, paternalistic, judgemental and non-informative"'.[81] Similarly, in the British context, feminist campaigners also protested against the medical profession's control of women's access to reproductive health services, highlighting concerns about a lack of attention to the alleged side effects of contraceptive drugs.[82] However, for many middle-class Irish women, because of the ban on contraceptives, the pill was the only contraceptive option available to them on prescription in the late 1960s and 1970s. According to Roisin Boyd, writing in Irish feminist magazine *Wicca* in 1977:

Because of this lack [of information on contraceptive choices], many women are using the Pill when it is unsuitable for them. Also the unavailability of contraception in country areas, means that women are dependent on sympathetic doctors or chemists. The situation at the moment is intolerable. There is an attitude prevalent among many doctors that you're lucky to be getting any contraception at all and they are reluctant to advise women on which is the best available method.[83]

As discussed in Chapter 4 the pill was heavily prescribed in Ireland during the 1960s and 1970s as it was the only contraceptive available

---

[78] Teresa Ortiz-Gómez, Agata Ignaciuk, 'The Fight for Family Planning in Spain during Late Francoism and the Transition to Democracy, 1965–1979', *Journal of Women's History*, 30:2, (Summer 2018), pp. 38–62, on p. 39.
[79] Statement by Irishwomen United, undated [RCAPA, BL/F/AP/1177/23].
[80] Watkins, *On the Pill*, p. 119.   [81] *Ibid.*, p.104.
[82] Jennifer Dale and Peggy Foster, *Feminists and State Welfare* (London, 2012), pp. 88–9.
[83] Roisin Boyd, 'Contraception: who to believe' in *Wicca* (1977), p. 10 [RCAPA, BL/F/AP/1498/3].

legally on prescription, albeit prescribed through 'coded language', as stated in an oral history interview with Ruth Riddick, an Irish feminist activist and founder of Open Door Counselling, an unplanned pregnancy counselling service. However, IWU members demanded that a greater variety of contraceptive methods should be made available to Irish women. Ruth Torode (IWU/CAP) explained:

I think it was assumed that the pill was the easiest for women to use though there were women who had difficulty with it. I think the demands around contraceptives were for choice and information and care. To make sure that you were monitored. I think that was an important thing. I think this whole thing about taking care of your body and that people aren't identical.

While IWU members were certainly influenced by the American feminist movement in particular, they believed that their approach was shaped by the particularities of the Irish context. Uniquely, the Irish campaign around contraception focused strongly on class and geographical inequalities, whereas for British and American birth control activists the issues of race and the maintenance of the right to contraception and abortion access were paramount.[84] Barbara Murray (IWU/CAP) explained: 'you know we were too busy trying to get things going and then there was the Troubles in the north and there was all this kind of ... you know ... But, we did feel we were part of an international women's movement but we weren't spending our time in contact with women elsewhere. We were busy doing stuff at home'. Respondents distinguished the Irish approach as being more practical than that of American feminists. Taragh O'Kelly (IWU/CAP) explained that American feminists 'were on a completely different plane. [They were engaged in] consciousness-raising and ... We were saying "We're trying to get contraception legalised". There was sort of, shall we say, an academic esoteric view and then a down to earth view of what is feminism'. While Anne Speed (IWU/CAP) recalled being inspired by the scholarship of Sheila Rowbotham and the American socialist writer Mary-Alice Waters, she felt that: 'a lot of our activity, we designed it ourselves, do you know what I mean? It was our own determination to keep momentum and it was our own anger and our own ... Yeah, our determination and our anger that kept us going'.

---

[84] In the words of Dorothy Roberts, 'reproductive politics in America inevitably involves racial politics. Dorothy Roberts, *Killing the Black Body: Race, Reproduction and the Meaning of Liberty* (London, 1998), p. 9).

7.3   The Contraception Action Programme

The Contraception Action Programme (CAP), established in spring 1976 to campaign specifically for the legalisation of contraception, emerged from the IWU Contraception Workshop. The organisation also included members from other interested groups. For instance, at a meeting of CAP at Buswell's Hotel, Dublin, in June 1976, attendees included members of Women's Aid, the IFPA, North Dublin Social Workers, Irish Women's Liberation Movement, Women's Progressive/Political Association, FPS, the Labour Women's National Council and IWU, all of whom were women, with the exception of Robin Cochran, representative of FPS.[85] However, the driving force behind the campaign were predominantly members of IWU. According to Anne Speed, a key figure in CAP, the group mainly consisted of 'about five or six of us really, holding the fort. Now there'd be momentum at certain times. You'd have a public event and then you might have twenty people coming to a meeting and then you know, a year later it might be back down to five'. At the June meeting, it appears that there was disagreement over the whether the campaign should demand free contraception. Women's Aid argued that that this demand would 'be seen by the general public as a demand for 'sex on the rates', while FPS contended that the demand for free contraception 'would be too great a leap to make at present'.[86] IWU argued strongly in favour of the demand for free contraception. The meeting ended with a resolution that the campaign would request contraception to be made available free of charge at health services and at a minimum cost through pharmacies and voluntary family planning services.[87] However, with the benefit of hindsight, Anne Speed (IWU/CAP) reflected that perhaps a different approach might have been more successful:

Now retrospectively, I'm thinking, would today, would you take the same view [regarding free contraception]? Maybe not. Because we might have actually affected reform quicker if we had understood how to fight for reform and how to build a broad front based on one or two key demands ... Maybe look for the legalisation of contraception, thereafter talking about how it would be available and how poor women would get access to it? In other words, you know. But we threw everything into that goal that we had.

CAP members were predominantly female, yet Anne Speed believed it was the age of IWU members in CAP that distinguished them from other

---

[85] Minutes of a CAP meeting, 22 June 1976 [RCAPA, BL/F/AP/1177/21].   [86] *Ibid.*.
[87] *Ibid.*

activist groups: 'We were 18, 19, 20. But like from the age of 18 … I and the oldest servers [in CAP] might have been 26, 27. You know what I mean, we were young. That really was very significant'. In comparison, an older and in some cases, arguably more conservative individuals were involved in organisations such as the IFPA. Oral history respondents expressed the sense of determination they felt through involvement in the CAP campaign. According to Taragh O'Kelly (IWU/CAP), "I think anybody that was on the ground in those days recognised that this was an issue and it was an issue we had to take by the horns and we had to win'. Betty Purcell (IWU/CAP) remarked similarly that 'The campaign was to absolutely embarrass the politicians and put the focus on making contraception an unstoppable force'.

CAP members also emphasised the health concerns relating to contraception, evidently drawing on fears raised by American feminists. Alicia Carrigy, CAP secretary in 1977, explained: 'We believe that people should have available adequate information on all methods of contraception, so that they may make an informed decision as to how best they can plan their families'. Carrigy drew attention to the fact that the contraceptive pill was the most widely used method of contraception in Ireland and that it 'appears to have inherent risks, especially to women over the age of 35'.[88] CAP activists were particularly motivated by the difficulties which faced working-class women who wanted to access contraception, another feature of the Irish movement which differentiated them from their British and American counterparts. Members of CAP were aware of the fact that many Irish people did not have access to contraception, in spite of the existence of several family planning clinics in Dublin by the late 1970s. Anne Speed linked the emphasis on class and the more militant approach of CAP to the youth of the group's membership:

I mean it was very evident that the people who went to the clinics were either women who had started to enter the workforce and were beginning to try and plan their life and control their fertility and as you say, women with money and confidence even to make, to go to these clinics. So that was a big part of the reason why we felt that we had to take a more militant and radical approach, because we could see that as young feminists.

Moreover, there were limited ways of accessing contraception in more rural areas. According to members of the Labour Party's Women's Council, writing to the *Irish Times*, CAP addressed an important gap. The family planning clinics in existence only provided 'for the population of the larger urban areas' and 'its clinics are frequented mainly by the

---

[88] *Irish Independent*, 13 October 1977, p. 14.

more affluent, giving little help to those less well off or to those living in rural areas'.[89] Labour councillor, Mary Freehill (CAP), remarked on the difficulties working-class women had in accessing family planning services:

Certainly getting to family planning clinics was not something that somebody from Ballyfermot would quite easily come into town, and it was a brave thing for women in less well off areas. There was quite a divide. That was a big part of what we were trying to do ... That's why we were out in places like Ballyfermot ... They [working-class women] were listening to the priests more seriously than middle-class women who had been in a position to have their own kind of ideas.

Similarly, Barbara Murray (IWU/CAP) remembered the problems that women in rural areas had in accessing contraception:

You would go down to the Irish Family Planning Services, you could. But, you see the trouble really was for people in country areas because nobody knew ... I just lived up the road so you could do what you wanted really. But, it was really the women in rural areas or in certain parts of Dublin. Where were they going and what were they doing, that kind of thing and they might not have known where to go so ... That was a concern as well. It was women in Dublin had a way ... but although some parts of Dublin, how could women get away to get access because they're minding their children at home and why did they want to go off on their own to somewhere? You know, that kind-of thing.

In 1978, a CAP statement argued that while a limited contraceptive service was available to middle-class Irish women through family planning clinics run by the IFPA and FPS, 'the large numbers of women who most need access and advice are just not getting it. O.K., so we here can ... understand how our bodies function, of what can go wrong. But what about other women? What about sisterhood and solidarity now? And it isn't a question of being charitable do-gooders. While one of us is oppressed – we are all oppressed.'[90] CAP also stressed the absence of women's voices in debates over contraception. CAP members regarded the Catholic Church and the 'capitalist state' as being a 'double barrier' in the campaign for the right to control one's own fertility. In their view, 'The Church has a very strong influence on people – firstly through organised religion, and secondly through the capitalist state which believes in the family unit but does little to help, and has little regard for women because it is so male dominated and petit bourgeois.'[91]

---

[89] *Irish Times*, 30 October 1976,
[90] CAP statement, undated, but probably February or March 1978 [RCAPA, BL/F/AP/ 1294/15].
[91] 'The Contraception Issue in Ireland', statement by CAP, undated [RCAPA, BL/F/AP/ 1177/3].

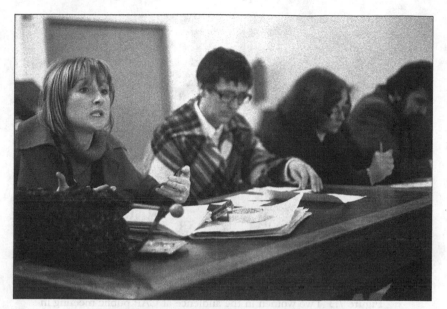

Figure 7.2 Anne Speed speaking at a Contraception Action Programme (CAP) public meeting in Ballyfermot, Dublin on 21 March 1978.
Photograph by Derek Speirs.

More specifically, CAP members believed that women's voices had been missing from discussions over legislation. Leading up to the drafting of the Family Planning Bill in 1978, Minister for Health Charles Haughey had met with groups such as the IFPA, the Irish Medical Association, Irish Nurses Organisation, representatives of health boards, church hierarchies and Catholic interest groups to discuss their views.[92] This was condemned by IWU, who complained that Haughey was 'busy asking BISHOPS, Medics and other Male bodies their opinions on contraception' rather than women.[93]

In order to remedy this, a meeting was organised by CAP at Ballyfermot Community Centre in March 1978 in order to 'give women a chance to make their voices heard'[94] (Figures 7.2 and 7.3). The Ballinteer branch of CAP also organised a survey among 540 predominantly female respondents in 1977. The survey highlighted the demand for family planning services in the area and received significant coverage in

[92] Girvin, 'An Irish solution', pp. 16–18.
[93] 'Legalise contraception now' in *Wicca* (1977 or 1978, undated), pp. 15–16.
[94] *Irish Independent*, 21 March 1978, p. 6.

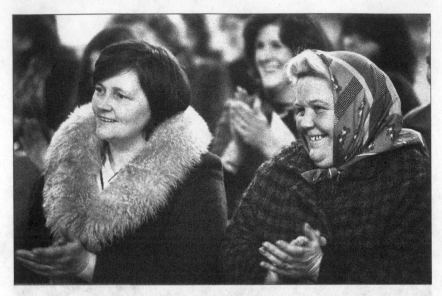

Figure 7.3 Two women in the audience at CAP public meeting in Ballyfermot, Dublin on 21 March 1978.
Photograph by Derek Speirs.

the Irish press.[95] Signature campaigns were also utilised by the group. CAP members remarked in *Wicca* magazine that in the course of collecting signatures for a national campaign, they were 'saddened and shocked at the appalling ignorance because of lack of access in information and education and unavailability of Family Planning'.[96]

Direct action also took the form of contraception provision. Evelyn Conlon (IWU/CAP) recalled that she and other CAP members sold condoms at the Dandelion Market at the top of Grafton Street, Dublin at the beginning of the CAP campaign. However, Conlon explained that members soon came to an awareness that 'we couldn't just be doing it on Grafton Street in the really hip sort of Dandelion Market area ... that we had to go into the suburbs as well and working-class places'. CAP literature also emphasised this point. CAP therefore employed radical strategies such as distributing contraceptives in housing estates.[97] Ballymun became a focus of CAP activism and a caravan was utilised to sell condoms and distribute leaflets, while information on 'sympathetic doctors' was also

[95] *Sunday Independent*, 13 November 1977, p. 4.
[96] 'Legalise contraception now' in *Wicca* (1977?), pp. 15–16.
[97] Connolly, *The Irish Women's Movement*, p. 144.

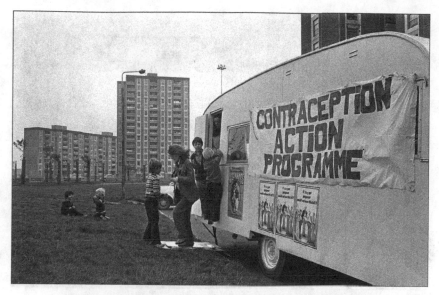

Figure 7.4 CAP caravan, Ballymun, Dublin, 13 October 1979.
Photograph by Derek Speirs.

provided (Figures 7.4 and 7.5). Betty Purcell (IWU/CAP) recalled that the caravan had the aim of providing 'service provision but also highlighting the issue and embarrassing the local politicians'. Historically, caravans have been utilised by birth control activists and had both practical and symbolic functions. In 1928, the British birth control campaigner Marie Stopes purchased two horse-drawn caravans which she used to provide information to communities in England and Wales without access to birth control clinics between 1928 and 1930.[98] Caravans were also utilised by the Vancouver Women's Caucus in 1970.[99] However, for CAP activists, the caravan was chosen for different reasons. In Ballymun, a working-class area of Dublin, where purpose-built flats had been erected in the 1960s, there were few local premises where the group could have set up a shop. According to Anne Speed (IWU/CAP):

[98] Fisher, p.29.
[99] The caucus travelled from Vancouver to Ottawa in a caravan which bore a coffin filled with coat hangers to represent the deaths of women from botched abortions, in order to protest against the restrictive nature of Canadian abortion law. Christabelle Sethna and Steve Hewitt, 'Clandestine operations: The Vancouver Women's Caucus, the abortion caravan, and the RCMP', *The Canadian Historical Review*, 90:3, (September 2009), pp. 463–95.

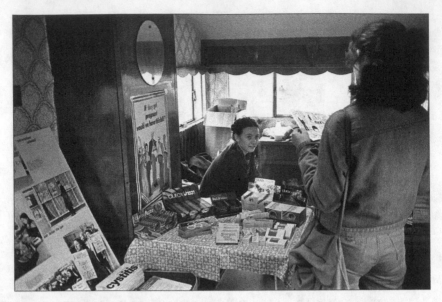

Figure 7.5 Interior of CAP caravan, Ballymun, Dublin, 13 October 1979. The woman facing the camera is Jacinta Deignan.
Photograph by Derek Speirs.

There were no shops. So we wouldn't have been able to hire any premises anyway … So that's why we thought the caravan would work. And we wouldn't be accountable or answerable to any landlord who might decide they didn't like what we were doing. But what we were doing was really publicly disseminating information. Where we were asked for specific help, we offered that help.

CAP activities brought some women into direct conflict with members of the Catholic Church, particularly during their work in disadvantaged areas. All CAP interviewees recalled receiving abuse from Father Michael Cleary, a well-known Dublin priest with a strong media presence.[100] Betty Purcell (IWU/CAP) recalled: 'I remember, actually, at one stage, going to a flat in Ballymun and knocking on the door and the person who opened it was Father Michael Cleary. He was living in the community and he was so abusive. I was very young; I was only sixteen or seventeen. I had an uncle who was a priest and I always thought a priest is a very respectable, decent person and he came out and he was just, "Fuck you".' Similarly, Taragh O'Kelly (IWU/CAP) recalled:

---

[100] Fuller, *Irish Catholicism*, p. 252.

Mary and I were out in Ballyfermot out doing the petitions one day and the local priest who is that Father Michael Cleary, came up and he basically threatened us. 'Are you doing this here?' and we said, 'How are you Father, would you like to sign?' and it was sort of, 'Get the F out of my area'. He pretty much said if we didn't F off out of his patch, there were fellas around here who wouldn't like their wives getting involved in that stuff.

In 1995, it emerged that Cleary and his housekeeper, Phyllis Hamilton, had been living as man and wife and that he had fathered two children, one of whom was given up for adoption. This, along with other scandals such as that of Bishop Eamonn Casey in 1992, were disastrous for the Catholic Church which 'needed all the moral authority that it could muster to influence Irish Catholics' in the particularly fraught period of the 1990s.[101] Given the hypocrisy of Cleary's moral outrage concerning CAP's campaigns in Dublin, the memories of their activists' interactions with him were vividly recalled.

Anti-contraception campaigners were also active in writing to the press to complain about IWU and CAP activities. Mary Kennedy, a member of Irish conservative group, the Irish Family League, remarked in a letter to the *Irish Times* in 1976: 'Just as at the beginning of Time Eve was used to bring about the downfall of Adam, so today the feminists are being used knowingly or otherwise to bring about their own degradation and the destruction of the family'.[102] In a letter to the *Sligo Champion* in 1976 (which also appeared in several other newspapers), Bridget Bermingham, secretary of Catholic group Parent Concern, outlined some of the group's anxieties about CAP. She pointed out that the legalisation and unrestricted availability of contraception would 'introduce counter and supermarket sales, purchases from slot machines, mail orders by school-children etc., making it impossible to restrict inquisitive teenagers from the advertising of devices, techniques, pornographic and debasing sex books, some of which are already on sale, despite numerous protests'. The 'sex casualties' that had occurred in England, as well as statistics relating to numbers of teenagers on the pill, having abortions, and suffering from sexually transmitted diseases, were also referred to.[103]

As well as actively writing to newspapers, campaigners against the legalisation of contraception would sometimes disrupt CAP meetings. Betty Purcell (IWU/CAP) recalled:

Where we were, they turned up. They would just be often quite angry, and not violent but certainly with the intention of breaking up meetings and that sort of thing, and shouting people down and that kind of thing. It was quite hostile

---

[101] *Ibid.*.   [102] *Irish Times*, 24 December 1976, p. 9.
[103] *Sligo Champion*, 10 December 1976, p. 14.

and disrespectful, definitely, and quite intimidating to younger women who were involved.

In spite of the potential for disruption, CAP members agreed that public meetings were an important means of disseminating information and generating discussion on the contraception issue. Their first major event was a public rally, held at the Mansion House in Dublin in November 1976, with speakers including Dr Patrick J. Crowley, chairman of the Health Committee of the South Eastern Health Board, Limerick councillor Jim Kemmy and Dr. James Loughran, one of the founders of the IFPA.[104] According to one report, the speeches at the rally were 'drowned by the shouts and jeers of about 20 hecklers'.[105] Another CAP meeting of over 300 people in Dublin in 1977 was disrupted by a group of six protesters led by Mena Bean Ui Chriblin, a postmistress and Catholic conservative campaigner.[106] These incidents highlight not only how divisive the issue of contraception was but also the generational divide between the CAP activists and those who were campaigning against their activities.

The efforts of CAP intensified following the publication of minister for health Charles Haughey's Health (Family Planning) Bill in 1978.[107] At a public meeting at TCD to discuss the bill in January 1978, CAP members argued that it would transfer power from family planning clinics to doctors and make contraception expensive. It would also put an end to mail order services for contraceptives, thereby further restricting access, especially for men and women who lived in rural areas.[108] The increase in power being given to doctors with regard to contraception was also a focus of concern. CAP stated in December 1978 that they 'totally rejected the suggestion that doctors should have the right to decide on "bona fide" family planning cases. The medical profession has only the responsibility to make all medical information available so that the patients may then make their decision.'[109] Furthermore, they argued that:

instead of expanding the limited voluntary service, he [Haughey] intends to hand over to a male dominated elitist profession, which obscures and mystifies women's sexuality, our right to choose. What is "bona fide" anyway and don't you already know that many male doctors and female doctors (it is a male defined profession) haven't got much of an understanding of women anyway. The right to know about our bodies will be strictly controlled, there will be little or no research into contraception and we do want to know about safety.[110]

---

104 *Irish Times*, 29 November 1976, p. 11.   105 *Irish Times*, 1 December 1976, p. 9.
106 'Protestors ejected from meeting on contraception', *Irish Times*, 18 October 1978, p. 5.
107 Ferriter, *Occasions of Sin*, p. 423.
108 CAP public meeting statement, T.C.D., 29 January 1978 [RCAPA, BL/F/AP/1139/9].
109 *Irish Times*, 16 December 1978, p. 6.
110 CAP statement, undated, but probably February or March 1978 [RCAPA, BL/F/AP/1294/15].

Some critics feared that not all chemists would necessarily comply with the legislation. According to Sally Keogh, IFPA information officer and CAP member, 'You could have a whole group of chemists in one town deciding yes they would stock them [contraceptives] or, no, they wouldn't, because some customers might decide to boycott a chemist shop because of their practice regarding contraceptive sales. We have not had a precedent like this before.'[111] A poster produced by CAP (Figure 7.6), illustrates the figures that CAP viewed to be standing in the way of contraception legislative reform: the archbishop of Dublin, politicians Charles Haughey, Jack Lynch and Garret FitzGerald, and a generic cartoon doctor, all drawn with pregnant bellies. The caption of the cartoon reads 'If they got pregnant would we have this bill?'

In reaction to the proposed legislation, which CAP described as 'repressive, regressive, restrictive and moralistic', a CAP-run shop, Contraceptives Unlimited, was opened on Harcourt Road, Dublin in November, 1978.[112] (Figures 7.7–7.9). The shop sold non-medical contraceptives such as condoms, jellies, creams and caps. Profits from the sale of contraceptives went towards the cost of fighting a court case over the confiscation of contraceptives imported by Family Planning Distributors.[113] According to Taragh O'Kelly (IWU/CAP), 'It was just blow the whole thing open was pretty much what our idea was'. The shop was following in a history of illegality with regard to contraception provision in Ireland, however, what distinguished it was that the women openly sold the contraceptives, rather than asking for a 'donation', as was done in the family planning clinics.[114]

Women who worked in the CAP shop recalled the anxiety that was felt when it opened, based on a fear that there would be no customers or a fear that they would be arrested. Joanne O'Brien (IWU/CAP) recalled: 'I remember Anne [Speed] saying to me just before we opened the shop, "Joanne, you will buy some" because she was so worked up and anxious that we would actually sell some. I remember saying to her, "Anne, I don't need them." She was just so funny, she was so worked up about it all. We didn't know what was going to happen, whether we were going to be all arrested'. Similarly, Taragh O'Kelly (IWU/CAP) recalled:

We opened up there with a clear view that we were openly selling. We were openly breaking the law, with a view to being arrested, essentially. We made a rule

---

[111] *Irish Press*, 3 January 1979, p. 9.
[112] 'The contraception issue in Ireland', undated [RCAPA, BL/F/AP/1177/3].
[113] Barbara Murray, unpublished booklet on Irishwomen United, Sept. 1995, p. 62 (MS in the possession of Barbara Murray).
[114] Cloatre & Enright, 'On the perimeter of the lawful', p. 473.

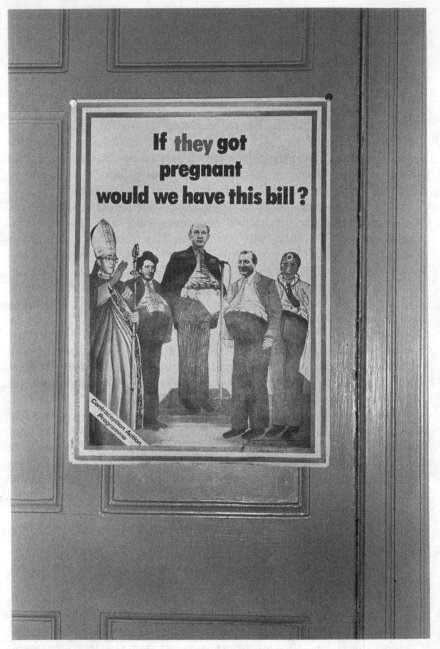

Figure 7.6 CAP poster, Limerick Family Planning Clinic, July 1981.

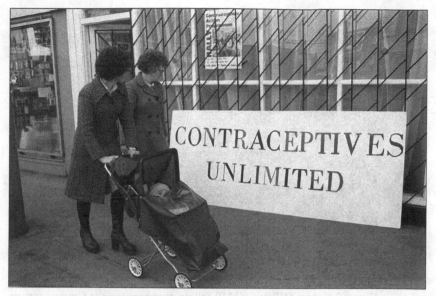

Figure 7.7 Front of Contraceptives Unlimited shop, Dublin,
28 November 1978.
Photograph by Derek Speirs.

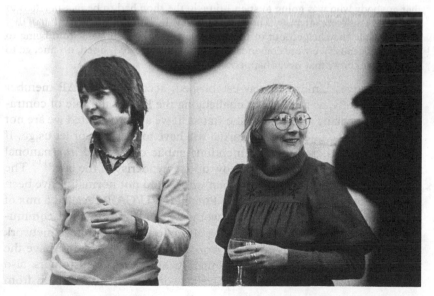

Figure 7.8 Anne Connolly (left) and Anne Speed (right) of CAP
celebrate the opening of Contraceptives Unlimited, 28 November 1978.
Photograph by Joanne O'Brien.

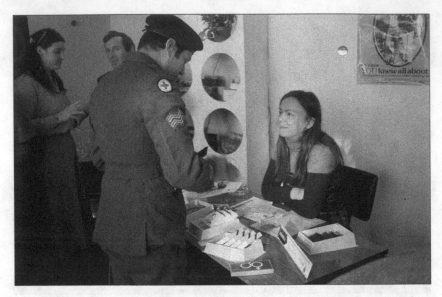

Figure 7.9 Ann O'Brien (CAP) selling contraceptives at Contraceptives Unlimited, Dublin, 28 November 1978.
Photograph by Derek Speirs.

that anybody who was going to spend time in the shop had to be in a position to go to jail. Therefore anybody who had parental responsibilities or anything of that nature, while they helped out of the back, they were discouraged from being to the front, because we were convinced, we would be arrested, fined, no fine, go to jail. As you know, that never happened.

Contraceptives Unlimited was established, according to CAP member Anne Connolly, as a means of challenging the law on the sale of contraceptives. Speaking at the time, she stated 'If we are prosecuted we are not going to pay the fines ... The Gardaí will have to arrest us or let us go. If they arrest us, there'll be a tremendous public outcry and international outrage. If they let us go it will show up the hypocrisy of the law.'[115] The shop also provided access for women who would not normally have been able to obtain contraception. Betty Purcell (IWU/CAP) recalled a mix of customers that included 'a lot of women from disadvantaged communities would come in who didn't have the amount of, I suppose, network support that middle-class women would have, and also didn't have the access to travel that a lot of women would have'. Customers also included members of the Irish Traveller community and women from

---

[115] *Irish Independent*, 29 November 1978, p. 12.

rural areas 'who were coming up from the country, it might be ostensibly doing a day's shopping but they'd come into us and say, "Where could I go and what could I" … It would be that they would be women who'd be fearful of opening up to their GP' as well as women who 'didn't want to tell their husband that they wanted to limit their families'. Purcell explained that the role of the shop was not only the sale of non-medical contraceptives such as condoms but also information provision about where women could obtain the contraceptive pill: 'It was helpful just to give them that very basic advice, to women, that this was where they could get a fair hearing and without the fear of an individual GP turning them down'.

There was some backlash from members of anti-contraception groups. Taragh O'Kelly (IWU/CAP) remembered protestors 'who came in and threw the holy water at us and things like that'. Other interviewees recalled pickets and intimidation by anti-contraception groups. Betty Purcell (IWU/CAP) remembered:

Then, yeah, we were distributing and then sometimes there'd be pickets on it, which were quite intimidating … Of course no one had mobile phones then or anything, so if you were on shift in the shop and the next thing 15 angry vociferous people were outside. They also used to take notes of people who were going in and that sort of thing.

The issue of young people potentially gaining access to contraception was one of concern to conservative groups when the shop opened. When asked by RTÉ reporter, George Devlin, if individuals would be asked their age when purchasing contraceptives, Anne Speed replied: 'No, we do not, we consider that an infringement on the individual right of people, because that is irrelevant to people. People have the right to engage in sexual activity irrespective of their age or their marital status. We will not be asking that question. We will, if very young people come into the shop obviously in need of advice be referring them to family planning clinics where we feel that trained counsellors and medical staff can help'.[116] Betty Purcell (IWU/CAP) also recalled attempts at entrapment where teenagers were sent into the shop to buy contraceptives. Despite the illegality of their activities, no legal action was taken against CAP members and no arrests were made. According to Joanne O'Brien (IWU/CAP): 'We thought we were going to be arrested. I think at that stage people must have felt that the issue, we had been campaigning for

---

[116] RTÉ news report on Contraceptives Unlimited, broadcast on RTE, 28 November 1978. Accessed: https://www.rte.ie/archives/2013/1127/489465-contraception-unlimited-1978/

quite some time at that point. I think people were starting to feel, well, you know, people have a right to this'. O'Kelly suggested that the lack of arrests was due to

pragmatism on the part of the government. There was an awful lot of international publicity. We were getting publicity from Germany, from France, from Holland and all of the rest of it, and bear in mind, on a business side of things, they wanted to prove themselves, be good Europeans and forward moving and the rest of it. The last thing they need or wanted was a bunch of women going to jail ... For what? For selling condoms?

By December, the shop was still open, and CAP stated that they would continue to keep it open 'in continuing defiance of the present laws'. In spite of reports that the Gardaí were planning on closing the shop down, the group stated that they had made plans 'for the immediate reopening and restocking of the shop in the event of a raid and confiscation of stock or arrest of members'.[117] The shop was never raided.

A CAP rally was held in Dublin on 3 December 1978. As well as the shop Contraceptives Unlimited, CAP activists also organised spontaneous sales of contraceptives, for instance, at Ballymun shopping centre in January 1979.[118] In March, 1979, CAP picketed the Fianna Fáil Ard-Fheis. The same month, six student CAP members who had organised a stall illegally selling contraceptives at UCC, were instructed by university staff to remove them.[119] The following month, the Gardaí seized contraceptives at stalls in Knocknaheney, Cork, and Princes Street in Cork.[120] CAP, nevertheless, continued with their activities, and organised a 'Festival of Contraception' in May 1979 at Wynn's Hotel in Dublin with films, lectures, stalls and a workshop on 'Contraception, health and women's sexuality' which included talks by female speakers.[121] In further defiance of the Health (Family Planning) Act, the CAP caravan took to the road to sell contraceptives in October 1979 and, over several weekends, it visited disadvantaged parts of Irish cities such as Rahoon in Galway, Ballymun in Dublin and Knocknaheney in Cork, as well as Shannon in County Clare and rural areas where people had difficulties getting access to contraception.[122] In November, the caravan visited Tuam, Co. Galway where the chair of the local community council, Cora McNamara, apparently complained that 'the intelligence of the people of Tuam was undermined' by the visit of the CAP caravan.[123]

[117] *Irish Times*, 18 December 1978, p. 5.   [118] *Irish Times*, 27 January 1979, p. 4.
[119] *Irish Examiner*, 30 March 1979, p. 5.   [120] *Ibid.*, 23 April 1979, p. 7.
[121] *Irish Times*, 4 May 1979, p. 12.   [122] *Irish Independent*, 11 October 1979, p. 12.
[123] *Irish Times*, 11 November 1979, p. 12.

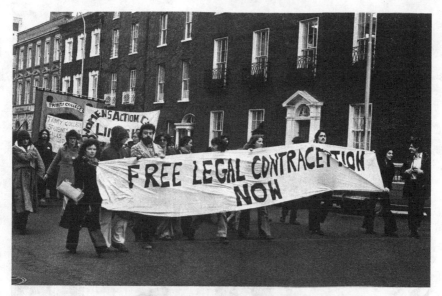

Figure 7.10 CAP march in Dublin, 3 December 1978.
Photograph by Joanne O'Brien.

Evidently, in spite of the introduction of the Family Planning Act in 1979, the issue of contraception remained controversial and divisive.

As had been predicted by CAP, access to contraception remained restrictive into the 1980s. According to a survey conducted by CAP in 1981, of 100 chemists who were asked if they stocked contraceptives, 46 said they did not; 39 refused to cooperate with the survey and 15 said they did stock contraceptives. Of the chemists who stated that they did not stock contraceptives, 39% said they were 'conscientious objectors', 26% claimed there was no demand and 17% stated they were prohibited because they were limited companies.[124] CAP continued to defy the law. Another shop, called the Women's Health Information Shop, was set up by CAP in December 1981 in Dublin, and opened from Wednesdays to Saturdays. The shop provided information on health and contraception, as well as selling non-medical contraceptives, 'to put pressure on the Government to change the Family Planning Act, which is ridiculous'.[125] In addition, CAP continued to sell contraceptives at the Dandelion Market in Dublin, until it was closed in 1981.[126]

[124] *Irish Independent*, 17 July 1981, p. 3.
[125] Untitled article in *Wimmin*, 1:1 (December 1981), p. 25.
[126] *Irish Times*, 12 October 1981, p. 7.

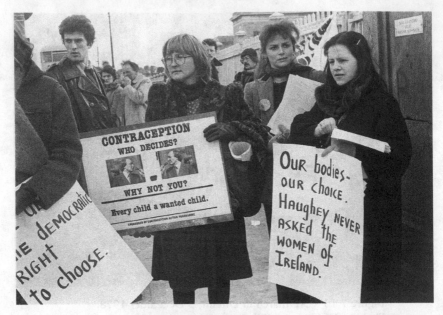

Figure 7.11 CAP picket outside Fianna Fáil, Ard Fheis, RDS, Dublin.
The three women are Anne Speed, Roisin Boyd and Geraldine
O'Reilly, 24 February 1979.
Photograph by Clodagh Boyd.

By the end of 1981, CAP had dismantled.[127] According to the *Irish
Feminist Review* in 1984, CAP 'collapsed because the effort that had been
put into the campaign over three years resulted in nothing but a miserable bill'.[128] According to Anne Speed, 'You can only take something so
far. You just become tired. And we just became tired then. And so we
didn't have any formal burial of CAP. CAP just kind of slipped into the
distance.' Following the legalisation of contraception, some members of
IWU and CAP became involved in the newly founded Women's Right to
Choose Group and Anti-Amendment Campaign which both opposed
the proposals for the eighth amendment of the Irish constitution, which
had been put forward by an active pro-life movement which mobilised
after the legalisation of contraception.[129] As Anne Speed explained:

Our main issue was as young militant feminists was, to get the break in the law, and
then we were looking for the next fight. You know what I mean? And the next fight

---

[127] 'The life and death of the contraception campaign' in *Irish Feminist Review* (1984),
p. 35.
[128] *Ibid.*.   [129] See Connolly, *The Irish Women's Movement*, pp. 162–9.

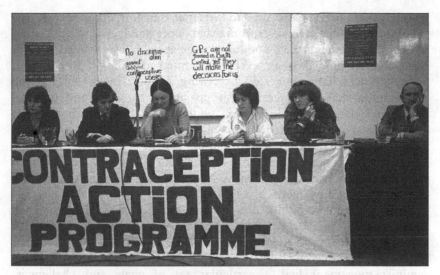

Figure 7.12 CAP public meeting in the Mansion House, Dublin,
31 May 1979. On the platform, L to R, unknown, Frank Crummey,
Ann O'Brien, Mary Freehill, Jane Dillon Byrne and Matt Merrigan.
Photograph by Derek Speirs.

was termination. So we didn't see ourselves ... Because we weren't the doctors, we weren't the counsellors, we weren't the nurses, we weren't the professional people. We were the political agitators that moved on. Individually, moved on. And we all went our separate ways.

7.4   Conclusion

As Diarmaid Ferriter has asserted 'Irish feminists were facing a 1980s that would, in many respects, seek to vehemently push them back down'.[130] Indeed, several respondents compared the idealism and enthusiasm they felt in the 1970s with later feelings of despondence and disappointment in the 1980s following the introduction of the eighth amendment of the constitution, and the cases of Ann Lovett (1984) and the Kerry babies (1985).[131] As Raewyn Connell has argued in relation to the women's liberation and gay liberation movements, the 'surge in the pace and depth of sexual politics and the power of theory opens the

---

[130] Ferriter, *Ambiguous Republic*, p. 679.
[131] Hug, *The Politics of Sexual Morality*, p. 121; Nell McCafferty, *A Woman to Blame: the Kerry Babies Case* (Dublin, 1985).

possibility of conscious social and personal transformation in a degree unthinkable before'. However, somewhat depressingly, she adds 'Yet the liberation movements have nothing like the social power needed to push this transformation through, except in limited milieux.'[132] In addition, some scholars have suggested exercising caution in overstating the contribution that these feminist groups made to social and political change in Ireland.[133] While it is difficult to quantify the contribution that Irish feminist groups made in terms of changes in the law on contraception, it is clear that they had an important role in opening up the public discourse on contraception and highlighting class and geographical inequalities that were not being assessed by other groups within the family planning movement.

While there are commonalities between the arguments made by Irish feminists and their British and American counterparts, such as, for example, in relation to the medicalisation of women's bodies, Ireland's distinctive religious and social climate, and laws, meant that the Irish feminist movement had a particular set of goals and challenges. Moreover, class became a central concern of their campaign to legalise contraception. Ultimately, Irish feminist campaigners believed in a women's movement that allowed for the equal distribution of sexual knowledge and access to contraception and, in this way, foregrounded the interconnection between health and economic rights. The feminist campaigns of IWU and CAP also illustrate the significance of informal women's networks in successfully navigating legal barriers to reproductive health in Ireland. In addition, it is important to note that CAP activities had an important legacy for future reproductive rights campaigns in Ireland.

Participation in direct action activities, such as the illegal import and sale of contraceptives could be personally challenging and not only put women activists in danger of being arrested, but also face-to-face with adversity and, occasionally, abuse. Irish feminist campaigners helped to publicise the hypocrisy and social disparities of the contraception issue. Moreover, through their demonstrations, meetings and service provision, in unconventional spaces, such as shops, markets, community centres and caravans, these women challenged the hold of both religious patriarchy and medical expertise in Ireland.

---

[132] Connell, *Gender and Power*, p. 279.   [133] Galligan, *Women and Politics*, p. 157.

8   Campaigns against Contraception in 1970s and 1980s Ireland

Writing to the *Irish Independent* in 1976, 'as parents and members of concerned organisations', a number of representatives of Irish conservative groups stated that in opposition to the 'desires expressed' by politicians such as Garret FitzGerald:

we do not want contraception, abortion, divorce, homosexuality, secular schools or any of the trappings of an uninspiring secular Ireland. Ireland suffered many centuries of persecution before regaining the freedom to express our religious and national ideals. Are we to discard some of our guiding principles so lightly after less than fifty years of being free to be ourselves?

This joint letter from conservative groups, including the League of Decency, Parent Concern, Irish Family League, Nazareth Family Movement, Pro-Fide Movement, Save our Society, and Mná na hÉireann (Irish for 'Women of Ireland'), highlights their concerns regarding the modernisation of Ireland, but also shows how groups used their authority as parents to justify speaking out on moral issues. The infusion of nationalist rhetoric suggests concerns about Ireland's changing identity, while the letter also illustrates anxieties around individualism, suggesting that 'it appears as if institutions of State are helping the attempt to pervert Irish society'.[1]

The contraception debate was an extremely polarising one. The previous two chapters have explored activist-led campaigns in favour of the legalisation of contraception. But, simultaneously, from the early 1970s, several groups also formed which actively campaigned against the legalisation of contraception.

The Catholic hierarchy continued to emphasise the Church's line on contraception in the wake of continuing debates. However, from the 1970s, bishops had encouraged individuals to follow their conscience in relation to matters of personal or sexual morality but 'reserved the right to voice their opinion on issues of morality, where legislation or constitutional reform had

---

[1] 'Efforts to "pervert" Irish society', *Irish Independent*, Friday, 21 May 1976, p. 10.

implications for the good of society, as they saw it'.[2] This meant that the policing of sexual morality and active campaigning on issues such as contraception, divorce and abortion were taken up by a number of lay conservative groups. Or, as Chrystel Hug has put it, 'these people had effectively taken over from the Church' and were unafraid to defend Church teachings and 'say loudly and clearly what kind of society they wanted to live in'.[3]

The foundation of Irish pro-life groups stemmed from the anti-contraception campaigns, in contrast to Britain where, as Olivia Dee has shown, pro-life groups such as Society for the Protection of Unborn Children (SPUC) (founded in 1967 to oppose the legalisation of abortion), and LIFE (founded in 1970), were primarily lobbying organisations which were set up to combat abortion.[4] While scholarship by Tom Hesketh and Cara Delay has illuminated elements of the Irish pro-life campaigns, there has been little research done on the anti-contraception campaigns that preceded them and which were integral to their foundation.[5] Moreover, as Diarmaid Ferriter has recently suggested 'there is a tendency to regard some of the individuals leading such groups as almost comic', but such views tend to underestimate 'how well connected and determined they were'.[6] Aidan Beatty has complicated the picture and shown how those who campaigned against contraception presented a vision of Ireland which 'represents a historically discrete modernist phenomenon'. In his view, conservative campaigners 'saw themselves as the defenders of a traditional social order' but these ideas owe their roots to the nineteenth century and 'centred on relatively specific notions about land ownership, gender roles, public respectability, religious belief, attitudes towards "foreign" culture, and the role of the centralized state in enforcing these ideas'.[7] As Chapters 2 and 3 showed, England was often portrayed as a permissive country in relation to matters of sexuality, and a threat to Irish womanhood.

As this chapter illustrates, it is also crucial to place Irish groups within the wider international context. Activists' rhetoric drew on a complex web of arguments which incorporated scientific evidence (such as the potential health risks of the pill) and sociological and statistical evidence

---

[2] Fuller, *Irish Catholicism*, p. 240.   [3] Hug, *The Politics of Sexual Morality*, p. 110.
[4] Olivia Dee, *The Anti-Abortion Campaign in England, 1966–1989* (New York: Routledge, 2019), pp. 41–4.
[5] See: Tom Hesketh, *The Second Partitioning of Ireland: The Abortion Referendum of 1983* (Dublin: Brandsma Books, 1990); Cara Delay, 'Wrong for womankind and the nation: anti-abortion discourses in Ireland, 1967–1992', *Journal of Modern European History*, 17:3, (2019), 312–325. The IFL is discussed briefly in journalist Emily O'Reilly's *Masterminds of the Right* (Dublin: Attic Press, 1988), p. 30.
[6] Ferriter, *Occasions of Sin*, p. 465.
[7] Beatty, 'Irish modernity and the politics of contraception', on p. 101.

in relation to the impact of 'the permissive society' in other contexts. As Jennifer Crane has argued in relation to child protection in 1970s Britain, emotional and experiential expertise (in particular motherhood) came to be more valued in public debates around the issue.[8] In the Irish context, anti-contraception campaigners also drew on their expertise as parents in order to give weight to their arguments. The chapter also shows how international networks, particularly links with conservative groups in the United States and the United Kingdom, assisted activists in developing their campaigns but also provided ideas which helped to set the foundation for the anti-abortion campaign in Ireland in the 1980s. Through the use of oral histories, archival material, newspapers and the publications of conservative groups, this chapter reveals campaigners' concerns about the modernisation of the country and legislative change.[9] The chapter more broadly highlights the value of exploring the history of conservative groups, which to date, have received little historical attention, in contrast with surveys of social movements which tend to focus on environmental or feminist activism.[10]

8.1   Early Activism: The Nazareth Family Movement and Mná na hÉireann

As Jeffrey Weeks has argued, the dramatic social changes and events of the late 1960s and early 1970s in Britain, such as the student revolts, economic crisis, industrial militancy, and the rise of the women's movement and gay liberation movements, came to be seen by more conservative members of society as being 'signs of breakdown or transformation in the old order'.[11] In Britain in this period there was a growing sense of social crisis and moral authoritarianism was perceived to be a solution to these crises. One of the leaders of this movement was Mary Whitehouse, who succeeded in mobilising significant cross-class support for her Clean Up TV Campaign and National Viewers' and Listeners' Association.[12]

---

[8] Jennifer Crane, *Child Protection in England, 1960–2000: Expertise, Experience and Emotion* (Basingstoke: Palgrave, 2018).

[9] Unfortunately, the majority of campaigners involved in Irish anti-contraception campaigns have passed away. This chapter draws on oral histories with surviving campaigners, John O'Reilly and Bernadette Bonar.

[10] Lawrence Black, 'There was something about Mary: The National Viewers' and Listeners' Association and Social Movement History' in Nick Crowson, Matthew Hilton, and James McKay (eds.), *NGOs in Contemporary Britain: Non-state Actors in Society and Politics since 1945* (Palgrave, 2009), pp. 182–200, on p. 182.

[11] Jeffrey Weeks, *Sex, Politics and Society: The Regulation of Sexuality since 1800*, 4th edition (Abingdon: Routledge, 2018), p. 312.

[12] See Black, 'There was something about Mary'.

In Ireland, similarly, a number of conservative groups emerged in the early 1970s which were concerned with changes in Irish society, in particular, the potential advent of the legalisation of contraception and the impact that this might have on the traditional family. The earliest of these appears to have been the Nazareth Family Movement which was formed in response to Pope Paul's 'call for a family apostolate' in *Humanae Vitae*. During the months that followed the publication of the encyclical in 1968, two of the founder members met to attempt to have the Rosary on television 'as a means of renewing and strengthening traditional family prayer' and out of this grew the Weekly Public Rosary Movement.[13] Writing to the *Evening Herald* in October 1970, founder member Marie Dunleavy MacSharry expressed her desire 'to establish a movement similar to the one initiated by Mrs. Mary Whitehouse' arising out of concerns from parents 'about the permissiveness in our midst', who were 'anxious that something be done about it'. She requested that interested parties contact her so that she could arrange a meeting.[14] The subsequent meeting was attended by twenty-two people and a committee was elected with Donal J. Cullinan as chairman and MacSharry as secretary.[15] In a small card which survives in the Dublin Diocesan Archives, the group listed their objectives as 'to voice lay support for the Church's teaching on marriage and the family; to combat the attacks on marriage and the dignity of man such as artificial contraception, abortion, divorce and euthanasia; to work to encourage and restore family prayers especially the Rosary; to express lay support for the magisterium of the Church and to help to restore all things in Christ'. The group was described as 'lay inspired and promoted' and membership was open to those who could actively participate in the work of the organisation, with all members asked to recite the Rosary, if possible with their family, at least once a week for the intentions of the movement.[16]

The group appears to have piqued Archbishop John Charles McQuaid's interest, or concern. His secretary wrote to Donal Cullinan, in June 1971, stating that he needed 'fairly urgently an account of the origins of the Nazareth Family Movement' and further detail of its activities.[17] Cullinan responded promptly the next day with an account

---

13 Nazareth Family Movement: report to Rev J.A. McMahon [DDA: Nazareth Family Movement, XXI/94/4/3].
14 'Move to organise parents', *Evening Herald*, 29 October 1970, p. 10.
15 Nazareth Family Movement: report to Rev J. A. McMahon.
16 Nazareth Family Movement card listing objectives. [DDA: Nazareth Family Movement, XXI/94/1/2].
17 Letter from Rev. McMahon, secretary, to D. J. Cullinan, 22 June 1971. [xxi/94/4/1].

of the origins of the group. In this he stated that the Nazareth Family Movement had been concerned with 'the wave of pornography sweeping the country'; but their efforts were soon focused on the contraception issue, particularly from 1971 when it became apparent that a bill would be introduced by Mary Robinson.[18] In March 1971, the group had defended the archbishop's statements in relation to *Humanae Vitae* against claims by IFPRA that these teachings were unorthodox.[19] The group also engaged in exchanges of letters with the Chairman of the IFPRA, were interviewed by printed media as well as the BBC and NBC, and printed and distributed a 'Prayer in Defence of Human Life'.[20]

The group then decided that it was 'inappropriate to act in a manner which would identify the Nazareth Movement as nothing but an anti-contraceptive pressure group' and instead decided to form the Association for the Protection of Irish Family Life at the end of March 1971. The aim of this organisation was to address youth and adult groups and ask them to voice their opposition to any change in the law on contraception.[21] The group claimed to take a non-militant approach, stating that 'we do not see the fight in terms of emotive debate, demon-strations or similar activities but in a call to our fellow lay-folk to bear witness in a practical manner to their Catholic life which is the only road to true happiness'. As such, the group was most concerned with the organisation of prayer vigils, the establishment of a perpetual novena of prayers in defence of human life, and visits to shrines, as well as the publication of a private newsletter.[22] McQuaid's secretary used the infor-mation provided by Cullinan to devise a report and also privately enquired with MacSharry and Cullinan's priest in Walkinstown. He wrote in his report to McQuaid that the parish priest had affirmed that MacSharry was 'a zealous, enthusiastic Catholic, a housewife with several children', and that the Curate in charge of the district where Cullinan lived stated that he was 'a fine Catholic. He is a Salesman, married, with several children'.[23]

In a 1971 statement, the Nazareth Family Movement argued that legalisation of contraception would lead to the introduction of divorce and abortion, quoting the example of Italy: 'Just before Christmas they got divorce, now contraception and they are now considering abortion'. In response to these comments, Senator John Horgan, who was one of

---

[18] Nazareth Family Movement: report to Rev J. A. McMahon.
[19] 'Contraception argument challenged', *Irish Press*, 18 March 1971, p. 3.
[20] Nazareth Family Movement: report to Rev J. A. McMahon.   [21] *Ibid.*
[22] Nazareth Family Movement: report to Rev J. A. McMahon.
[23] Report on the Nazareth Family Movement, 25 June 1971. [DDA, XXI/94/4/4].

the senators backing Mary Robinson's bill, argued 'This vision of Irish society exists nowhere but in the heads of the people who think it is true. We already have a permissive society and people are exploited in other ways. This whole business of the floodgates opening is utterly ludicrous'.[24]

Marie Dunleavy MacSharry and Donal Cullinan were active in writing to the press in the early 1970s. For example, in March 1971, a letter by MacSharry published in the *Evening Press* argued that 'the responsible planning of children is an essential part of Catholic teaching which involves a man's being a man, and proving he is, by self-control, true love and consideration'.[25] These ideas were not always well-received by members of the public. In response to a letter by MacSharry, a woman called Anne Doyle wrote a letter in favour of the legalisation of contraception to the *Evening Press* in March 1971, and sent copies of the same letter to a range of politicians, Church hierarchy, journalists and RTÉ staff. In a postscript to the letter, she addressed MacSharry directly, stating:

It is very easy for you to talk from the comfort of your home in Limekiln Drive but how would you like to live in one or two rooms in our city slums with 10 or 12 children. You are entitled to have as many children as you wish but you should not be stuffing your views down other people's throats. Every woman should have the right to plan her family as she likes without people like you telling her what, in your opinion, is the right way to go to Heaven. It is pretty obvious that you have not got a large family because, if you had, you would not have so much time for writing to the papers and telling us what you consider is right, but of course you may have a daily who does your extra work.[26]

MacSharry, writing to Taoiseach Jack Lynch in March 1971, explained that she had received a copy of this letter and wanted to inform him that she was 'the mother of 12 children, 6 surviving and of schooling age. One of these is an autistic child. I do all my own housework together with some other charitable works. I am active member of a few committees and have other interests. I have never had the luxury of a daily help.'[27] MacSharry's need to defend herself in this way against Doyle's allegations suggests that she viewed her role as a mother of several children as an important marker of her authority to speak on the family planning issue. Cullinan and MacSharry wrote to Lynch again in June 1971 to state that they were strongly opposed to any change in the legislation

[24] 'Family protection V Family planning', *Irish Independent*, 30 March 1971, p. 10.
[25] 'The dignity of motherhood', *The Irish Catholic*, 18 March 1971. [NAI, 2002/8/459].
[26] Letter from Anne Doyle, March 1971. [NAI, 2002/8/459].
[27] Letter to Jack Lynch, 30 March 1971. [NAI, 2002/8/459].

relating to contraception, because they felt that it was contrary to 'Natural Moral Law' and that its introduction would lead to a 'lowering of moral standards'.[28] The group seems to have declined in activity from late 1971 onwards, however, they later appear to have emerged again as part of the umbrella group Council of Social Concern which was a member of the Pro-Life Amendment Campaign founded in 1981.

There were also conservative groups established outside of Dublin. Mná na hÉireann was a small but active group originally based in Cork, founded by Úna Mhic Mhathúna (chairman) and Áine Ní Mhurchú (vice-chairman) in 1971. Like the Nazareth Family Movement, they were strongly opposed to the legalisation of contraception. In 1977, the Irish feminist magazine *Wicca* characterised Mná na hÉireann's beliefs as 'reactionary and hysterical ravings', suggesting that what united conservative groups was their 'common denial of a human right to choose', placing them in opposition to the women's movement, which was united with 'pro-contraception forces' through 'our absolute defence of the right of women in particular to control our fertility and obviously our lives'.[29] Mná na hÉireann, conversely, were critical of the movement in favour of contraception, in one letter stating 'So much for "Women's Rights" and nothing at all for their dignity'.[30] In an interview with Mary Leland of the *Irish Times* in 1973, they stated that 'There is a handful of women in Dublin who claim to be speaking for the majority of women in Ireland and we believe that it's not a majority opinion at all. The same number of women are always involved and some of them, the most vociferous, are foreigners'.[31] Leland described the members of Mná na hÉireann as 'young women with young families. The familiarity of a shared Cork background indicates that they are idealistic and nationalistic, and they believe that the majority of Irish women are in their homes, rearing families, wanting family life to remain as it is'. In the interview, the group expressed the view that 'We don't believe that any person makes a conscious decision to use artificial contraceptives: they do it under pressure from propaganda', and argued that there was no distinction between contraception and abortion because 'they have the same aim, that of destroying new life'. There were also moral undertones to the statements made by the group. Leland reported that they 'spoke nostalgically of the Irish way of life "when Ireland was truly Ireland,

---

[28] Letter from Nazareth Family Movement, 1 June 1971. [NAI, 2002/8/459].
[29] 'Contraception: a four-page pull-out', *Wicca* (1977), p. 7. [RCAPA, UCC, BL/F/AP/1398/3].
[30] 'Family planning', *Irish Press*, 18 February 1974, p. 8.
[31] 'Women of Ireland', *Irish Times*, 24 November 1973, p. 6.

when we had our own language and culture and religion"; then, they said "we were a moral nation"'.[32]

Mná na hÉireann's key forms of action were letter writing to newspapers, the collection of signatures on petitions and the production of circulars outlining their aims and beliefs. The group claimed in 1973 that there was not public support for the legalisation of contraception. They alluded to influences from Britain, arguing that 'if the Government believes that it is the Government of a sovereign state it should legislate for the good of the people and without regard to the wishes or standards of a foreign state'.[33] A letter in the *Irish Examiner* praising the efforts of the group from Micheal Ua Maignneir, based in Leeds, commended the two women for 'making such stout and able defence of the Holy Father's teaching on this subject [...] May you yet win the day against the strangely voluble Slummi of anti-Catholicism and shoneenism'.[34] Writing to Taoiseach Liam Cosgrave in February 1974, Úna Mhic Mhathúna and Áine Ui Mhurchú set out their key arguments against Mary Robinson's bill on contraception. They referred to the fact that Senator Robinson was a Trinity College nominee to the Seanad and not an elected representative of the people, and therefore 'should not be allowed to impose her views on the people in a matter of such national importance'.[35] The group was concerned that the legalisation of contraception would lead to a 'promiscuous society' and would resent having to pay 'for abortifacient contraceptives' through rates and taxes when 'the whole anti-life idea runs contrary to our religious beliefs'. The letter also drew attention to biases in the media which they felt were pressuring women to use artificial contraceptives while also stating the potential physical and psychological ill-effects of these contraceptives on women.[36]

In 1974, Mná na hÉireann wrote to the *Irish Press* to express their concerns that the legalisation of contraception would lead to depopulation and 'a campaign for compulsory artificial contraception and sterilisation'. The group was concerned with the side effects of the pill and the actions of the IUD, arguing that women were being used 'as guinea pigs and guinea pigs are always in a very dangerous position'.[37] In April, 1974, the group collected over 250 signatures outside churches in Tralee, and claimed to have collected almost 10,000 signatures in Cork county and city alone.[38] Petitions were a common strategy by anti-contraception

[32] 'Women of Ireland', *Irish Times*, 24 November 1973, p. 6.
[33] 'Contraception less "trendy"', *Irish Independent*, 26 November 1973, p. 10.
[34] *Irish Examiner*, 5 December 1973, p. 8.
[35] Letter from Mna na hEireann to Liam Cosgrave, 13 February 1974.   [36] *Ibid.*
[37] 'Family planning', *Irish Press*, 18 February 1974, p. 8.
[38] 'Mna na hEireann canvass support', *Kerryman*, 12 April 1974, p. 4.

campaigners and helped to illustrate that others agreed with their beliefs. Mná na hÉireann was also concerned with the role that the IPPF had with regard to the workings of the IFPA clinics and raised concerns that there would be a push towards compulsory sex education in schools and that children would begin using contraceptives.[39] A circular produced by Mná na hÉireann and distributed to TDs and senators in Ireland alleged that the IPPF was 'spreading disease and destruction to millions' and suggested that the spread of contraceptives in Ireland had resulting in an increase in venereal disease.[40]

Mena Bean Uí Chribín (1928–2012) (often spelt Mena Cribben), an Irish conservative campaigner, joined the group as publicity officer in 1974.[41] Cribben had also written to the Taoiseach in 1973 with her husband Gus, to express her concerns about Mary Robinson's reintroduced bill on contraception, arguing that the truth about contraceptives was being concealed and that the 'dangers to health, spiritual and physical' should be explained to the general public. In their view, the introduction of 'uncontrolled drugs and devices' would 'reduce people to below the level of animals' and she felt that the pro-contraception lobby was 'not representative of the decent Catholic men and women of Ireland'.[42] In an interview with Emer O'Kelly for her 1974 book *The Permissive Society in Ireland?* the Cribbens argued that the media was biased in favour of contraception and 'foreign, anti-Irish influences'. Moreover, their views highlight the tensions between old traditions of Irish family life and new societal changes. They explained 'We think that it's the Irish standards which were always accepted which have made us happy. We're fighting to give our children the same chance of happiness'.[43] Illegitimacy was also deemed to be the result of foreign influences. Mena explained: 'Illegitimacy is not part of our Irish heritage. If you look at the Aran Islands, where Irish culture in its true sense is still alive, there's no illegitimacy problem. Foreign influences create the problems, which is why we've set our faces against things like foreign pop music'.[44] Evidently, for members of Mná na hÉireann, concerns about the influence of foreign (British) forces were paramount. Moving later into the 1970s, however, groups such as the Irish Family League were more strategic in how they framed their arguments, drawing on

[39] 'Queues grow at family planning clinics', *Sunday Independent*, 25 May 1975, p. 8.
[40] 'Contraceptive circular "inaccurate"', *Irish Press*, 27 March 1976, p. 4.
[41] 'Fighting the pill, porn, nudes and naughty foreign pictures', *Irish Press*, 10 April 1978.
[42] Letter from Gus and Mena Cribben to Taoiseach, 5 November 1973, [NAI, 2004/21/461].
[43] O'Kelly, *The Permissive Society in Ireland?* pp. 62–3.   [44] *Ibid.*, p. 64.

medical evidence relating to the side effects of artificial contraception, as well as concerns about what the introduction of contraception might lead to, in order to bolster their arguments.

8.2   The Irish Family League

The Irish Family League (IFL) was a group of Catholic campaigners founded in May 1973 and one of the most prominent organisations that campaigned against the legalisation of contraception. The key figures involved in the IFL were its chairman John O'Reilly, a married father of five children, who went on to be heavily involved in Ireland's Pro-Life Amendment Campaign in the 1980s, and Mary Kennedy, who acted as secretary to the group. The executive was composed of less than ten individuals who met on a weekly basis. The group positioned themselves as being concerned with 'promoting a Christian family atmosphere in Ireland, and fostering family welfare'.[45] The IFL was extremely active in writing to the press and lobbying politicians. By 1980 they claimed to have 2,000 members.[46] The IFL was formed following a visit from American pro-life campaigner, Father Paul Marx, to Ireland in 1973. Marx, a Catholic priest and Benedictine monk, was one of the leaders of the pro-life movement in the United States, establishing a number of organisations such as the Human Life Center (1971) and Human Life International (1981) and the Population Research Institution (1989).

Father Marx came to Ireland in January 1973 as part of a tour of talks in Ireland and Britain organised by the British SPUC. He gave a lecture at Power's Royal Hotel, Dublin on 15 January.[47] In his lecture, attended by about 150 people, Marx discussed abortion in the United States and advocated the education of young people in schools on the issue. He showed the audience a series of slides and film strips of normally developed foetuses and aborted foetuses as well as playing an audio recording of 'an ultrasound record of what was described as a foetal heart beating in the foetus of three months gestation'. Marx also drew attention to the family planning clinics that had been recently established in Dublin, stating: 'You have an organisation of family planning clinics paid for with outside money. I give you my word of honour that these people promote abortion – soon if not already', referring to the IPPF which 'you've got it right under your noses' as he waved a booklet on

---

[45] Irish Family League, *Is Contraception the Answer?* (Dublin: Irish Family League, 1974), p. 22.
[46] 'Fighting the "lobby"', *Irish Press*, 8 October 1980. [RCAPA, UCC, BL/F/AP/846/16].
[47] 'The protection of unborn children', *Sunday Independent*, 7 January 1973, p. 16.

family planning published by the IFPA. Marx also argued that contraception was not the solution to avoiding abortion, stating that 'contraception leads to abortion'.[48] In response to Marx's comments, the IFPA publicly stated that under no circumstances did they advocate abortion.[49] As part of his visit, Marx spoke to a group of hundreds of teenage schoolgirls at St. Marie's of the Isles School in Cork on the abortion issue, using slides of aborted foetuses to illustrate his talk as well as showing them a 14 week old foetus in a jar.[50] The showing of the foetus gained significant publicity and in response, the Archdeacon James Bastible of Cork stated that the foetus had been shown to the group without his foreknowledge and approval.[51] As Kathryn Slattery has shown, Marx and other American anti-abortion campaigners would go on to play an integral role in Irish anti-abortion campaigns in the 1980s, particularly in the development of constitutional activism.[52]

Following Marx's visit, the IFL was formally organised in May 1973. As James Jasper has argued, 'moral emotions are the core of political rhetoric. Indignation is the hottest of the hot cognitions; as a moral form of anger, it encourages action'. Social movements offer a means for activists to channel collective anger into collective protest.[53] John O'Reilly, who was a founding member of the IFL, explained to me that he felt the need to set up a group because 'things were happening and nobody seemed worried about them [...] I was amazed that there was so much approving publicity about contraception although it was illegal'. In a letter to the *Irish Independent* in November 1973, IFL secretary Mary Kennedy, summed up their key aims as being 'enshrining Christian values in our legislation, promoting Christian education of youth and family welfare; to oppose threats to the family and society such as violence, pornography, divorce, contraception and abortion' as well as the promotion of natural forms of family planning such as Billings Ovulation and the Temperature method.[54] IFL member Mavis Keniry founded the Dublin Ovulation Method Advisory Service, which later became the National Association of the Ovulation Method in Ireland

---

[48] 'U.S. priest says Ireland needs campaign against abortion', *Irish Times*, 16 January 1973, p. 1 and p. 5.

[49] 'Family plan group deny advocating abortion', *Evening Herald*, 16 January 1973, p. 5.

[50] *Irish Times*, 20 January 1973, p. 6.

[51] 'Archdeacon says he did not know of foetus', *Irish Times*, 20 January 1973, p. 13.

[52] See: Kathryn Slattery, *Building a 'World Coalition for Life': Abortion, Population Control and Transnational Pro-Life Networks, 1960–1990*, (PhD thesis, 2010, University of New South Wales), pp.109–121. Available online: http://unsworks.unsw.edu.au/fapi/datastream/unsworks:9072/SOURCE02?view=true

[53] James M. Jasper, *The Emotions of Protest* (University of Chicago Press, 2018), p. 149.

[54] 'Fr. Marx's campaign against abortion', *Irish Independent*, 22 November 1973, p. 17.

(NAOMI). As well as these aims, the IFL's objects were to 'promote the Christian education of youth and the welfare of the family' as well as opposing any permissive legislation. Euthanasia and secularism were also to be countered while amendments to the Irish Constitution and laws would only be accepted if they were in line with the Vatican II teachings 'to infuse a Christian spirit into the mentality, customs and laws and structures of the community'.[55] Hindering the legalisation of contraception was, however, the group's key goal. John O'Reilly explained:

The main thing was to try and stop the legalisation of contraception. We had, privately, a lot of other ideas about family life and all this sort of thing. As we visualised it, if contraceptives became freely available, you were going to have much more ... births out of wedlock and demands for abortion. At that time, we had a very, very low rate of births outside of marriage. It was something like about 2% or 3%. Where it's up to about 33% today. We thought flowing from that, there would be more sexual activity. Where you had more sexual activity, you're going to have more out of wedlock births and then you were going to have more abortions, one thing another. Also, we believed that human life should be protected from contraception. And the contraceptives now coming into use were abortifacient at times if not always e.g., the IUD, contraceptive pill etc.

Concerns about an increase in promiscuity and sexual activity among young people were not unique to Irish conservative groups like the IFL. In the 1960s, as Steven Angelides has noted, 'a moral panic erupted across the United Kingdom, North America and Australia over an apparent rapid rise in rates of premarital sex, promiscuity, immorality, illegitimate births, and venereal disease amongst young people.'[56] In these countries, sex education was usually put forward as the solution to this problem, although there was considerable debate over the form that this should take.[57]

John O'Reilly had spent five years in Canada in the late 1950s, first in Montreal and then Toronto, returning to Ireland in 1960. He recalled:

And Toronto then was a much looser society than Ireland for instance. And you could see the effects of certain behaviours actually there; the way they were coming out. So, I became convinced for instance like this on certain values, which incidentally at that time for instance contraception was forbidden in Canada, believe it or not. But, there was such an underground market, as a matter of fact, for it, that it didn't make any difference. Abortion was certainly

[55] *Is Contraception the Answer?* p. 22.
[56] Steven Angelides, 'The "Second Sexual Revolution", Moral Panic, and the Evasion of Teenage Sexual Subjectivity', *Women's History Review*, 21:5, (November 2012), pp. 831–47, on p. 832.
[57] Angelides, 'The "Second Sexual Revolution"', p. 834.

for instance *verboten* there. Nobody would think of abortion. Now, for instance, Canada is one of the leading lights in abortion and euthanasia. So, you can see the deterioration.

While some campaigners' visions of the permissiveness of other countries were not based on lived experience, for O'Reilly, it is clear that his time in Canada had a significant impact on his thinking. He explained his concerns at the time about the potential effects that the introduction of contraception would have on Irish society:

The Family Planning Association was founded in 1969, I think. They called themselves the Fertility Guidance Company, at that time. They were founded by and given a grant by the International Planned Parenthood Federation. And all of a sudden, there was propaganda all over the place. I was concerned that there was no adverse reaction to it, that there was nobody opposing it and giving an opposite view for instance to it and citing the effects of it on society. I didn't talk to anybody. There was nobody really that I knew talking about it either. I met an old friend. [...] He said, 'We should really try and do something about it'. I think the first thing we did, was write a circular to the Bishops, getting a few hundred signatures on it and saying that they should be speaking up about it. Then some of us got in touch, as a result of that and had regular meetings. We met other concerned people that were interested and we formed the Irish Family League. So that's about the genesis of it.

As with other groups, for the IFL, the use of petitions helped to demonstrate wider public support for their arguments. Members of the IFL were concerned by the open flouting of the law by groups such as the IFPA and FPS. In an open letter to the Irish government in July 1973, the IFL expressed their concerns about the illegal activities of groups distributing contraceptives in Ireland and requested that the government put a stop to these activities.[58] In an attached document, the directors of both FPS and the IFPA were listed in addition to the laws that they had contravened.

One of the IFL's major concerns was around young people and the potential for rising rates of promiscuity if contraception was legalised. In a 1973 letter from John O'Reilly and Mary Kennedy to the *Irish Press*, they asserted that the laws prohibiting the sale of contraception 'reflect a standard of Christian morality geared to protect the young and society at large'. They believed that a change in the law would have consequences that 'could only be inimical to public morality and render the rearing of children still more difficult'. Moreover, they raised concerns that some of the clinics did not differentiate between married and single clients. In the

---

[58] Open letter to the Government from the Irish Family League, 19 July 1973. [NAI, 2004/21/460].

group's view, 'we do not accept that contraceptive peddling is an altruistic business, engaged in from the highest humanitarian motives. It is a sordid business, involving money, big business, and new vistas for medical careers. It provides medicine with an instant, lazy, and wrong answer to a problem. Its end results are sordidness and death and any short-term good is bought at an eventual terrible price'.[59] Most notably the letter stated that the group had it on record that one of the family planning clinics had sold contraceptives to an 11-year-old. The 11-year-old in question was John O'Reilly's daughter Deirdre. According to O'Reilly, in an oral history interview:

They were both selling contraceptives, Family Planning Services and the Irish Family Planning Association ... So there was a bit of a entrapment involved. Writing letters into them, and they used to look for a voluntary contribution. But, when we were testing them out and they were a bit unsubtle about it. If you left out the contribution, they wouldn't send you anything. They'd just tell you to send a contribution. But, at least so much, you know?

On 26 June 1973, O'Reilly wrote a letter to FPS with a postal order for 75p requesting condoms and had his daughter Deirdre sign it. FPS sent back condoms in a plain envelope addressed to Deirdre. In his words:

Anyhow, there was a bit of entrapment involved. It was clearly in the Act, that that was illegal. That was an illegal activity. So we reported it to the Gardaí and gathered evidence, reported it to the Gardaí.

On 14 July, he made a subsequent draft letter to FPS enclosing £1.10 and had his 9-year-old daughter Eilish copy the letter word for word. A parcel containing a contraceptive was sent in return. In addition, the IFPA was charged with distributing the booklet *Family Planning for Parents and Prospective Parents* without a permit and for advertising an intra-uterine device for sale. Robin Cochran, secretary, and David McConnell, chairman, of FPS, were interviewed by the Gardaí and cautioned. In the court case that followed at Dublin District Court, the charges were dismissed.[60] In the court case, the defendants argued that they could not have been aware of the ages of Deirdre and Eilish O'Reilly.[61] And, as John O'Reilly explained 'Unfortunately, the DPP didn't act until the Supreme Court case had taken place. [McGee case which deemed the right to import contraceptives a matter of marital privacy]. And then the activity was no longer illegal. So that fell flat on its face. But it had a chance of winning, or we wouldn't have tried it. But,

[59] 'Breaking the law', *Irish Press*, 25 July 1973, p. 8.
[60] 'Family planning summonses fail', *Irish Press*, 20 February 1974, p. 5.
[61] 'Contraceptive charges dismissed', *Cork Examiner*, 20 February 1974, p. 5.

it didn't win.' However, through bringing the case to court, the IFL succeeded in raising concerns about the possibility that young people *could* gain access to contraception through significant coverage of the case in the media. There does not appear to have been unease in the press about O'Reilly's use of his children for the purposes of entrapment. Instead, O'Reilly used his position as a parent to claim authority. For example, in a letter from O'Reilly and Mary Kennedy to the *Irish Press* in July 1973, O'Reilly and Kennedy wrote 'As Irish parents, Christians and citizens, we take grave exception to the activities of certain organisations which are acting in open defiance of the laws of this State by distributing contraceptives and contraceptive literature and fitting contraceptives' and noted that 'we have on record that one of them supplied contraceptives to an eleven-year-old child'.[62] The same letter appeared in the *Evening Herald* on 17 August 1973.[63] Undoubtedly, the idea that children were somehow gaining access to contraception would have created concern among some readers.

The IFL's publications and letters to newspapers were rigorously researched and often included references to medical texts as well as statistical evidence in relation to issues such as abortion, venereal disease, and illegitimacy which were used to back up their arguments. This was a distinctive form of campaigning; perhaps activists were aware of the need to support their arguments with evidence rather than overly relying on moral arguments. The IFL self-published a booklet *Is Contraception the Answer?* in 1973, identifying themselves on the cover page as a 'Team of Catholic Parents' (Figure 8.1). 20,000 copies of the booklet were printed and circulated to doctors, pharmacists, nurses, all members of government, priests and nuns.[64] According to John O'Reilly, this coincided with Mary Robinson's Family Planning Bill which was put to the Senate on 14 November 1973. John O'Reilly stated:

We became very active at this stage. At that time Mary Robinson was pushing a Bill on contraception in the Senate. So we decided to circulate the booklet to people that we thought would be interested or affected by it. We sent a copy to every GP for instance. At that time, they were all in the Golden Pages. We sent a copy to every pharmacist. We sent a copy to some Churchmen here or there, and to people interested in the subject with a letter explaining the situation and explaining the legislation. We were asking for donations so that we could circulate to more people. That's the way it went on.

[62] 'Breaking the law', *Irish Press*, 25 July 1973, p. 8.
[63] 'Legalised murder', *Evening Herald*, 17 August 1973, p. 10.
[64] 'Postal campaign on contraceptives bill', *Irish Times*, 23 March 1974, p. 9.

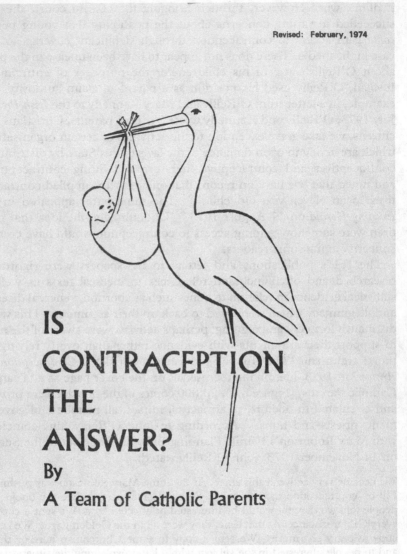

Revised: February, 1974

IS
CONTRACEPTION
THE
ANSWER?
By
A Team of Catholic Parents

Figure 8.1 Cover of *Is Contraception the Answer?* by the Irish Family League, 1974.
Courtesy of the National Library of Ireland.

O'Reilly recalled, to his surprise, receiving particular support from doctors and pharmacists who provided contributions to the IFL. In his view, 'There were a lot of doctors, as a matter of fact, at that time, who resented the idea of legalised contraception and a lot of pharmacists who feared that they might be forced to sell them'.

Is Contraception the Answer? emphasised a number of key points. Firstly, it argued that fundamentally, the use of artificial contraception went against the teachings of the Catholic Church. It claimed that since the publication of *Humanae Vitae* in 1968, the Irish public had been subjected to 'a barrage of brain-washing from the media in favour of contraception and its legalisation in Ireland', based on superficial reasons and hard cases, including 'the horde of hypothetical women with sixteen children, living in one room with a drunken, unemployed husband'.[65] The booklet drew on statistical evidence relating to illegitimate births in England in addition to quotes from medical professionals and campaigners such as Father Paul Marx. Fundamentally, the key argument of the booklet was that contraception would lead to 'increased promiscuity, increased illegitimacy, rocketing V.D. figures, and a demand for abortion'.[66] Links were made between contraception and abortion. The booklet argued that IUDs, which were available at family planning clinics in Dublin, were a form of abortifacient because 'their action is to abort the fruits of conception at an early stage. [...] Yet the I.U.D. is dishonestly described in the FGC's brochure as a contraceptive and is fitted at their clinics in Dublin. So abortion is actually taking place quite openly in Dublin.'[67] In addition, the booklet drew attention to the side effects of the contraceptive pill and IUD.[68] While the publication explained that the early form of the pill was purely contraceptive in action, the newer low-dosage pills were 'less successful in suppressing ovulation, but if they fail to do this, they will abort the fertilised ovum as does the I.U.D.'[69] Instead, the IFL encouraged readers to utilise Catholic Church-approved natural family planning methods such as the temperature method and Billings method. Advice on these methods could be obtained by writing directly to the group.[70] Moreover, it was argued that rather than reducing rates of illegitimacy, the introduction of contraception would result in an increase in births outside of marriage as well as leading to the legalisation of abortion.[71] In order to combat the issue of contraception, readers were encouraged to join the IFL, to make their views known to friends when the subject arose, to write to newspapers, TDs and senators, and 'become an activist. You are fighting to prevent murder and the slaughter of innocents'.[72] This wording clearly had pro-life connotations.

[65] *Is Contraception the Answer?*, p. 2.   [66] *Ibid.*, p. 3.   [67] *Ibid.*, p. 5.   [68] *Ibid.*, p. 7.
[69] *Is Contraception the Answer?* p. 6.   [70] *Ibid.*, p. 13.   [71] *Ibid.*, p. 7.   [72] *Ibid.*, p. 12.

An appendix at the back of the booklet contained details of the two key family planning groups, the FGC, and FPS, as well as listing names and contact details of individuals involved in the family planning movement in Ireland. These names were published 'not to cause embarrassment to the people concerned but so that if you hear any of these people advocating contraception on the media, you will understand the significance of their doing so'.[73] As well as reiterating earlier points about the illegality and perceived danger of the activities of the groups, the booklet also asserted that they had 'documentary proof that the squalid activities of this organisation include the posting of contraceptives to children. Any child can obtain contraceptives in this way provided that an appropriate "donation" is enclosed'. It was asserted that through the publication of their activities in publications such as *Nikki, Woman's Choice* and the *Sunday World* newspaper, family planning campaigners seemed 'to be seeking to develop a market for their wares among teenagers, some of whom are mere children'.[74]

In a letter accompanying a copy of the booklet sent to Taoiseach Liam Cosgrave in November 1973, Mary Kennedy stressed that the IFL was 'much distressed and alarmed by persistent rumours, and more than rumours of permissive legislation in regard to contraception and divorce' and their concerns regarding the breaches of the law by family planning groups. Kennedy asserted that the existing laws were positive ones if fully enforced, and that if family planning clinics were to be established, they should be based entirely on natural methods. She asked if Cosgrave would receive a deputation of four or five of their members to discuss the situation, emphasising that 'the question is most important to the real welfare of our country. We pray that God may guide our government'.[75] Cosgrave's secretary replied to say that the government had not taken any decision concerning changes to legislation relating to contraception. Furthermore, he wrote that the Taoiseach would be unable to receive a deputation to discuss this matter but that he would bring their letter to the attention of the Minister for Health.[76]

The IFPA produced their own response to the IFL booklet entitled *Facts on Contraception: An Answer to 'The Irish Family League'*, which was sent to members of government. In this, the IFPA refuted the IFL's claims around the links between contraception and illegitimacy, the idea that legalised contraception would lead to legalised abortion, links

---

[73] *Ibid.*, p. 14.   [74] *Is Contraception the Answer?* p. 17.
[75] Letter from the Irish Family League to Liam Cosgrave, 3 November 1973. [NAI, 2004/21/461].
[76] Reply to Mary Kennedy, 6 November 1973. [NAI, 2004/21/461].

between contraception and promiscuity, and claims that the pill and IUD were abortifacients. The IFPA claimed instead that 'effective contraception, provided for women who need it and who want it, is a means of reducing the toll of abortion. To change the laws is not to force women to use contraception, merely to allow them to meet their needs without breaking the law'.[77]

In a follow-up publication called *Whither Ireland?* the IFL discussed other trends that would follow the legalisation of contraception and the separation of heterosexuality from reproduction including homosexuality and test-tube babies.[78] The contraception issue continued to be conflated with concerns about the introduction of abortion in Ireland. Father Paul Marx returned to Ireland in November 1973 where he gave lectures on abortion at a number of locations, including TCD, UCD and Maynooth, with a total of 20 talks over two weeks organised by the IFL.[79] At a Dublin meeting attended by 300 people, Marx showed an anti-abortion film 'Abortion: A woman's decision' as well as numerous slides depicting aborted foetuses. He encouraged audience members to help the pro-life cause 'by joining the Irish Family League'.[80] The IFL began to intensify their activities. Mary Kennedy regularly wrote letters to Irish newspapers, and was often interviewed by the press. In one interview with the *Observer*, she stated that 'The group exists to protect Irish family life from contraception, which will be followed by abortion, divorce, and euthanasia. People should not be given something just because they want it. Some people want guns and drugs, but we don't give them guns and drugs. Contraceptives are even more dangerous.'[81] Given that family planning campaigners wanted contraception to be available to single as well as married people, Kennedy, in one letter, believed that they should perhaps be called 'Promiscuity Promoters'.[82]

By identifying themselves as 'parents' or individuals concerned with family welfare, conservative campaigners positioned themselves in direct contrast to feminist campaigners. Moreover, the age of conservative activists, who would have, for the most part, been middle-aged at the time of campaigning, meant that they contrasted with the youthfulness of

[77] *Facts on Contraception: An answer to 'The Irish Family League'* (undated but likely 1974), p.15. [NAI, 2005/7/345].
[78] *Whither Ireland? A Study (August 1974) of Recent Trends. Contraception and Associated Issues* (Irish Family League, Cahill and Co Printing, Dublin, 1974), p. 11.
[79] 'Father Marx hits Irish hypocrisy', *Evening Herald*, 15 November 1973, p. 6.
[80] 'An evening with Father Marx', *Irish Independent*, 19 November 1973, p. 8.
[81] 'Why the priests are calling Dublin "Sin City"', *Observer*, 10 March 1974, no page number. [NLI, Bruce Arnold papers, MS 41,428].
[82] 'Promiscuity promoters', *Irish Press*, 18 April 1974, p. 8.

members of feminist groups such as IWU and CAP. Yet, one aspect which both feminist campaigners and the IFL agreed on was their concerns about the side effects of the contraceptive pill. Writing to the *Irish Times* in 1975, Mary Kennedy referred to the American Food and Drugs Administration report on the contraceptive pill.[83] The following year, in another letter, she asked 'Have we so soon forgotten the thalidomide children and the tragedy of their lives?'[84] Kennedy also alleged that the contraceptive pill might have potential long-term effects on the third and fourth generation of users of chemical contraception, and cited the work of German doctor Siegfried Ernst while also commenting that 'genetic damage has also been noted in the USA'.[85] In her view, if groups such as CAP were successful in having contraceptives made available, the tax payer would not only have to pay for the provision of the services but would also 'have to provide compensation when the users suffer damage to their health'.[86] England was often portrayed in Kennedy's letters in a negative light, with statistics on rising rates of illegitimacy and abortion there often quoted. In 1975, she wrote: 'In England, abortion has debased the profession of medicine and of nursing to that of paid killer, highly profitable to those involved. However, the state of the profession there at the moment must be an example to us of what can happen when the selfishness of the contraceptive society is given free rein'.[87] Anti-British rhetoric was also common in anti-abortion discourse in the 1980s.[88]

The IFL's concerns over the side effects of the contraceptive pill were also discussed in detail in a subsequent publication in 1975 called *Alert: oral contraceptive*. The publication reminded readers of the thalidomide tragedy of the 1960s where the drug was made available without adequate testing of its effects.[89] A claims prevention letter which could be used by doctors in the US who were prescribing the pill was also included to illustrate the concerns over side effects and litigation.[90] The publication asserted that contraception was wrong for a range of reasons, which included the fact that contraception went against the purpose of 'the marriage act' as designed by God. The use of artificial contraception

[83] 'Letters to the editor: Family Planning', *Irish Times*, 3 November 1975, p. 9.
[84] 'Letters to the editor: the pharmacist's duty', *Irish Times*, 24 November 1976, p. 11.
[85] 'Letters to the editor: the pharmacist's duty', p. 11.   [86] *Ibid.*
[87] 'Students' call', *Irish Press*, 29 December 1975, p. 6.
[88] Delay, 'Wrong for womankind', p.323; Lisa Smyth, *Abortion and Nation: The Politics of Reproduction in Contemporary Ireland* (Ashgate, 2005), p. 49.
[89] Irish Family League, *Alert: Oral Contraceptive* (Dublin: Irish Family League, undated but c.1975), p. 2.
[90] *Alert: Oral Contraceptive*, pp. 8–9.

was also believed to result in selfishness which could cause unhappy marriages or their break-up. Contraception was believed to lead to 'psychic troubles' as a result of the 'frustration of the instinct of parenthood'. In addition, it was emphasised by the IFL that the legalisation of contraception would be followed by the legalisation of abortion. Concerns were also raised about how legal safeguards could be enforced to prevent young people from using contraception and about the impact of legalisation on Ireland's small population. Finally, the IFL believed that if contraception was legalised it could result in eugenic programmes to 'better' the population, arguing 'once the floodgates are opened, the tide will sweep through' and reminding readers of the practices which occurred during the Second World War. Finally, a focus on the legalisation of contraception also distracted attention from 'the real economic evils of society' such as housing and unemployment.[91]

A detailed section on the IUD emphasised the IFL's belief that this acted as an abortifacient because it interfered with the implantation of the fertilised ovum in the womb.[92] Readers were advised to be aware of 'humanist reformers' who had 'devised a very effective technique in altering social laws' which had been particularly effective in the United Kingdom and in Southern Australia. The tactics had three stages, the first being to promote public controversy in the media about the issue in question, the second to 'prove' that public opinion was in favour of reform of the law, and the third was a parliamentary phase with the introduction of a private members bill 'coupled with the isolation of opponents who are labelled fanatics or "Catholics who are trying to impose their moral views on the community"'. The IFL claimed that these tactics were being used in Ireland and that 'the unfortunate thing is that comparatively few people seem to be aware it is happening'.[93]

By 1976, the group's language around the contraception issue had become more pro-life in nature. In their publication *Why you should oppose contraception*, they focused on two reasons why contraceptives were wrong: the first being that 'many so-called contraceptives are in fact abortifacients and human life is so precious that nobody has the right to kill' and secondly that the introduction of artificial contraception would bring 'so many other evils in its wake', leading to rising rates of extra-marital sex, promiscuity, VD and illegitimacy and eventually the introduction of abortion in order to cover contraceptive failure.[94] The IFL was convinced that the majority of the population did not want contraception to be legalised and felt that a referendum would illustrate

[91] *Ibid.*, pp. 4–6.   [92] *Ibid.*, pp. 5-6.   [93] *Alert: Oral Contraceptive*, p. 10.
[94] *Why You Should Oppose Contraception* (IFL, 1976).

this. Contraception was viewed as being 'the wedge to break Ireland's Catholic heritage' and readers were advised to oppose it for the sake of their children.[95]

The IFL believed that family planning groups were concerned with the profits to be made from artificial methods of birth control rather than women's health. In a letter to the *Evening Herald* in 1974, Kennedy asked why family planning clinics in Dublin 'decry the reliability of the natural Billings Ovulation method, yet they claim to help women who have difficulty in achieving pregnancy, obviously they are able to identify the fertile time. What is the factor then which makes them push the artificial methods at all costs?'[96] In a 1976 letter to the *Irish Times*, Kennedy asserted that pills and devices were being 'pushed in this country by concerns whose motivation is purely commercial' and that such concerns were being supported by family planning groups, 'the young people in Irish Women United and by some in the universities'. This meant, in her view, that all publicity was being given to artificial methods and none to natural methods.[97] In addition, Kennedy believed that Irish doctors prioritised prescribing the pill over other forms of contraception:

We have been told by women seeking information on natural methods: 'He would not spend five minutes to discuss the problem with me, but just wanted to write a prescription for the Pill'. Other women have told us that doctors did their best to persuade them to take the Pill when they went for a post-natal check-up, even though these women had not asked for advice and were indeed already adequately spacing their families.[98]

In Kennedy's view, prescribing the contraceptive pill meant that doctors did not have to spend time advising on other methods which would take more explanation. Furthermore, in a letter later that year, Kennedy asserted that she believed there was opposition towards natural methods such as the Billings method because 'there is no money to be made from showing a woman how to learn and use this method'.[99] She also claimed in 1978 that the example of the 'married woman with 10 children and a drunken husband has been dropped in favour of contraceptives for the young and single' because the latter would 'provide a more lucrative market for the trade'.[100]

[95] *Why You Should Oppose Contraception* (IFL, 1976).
[96] 'Question of family planning', *Evening Herald*, 19 October 1974, p. 5.
[97] 'Letters to the editor: Availability of contraceptives', *Irish Times*, 13 February 1976, p. 6.
[98] 'Letters to the editor: Availability of contraceptives', p. 6.
[99] 'Letters to the editor', *Irish Times*, 29 December 1976, p. 9.
[100] 'Letters to the editor', *Irish Times*, 13 June 1978, p. 13.

The activities and letters of the IFL received significant attention. Mrs. Ann Collins from Finglas in Dublin, writing to the *Evening Herald* in 1973, stated that the group had 'a nerve trying to dictate to the Irish people on the very personal matter of family planning. It is the prerogative of myself and every other woman to have the number of children I desire and I don't mean fifteen or sixteen [..] People like Mary Kennedy and John O'Reilly nauseate me, with their puritanical attitudes'.[101] Another frequent opponent was journalist Hilary Boyle, who argued that as a single woman, Kennedy could have no understanding of the challenges facing disadvantaged, married couples. For example, in one letter to the *Irish Press* in 1978, Boyle argued 'if the amount spent by these single women on "false dogmas invented by men" was spent instead on helping the poor get proper homes and to limit their families to the number they can afford to feed and clothe, then one would consider them Christians and worth listening to.' Boyle argued that Kennedy and another advocate of the Billings Method, Sister Mary O'Sullivan, 'cannot fulminate on how wonderful the Billings method is unless they have tried both it and married life'.[102] Such comments clearly impacted on Kennedy. In an interview with the *Irish Press* in 1980, she remarked 'Because you are celibate or because you are not married does not mean you don't have feelings. You still have to get on with people'.[103] Others wrote to newspapers defending the IFL's activities. Following an interview between Mary Kennedy and Rodney Rice on an RTÉ radio programme in 1978, where Rice allegedly shouted down the interviewee, Maureen Fehily from Blackrock wrote to the *Evening Herald* to complain about Rice's impartiality and treatment of Kennedy. She hoped that Kennedy was 'not unduly discouraged; she can rest assured that the majority of people would endorse her views'.[104] Similarly, in August 1978, Marie Dunleavy MacSharry, former secretary of the Nazareth Family Movement, wrote to the *Irish Independent* to complain about Pat Kenny's treatment of Mary Kennedy in an interview on RTÉ radio.[105]

In 1978, the IFL undertook a survey of over 1600 homes in the Dublin (Raheny) constituency of the Minister for Health, which showed that 80% were against the legalisation of contraception.[106] The IFL suggested that the majority of people in the country were opposed to the legalisation of contraception and that a referendum on the subject should be held.

[101] 'Incensed by attitude of Irish Family League', *Evening Herald*, 27 August 1973, p. 10.
[102] 'Letters to the editor', *Irish Press*, 12 April 1978, p. 8.
[103] 'Fighting the lobby', *Irish Press*, 8 October 1980, p. 9.
[104] '"Unseemly display" in RTE interview', *Evening Herald*, 13 April 1978, p. 17.
[105] 'Manners on RTE', *Irish Independent*, 11 August 1978, p. 12.
[106] 'Irish Family League survey', *Irish Press*, 12 December 1978, p. 3.

The IFL met with Charles Haughey, Minister for Health and Social Welfare in July 1978 in order to put their medical, social and demographic objections to the legalisation of contraception.[107] The group was one of a number of groups that met with Haughey.[108] In their meeting with Haughey, the IFL argued that 'laws must be based on fundamental moral principles' and that the government was committed by the Constitution to protecting marriage and the family, both of which, they felt, would be threatened by the legalisation of contraception.[109] They also raised concerns about the power that the bill would place in the hands of the medical profession, arguing that 'in other countries it is the medical profession which performs the millions of abortions carried out'.[110] The IFL and their supporters were also concerned with biases in the media. In 1979, they aired their disappointment at being offered two audience seats for a discussion on the Family Planning Bill, rather than being invited to be on the discussion panel. The IFL stated that they would be boycotting the programme because they felt it would be 'biased toward the pro-contraception lobby'.[111] The IFL also claimed to have collected over 80,000 signatures against the legalisation of contraception.[112]

From 1977, the IFL became a member of the newly founded umbrella group the Council of Social Concern (later COSC) along with the Nazareth Family Movement., the League of Decency, Society to Outlaw Pornography, Parent Concern, Youth Alert, and Veritas Christi.[113] COSC was affiliated with the Knights of St. Columbanus, a Catholic fraternal organisation.[114] According to John O'Reilly, who joined the Knights in the early 1970s 'When the Charlie Haughey Bill on contraception came up, they decided they wanted to set up a committee to sort of reach a decision on stuff that arises'. COSC was chaired by Nial Darragh with O'Reilly acting as vice-chairman and it published a booklet, *The Gift*

[107] 'What we told minister', *Limerick Leader*, 29 July 1978, p. 7.
[108] Haughey met with representatives from the Medico Social Research Board, The Irish Medical Association, the National Health Council, The Pharmaceutical Society of Ireland, the Irish Pharmaceutical Union, The Catholic Hierarchy, the Church of Ireland, the Presbyterian Church, the Methodist Church, the Jewish Representative Body, the Health Boards, the Irish Nurses Organisation, the Association of Social Workers, the IFPA, the Irish Congress of Trade Unions, and representatives of organisations such as NAOMI which promoted the Billings method of family planning. Dáil Éireann debate, 24 October 1978, 308:6, Questions: Availability of Contraceptives.
[109] 'What we told minister', *Limerick Leader*, 29 July 1978, p. 7.
[110] 'Family planning bill', *Irish Press*, 10 April 1979, p. 8.
[111] 'Boycott of RTE by Family League', *Irish Independent*, 18 May 1979, p. 8.
[112] 'No swing to contraception', *Irish Independent*, 26 February 1979, p. 6.
[113] ''Legalised abortion' warning to Haughey', *Irish Independent*, 25 March 1978, p. 9.
[114] O'Reilly, *Masterminds of the Right*, p. 48.

of Life in 1978 which was edited by O'Reilly. The booklet was sent to bishops, politicians and members of the medical profession. Similar to other publications O'Reilly had been involved in, it outlined a number of key arguments against artificial contraception. Conception was deemed to take place at the moment of fertilisation with prevention of this union classed as abortion. Only natural forms of family planning were advocated. Artificial contraceptives were deemed to be damaging to health, unreliable, 'damaging to personality, interpersonal relationships and personal dignity', and 'pushed by profit', while they were also said to cause increases in VD, promiscuity, illegitimacy, abortion and marital breakdown.[115] In relation to the proposals to legalise contraception, the publication argued that the government 'should legislate against the importation of contraceptives for 'free' distribution' and instead provide sponsorship for natural methods of family planning.[116] John O'Reilly explained that 'it was through the Council of Social Concern that we ruminated for instance what was going to happen to stop the further deterioration for instance, after the contraceptive period'.

Members of the IFL, in common with family planning and feminist activists, were disappointed with the 1978 Health (Family Planning Bill). A December 1978 statement read as follows:

The Bill is a nasty offering to the people at the Christmas season, reminding us of Herod and the massacre of the innocents, as Fianna Fail like Judas prepares to betray innocent blood. The Bill is a shamelessly cynical sell-out to the contraceptive trade. There is no pretence of providing any safeguards whatsoever against contraceptives for the unmarried, or to children without the knowledge of their parents. No steps have been taken to ban abortifacients masquerading as contraceptives and in use by the medical profession engaged in contraceptive work.[117]

While the IFL ultimately did not succeed in its key aims around contraception, it did, in John O'Reilly's view, have some success:

I think our main contribution, in hindsight, is very difficult. We obviously didn't fail in the purpose, in its ultimate purpose. The only thing is, I'd say, we did expose a lot of objections to it. That the advantages being touted weren't there. Then I think probably the Taoiseach at the time, actually voting against it, gave it a respectability then, that there are a lot of other people against this as well. The church did speak out afterwards. They published four pamphlets on family planning. I suppose, we found a basis for opposing abortion when it did come along. Doing it at a different level, getting doctors involved and getting lawyers involved.

---

[115] *Gift of Life* (Dublin: Order of Knights of St. Columbanus, 1978), p.1.
[116] *Ibid.*, p. 3.
[117] 'Family plan bill is 'undemocratic', *Cork Examiner*, 29 December 1978, p. 4.

In a letter to the *Irish Independent* in 1979, the IFL was one of a number of groups under the banner of COSC which expressed its indignation at the operation of the illegal CAP shop detailed in Chapter 7, Contraceptives Unlimited. Although a complaint had been lodged about the shop the week it opened, seven weeks later, it continued to operate 'with impunity, despite the fact that those responsible for the operation have stated, in the press, that they are knowingly breaking the law'. Chairman of COSC Nial Darragh expressed his frustration that 'the law should be fragrantly broken, our Constitution violated and the responsibility passed from one to another without any action being taken in the matter is, to say the least, scandalous.'[118] By 1979, the organisations affiliated with COSC also included STOP, Christian Political Action Movement, Mná na hÉireann, Pro Fide and the Concerned Doctors Group.[119] It later became a member of the Pro-Life Amendment Campaign to push for the eighth amendment.

8.3   The Responsible Society

Following the legalisation of contraception for *bona fide* family planning purposes in 1979, conservative groups began to mobilise on the abortion issue. One such group was the Irish branch of the Responsible Society, founded in 1980. The Responsible Society had originally been established in England in 1971 and its key concerns were around issues of sexual morality, and in particular sex education and the morality of young people.[120] The Irish branch was founded following a public meeting in March 1980 where Valerie Riches, of The Responsible Society in England, gave a talk on the theme of 'The Permissive Society and its Lessons for Ireland'. Riches' paper was followed by talks by Professor John Bonnar and Dr. Austin Darragh. Following this event, the group who organised it decided to form an Irish branch of the society. John O'Reilly, who had been chairperson of the IFL, was secretary of the Responsible Society and Bernadette Bonar, a pharmacist, was chairperson, with other committee members including John Lee, Julia Lane, Denis Barror, Brian Forbes, Helen O'Donnell and Sheila Killian.[121] The organisation published a newsletter called *Response* which it sent to members along with the newsletter of the British organisation. According

---

[118] 'Law being held up to ridicule', *Irish Independent*, 25 January 1979, p. 10.

[119] *Ibid.*, p. 10.

[120] Valerie Riches, 'The responsible society', *Journal of the Institute of Health Education*, 11:4, (1973), pp. 20–5.

[121] *Response: newsletter of the Irish Branch of the Responsible Society*, 1:1, Spring 1982, p. 1. With thanks to John O'Reilly.

to John O'Reilly, 'We published about 1500 copies of our *Response* that we sent every quarter. But, we sent them actually to certain politicians and to bishops. We also sent them to some prominent lay people. We'd send round to the people who were on the mailing list'. The Responsible Society focused on a range of moral issues including primarily abortion, sex education, divorce, and later AIDS and IVF but for the purposes of this chapter, I will focus on their work on the contraception issue.

In common with the previous groups, the Responsible Society was inspired by the work of conservative campaigners both in the United Kingdom and United States. Bernadette Bonar, the chairperson of the Irish branch of the Responsible Society, explained to me:

That was an English organisation and they were very concerned about what was happening there. Increase in promiscuity and that which was being promoted and dishing contraceptives to young people. If you're dishing out contraceptives for young people, for youth isn't it? Promiscuity, yeah. They were very concerned about that. They were also terribly concerned about sex education in the schools. The parents were really conned there. Parents thought it was teaching them to be chaste and to be self-respecting and so on and so forth. It was about how to use the condoms. Just so ugly. So evil. That was all coming from Planned Parenthood.

Bonar was concerned that similar practices could occur in Ireland. When I asked if she was worried about this, she told me, 'Oh, we'd no doubt. We had no doubt, no. No doubt in the world'. Moreover, her testimony raises concerns about individualism and the power of governments to introduce legislation relating to moral issues. Using the example of abortion, she stated, 'But you see the English people had no say, that's the important thing there. Neither had the American people. It was foisted on them'. In addition, Bonar expressed her concerns about the increasing liberal attitudes of the medical profession and the impact of the secularisation of Irish society:

I was elected to the Eastern Health Board, as a pharmacy representative. Many a rows there of course about it. Some of the doctors were great, they were very anti-contraception as a conscience issue. It was morally wrong and that. Then as the years go by, you get different doctors in and they kind of go with the flow. There's a decline in religious practise, of course, as well. I suppose you'd have to say that's what guides people, your beliefs. As G.K. Chesterton said, "If you don't believe in God you can then believe in anything".

Father Paul Marx was also invited by the group to give a talk in September 1980 during which he referred to abortion in the United States and Britain, particularly drawing attention to how 'children were encouraged to experiment with sex as a result of lurid sex education courses financed by the State' and how, as a result, 'the incidence of VD, unwanted pregnancy and abortion soared among adolescents'.[122] Professor Charles Rice, of Notre Dame University, the author of a number of pro-life books, provided a lecture on pro-life constitutional amendments to the group in June 1981.[123] Valerie Riches also regularly visited Ireland to give talks on topics such as sex education.[124]

While most of the Responsible Society's energies were focused on the Pro-Life Amendment Campaign in the early 1980s, their newsletters, letters to the press, and public talks also addressed their concerns regarding the liberalisation of the law around contraception. For instance, in 1984, they reported on the government's plans to amend the Family Planning Act so that condoms would be made available in chemists to persons over aged 18 rather than on prescription. The Responsible Society argued that the proposed bill 'would be society's seal of approval on sexual relations outside marriage and all the evils which flow therefrom, illegitimate births, abortions, venereal disease et cetera' and that if the bill passed, 'other 'reforms' such as illegitimacy, adoption and finally Divorce would be considerably easier'.[125] In a talk given to the Women's Political Association in Waterford in 1984, Bernadette Bonar echoed these sentiments and stated that politicians 'have an enormous responsibility to represent the views of the electorate and not be influenced by minority pressure groups who for ideological or commercial reasons seek to destroy the traditional moral values of our Society'.[126] The Responsible Society members were clearly concerned with the issue of young people and promiscuity, believing that the passing of the bill and 'the diversification of outlets is such as to amount to an uncontrollable situation and it is widely admitted that contraceptives for 18 year olds, in practice means 13, 14, 15, 16 and 17 year olds as well.'[127]

It is important to note here that the views of conservative groups were not unusual and were mirrored in the responses of many members of the general public. Surviving correspondence sent to the Irish government indicates that many agreed that the amendment to the Family Planning Act would be a step too far. Nora Hurley, writing to the Taoiseach Garret FitzGerald in 1985, stated that 'this bill can only promote fornication' and 'if this bill is passed, and I hope and pray that Our Blessed Lady will not allow it as it will bring a curse on our beloved country, your chances

---

[122] 'Heartbreak of girls on the abortion trail', *Irish Independent*, 23 September 1980, p. 16.
[123] *Response*, 1:1, Spring 1982, p. 1.   [124] *Ibid.*, 1:2, Summer 1982, p. 1.
[125] *Ibid.*, 3:4, Winter 1984, p. 2.
[126] 'Majority want no change in Contraceptive law', *Munster Express*, 28 December 1984, p. 5.
[127] *Response*, 4:1, (Spring 1985), p. 3.

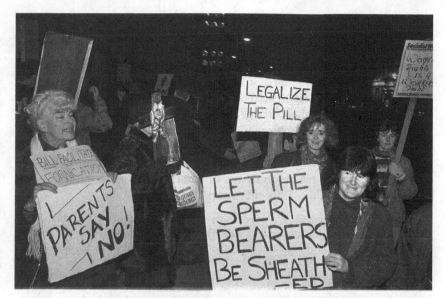

Figure 8.2 Protest at Leinster House/Dáil Éireann during the debate
inside Dáil Éireann on the Health (Family Planning) Amendment.
Protestors from the Socialist Workers Movement came face-to-face with
anti-contraception activists.
Photograph by Derek Speirs.

of winning the next election are nil'.[128] Jerry Gallagher, a retired teacher,
writing to Garret FitzGerald, used stronger language, stating in a typed
letter with the subject 'Re: Family Planning Bill' the brief statement
'Next time I hope Maggie Thatcher disembowels you. Out * Out * Out
*'[129] Similarly, writing to then President Hillery, Maureen Kennedy, the
mother of six children, pleaded for him not to sign the 1985 amendment
to the Family Planning Act, believing it 'will destroy the fabric of our
society and weaken the moral behaviour of our young people, and so,
also undermine the family'.[130] Writing to the Taoiseach in February
1985, Sheila Diskin stated 'I do not consider that young girls should
have use of contraceptives and I think they should only be given by G.P.s
to married people. We have seen the rise in syphilis and V.D. in other

---

[128] Letter from Nora Hurley to Garret FitzGerald, 15 February 1985. [NAI, 2015/88/611].
[129] Letter from Jerry Gallagher, 22 February 1985. [NAI, 2015/88/611].
[130] Letter from Maureen Kennedy to President Hillery. Undated but likely February 1985.
[NAI, 2015/77/94].

countries where they are readily available'.[131] A letter to Minister for Health Barry Desmond from the Society of St. Vincent de Paul Foxrock Conference stated that 'We are greatly concerned and believe that this proposition of yours if implemented, would seriously demoralise our youth and lower the standard of their social behaviour.'[132]

It is clear that the Responsible Society and other conservative groups in the 1980s came together on the issue of abortion. Bernadette Bonar explained that, 'We went completely behind the SPUC. We were clubbed up with them. Joined forces. We had great meetings. Tremendous meetings. Everyone was just ... Marvellous really.' Similarly, John O'Reilly's testimony regarding his involvement in conservative organisations shows the overlap between the different groups:

We were really interlocked. We were really very much interlocked. And later on, not in the beginning for instance, I was Vice Chairman of SPUC Ireland. And I was Secretary of the Responsible Society. And then Vice Chairman of The Council of Social Concern. So, we were very much interlocked.

Ultimately, the campaigns against contraception in the 1970s provided campaigners with the skills, experience and networks which would be crucial to campaigns against abortion in the early 1980s and beyond.

8.4   Conclusion

Anti-contraception campaigners represented an important social movement in 1970s and 1980s Ireland. The arguments put forward by conservative groups are revealing and highlight new ways of thinking about popular individualism in Ireland in this period, illustrating how, as in Britain, by the 1970s, people were becoming more insistent in 'defining and claiming their individual rights, identities and perspectives'.[133] Tools such as petitions and statistical evidence were used to back up activists' arguments, while they also drew on a rhetoric of moral decline and otherness in their publications. They not only indicate deep-rooted tensions around the modernisation of Ireland but also highlight the persistence of early twentieth-century postcolonial ideas that Ireland was under attack from 'foreign' influences, usually Britain.

---

[131] Letter from Sheila Diskin to the Taoiseach Garret FitzGerald, undated, [NAI, 2015/88/611].

[132] Letter from St. Vincent de Paul Foxrock Conference to Barry Desmond, Minister for Health, 11 December,1984. [NAI, 2015/88/611].

[133] Emily Robinson, Camilla Schofield, Florence Sutcliffe-Braithwaite, Natalie Thomlinson, 'Telling stories about post-war Britain: popular individualism and the "crisis" of the 1970s', *Twentieth Century British History*, 28:2, (2017), 268–304, on p.302.

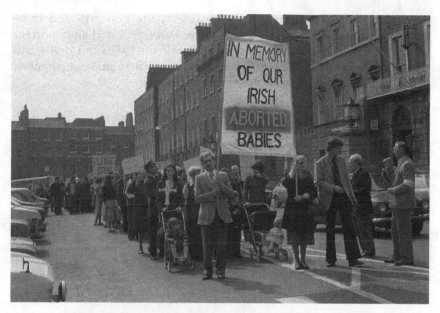

Figure 8.3 Pro-life march and rally, GPO, Dublin, 12 May 1979.
Photograph by Clodagh Boyd.

Anti-contraception groups in Ireland which emerged in the 1970s were
concerned with a number of issues. Earlier groups such as Mná na
hÉireann and the Nazareth Family Movement focused on a nationalist
rhetoric that prioritised Catholic values and a vision of a morally pure
Ireland, in contrast with Britain. As such, their campaigns had echoes of
the anti-contraception rhetoric of the 1930s which classed contraception
as a 'foreign' influence. With the establishment of the Irish Family
League and engagement of individuals such as John O'Reilly, the anti-
contraception arguments focused on the health risks of artificial contraception and concerns that its legislation would lead to other perceived
social evils, in particular abortion. Yet, groups such as the Irish Family
League and the Responsible Society were also influenced by the work of
conservative groups in the United States and United Kingdom and these
transnational networks were important to the trajectories of these groups.
    Moving into the 1980s, the perceived moral decline of young people was
an important theme in campaigners' propaganda, reflecting fears about
the expansion of access to contraception which they believed would
result in increased promiscuity. However, at the heart of campaigners'
concerns was a fear that following the legalisation of contraception, abortion would follow. While the Family Planning Act of 1979 was a significant

disappointment to conservative campaigners, the networks and campaigns formed against contraception in the 1970s provided an important bedrock for anti-abortion campaigns to follow in the 1980s and 1990s, and also enabled activists to form key alliances with international campaigners, which would prove crucial to these later campaigns.

9 Family Planning after the Family Planning Act
Access to Contraception in 1980s and 1990s Ireland

In November 1980, Margaret Farrelly was interviewed for the RTÉ programme 'Today Tonight'. Farrelly, who lived in Ballyfermot, Dublin, had married at 16, and had fourteen children between the ages of 4 and 24. It was reported that Margaret had seventeen pregnancies in twenty years, with three of the children not surviving. Farrelly had tried to use the safe period, unsuccessfully, stating 'There are still a few safe period babies there, it doesn't work for everybody'. Speaking to the reporter Joe Little, she explained, 'It's not something you're looking for, to keep having babies every year. No break at all for yourself. Social life ... always in the kitchen with them, going after them, you know?' Farrelly also spoke about the economic toll of raising so many children, stating, 'That takes me out to the pin of my collar, you know. And there are waiting days, when you're waiting for your husband to come in with the few bob'. She also reflected on the emotional toll fear of pregnancy had on a marriage, stating, 'it would cause a lot of discomfort in the home, and trouble, it would. You know, like, you'd be frightened every month, let's face it, that you're going to become pregnant'. Farrelly's statement echoed the accounts of Irish women throughout the twentieth century, but unlike these women, from 1980, she could legally access contraception as a result of the 1979 Health (Family Planning) Act which made contraception legal for *bona fide* family planning purposes, although access remained patchy. Farrelly was prescribed the pill by her GP, Dr. Paddy Leahy, and justified her decision for economic reasons, recognising that she could go on to have four or five more children.[1]

The same month as Margaret's interview, Charles Haughey delivered the opening address at the national forum organised by the Council for the Status of Women on the United Nations Decade for Women. A group of women protestors, including members of CAP, announced

[1] 'Today Tonight', broadcast on RTÉ, 8 November 1980. Accessed : https://www.rte.ie/archives/2020/1029/1174622-family-planning-access/

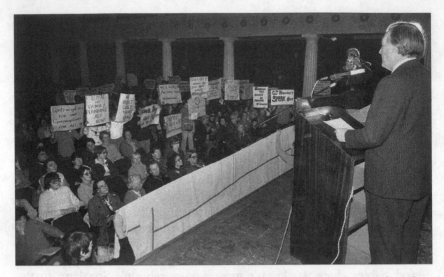

Figure 9.1 Protest during Taoiseach Charlie Haughey's speech at the opening of the National Forum on the UN Decade for Women 1975–85, Dublin, 15 November 1980.
Photograph by Derek Speirs.

earlier in the day that they planned to protest when Haughey arrived by throwing condoms at him. Haughey instead entered through a side door and the protest was abandoned. However, as soon as he rose to speak, a group of thirty female protestors stood up in the audience with posters relating to contraception (Figure 9.1). A CAP banner was unfurled as well as another printed on clear plastic which read 'Women's right to choose – clingfilm, Irish solution to an Irish problem'. Other placards called for the repeal of the Family Planning Act, with slogans such as 'Keep your filthy laws off my body' and 'Article 44 is alive and well and living in the Family Planning Act'. A newspaper account stated that Haughey ignored the protests and 'read straight through his script' despite some heckling at certain points.[2] While Haughey was apparently unfazed by the demonstrators, these protests drew attention at an early stage to the clear problems with the Family Planning Act, which would have implications for Irish men and women across the country trying to access contraception in the 1980s.

As this chapter will show, in agreement with Brian Girvin, the Family Planning Act of 1979 was not a turning point in the history of

[2] Forum on the status of women: Haughey heckled', *Irish Times*, 17 November 1980, p. 6.

contraception.[3] The Act was restrictive and its stipulation that contraception could only be obtained for *bona fide* family planning purposes, was widely interpreted as meaning that only married couples could access it. Chrystel Hug has suggested that the act 'seems to have closed more doors than it opened, on paper anyway', pointing also to the doubling of the price of condoms overnight from £1.60 to £3.45.[4] Notably, the Act did not contain any provision relating to male and female sterilisation, an issue raised by TDs Dr. Noel Browne and Dr. John O'Connell during the debates over the bill.[5]

More widely, if anything, the 1980s and early 1990s represented a period of intense sexual repression in Ireland including divisive referendums over abortion (1983; 1992) and divorce (1986; 1995).[6] As mentioned in Chapter 7, 1984 was witness to two painful cases in Ireland which exemplify the impact of the sexually repressive environment. The first was the death of Ann Lovett, a 15-year-old schoolgirl, who died after giving birth to a stillborn baby at a grotto in Granard, Co. Longford, in January 1984.[7] The second was the Kerry Babies case, a 17-week inquiry after two new-born babies were found dead within 100 km of each other in April 1984. Joanne Hayes, the mother who had concealed one of the babies, was arrested and charged with murder of the other baby. It was claimed erroneously during the case that she was also the mother of the second baby.[8] More broadly, AIDS was first reported in Ireland in 1982, but as Ann Nolan has shown, and as was the case in the UK and US, the Irish government was very slow to address the AIDS issue. In Ireland, it was activist groups such as Gay Health Action who first responded to the AIDS crisis; there were no substantial government AIDS public health campaigns until the 1990s.[9]

This chapter shows that following the introduction of the Family Planning Act, very little changed in relation to access to contraception. Individuals were still reliant on a sympathetic doctor and a chemist that would stock contraceptives. Moreover, into the 1980s and 1990s, class, location, and age had a significant impact on access. As the case of tubal ligation shows, the UK continued to be relied upon for Irish women's reproductive healthcare. This chapter argues that direct challenges to the

---

[3] Girvin, 'An Irish solution', p. 3.   [4] Hug, *The Politics of Sexual Morality*, p. 114.
[5] Health (Family Planning) Bill, 1978: Committee Stage, Dáil Éireann Debate, 9 May 1979. Accessed: https://www.oireachtas.ie/en/debates/debate/dail/1979-05-09/8
[6] Diarmaid Ferriter, *Ambiguous Republic, Ireland in the 1970s* (London, Profile Books, 2012), p. 679.
[7] Hug, *The Politics of Sexual Morality*, p. 121.
[8] See: Nell McCafferty, *A Woman to Blame: The Kerry Babies Case* (Dublin, 1985).
[9] Ann Nolan, 'The Gay Community Response to the Emergence of AIDS in Ireland'.

law by activists such as Condom Sense and the IFPA youth group highlighted the problems with the law and ultimately helped to act as a catalyst for its liberalisation in 1993.

9.1   Problems with the 1979 Act

The Family Planning Act undoubtedly strengthened doctors' authority over the provision of contraception and further cemented the class divide with regard to access. Writing in *Socialist Republic* in 1980, CAP member, Jacinta Deignan, commented that:

the new law will make it harder to get contraception and advice. For condoms, cream, etc., you will need a doctor's prescription. This will cost money and so will the chemist's fee. Medical card users will not be able to obtain contraceptives free under the new law.[10]

Yet, many members of the medical profession were also unhappy with the legislation. In the *Journal of the Irish Medical Association* in January 1979 it was reported that 'doctors feel affronted by the provision that the use of contraceptives has to be authorised by a registered general practitioner', and that the proposed law would make the medical profession 'the sole instrument of the State in the regulation of the supply of contraceptives'. They noted that the decision to use contraceptives had 'nothing to do with medicine'.[11] Writing to the *Journal* later that year, Arthur Barry stated that 'doctors are to become common hucksters of contraceptive devices, etc.'.[12]

Some doctors also refused to provide contraception on moral grounds. Section 11 of the 1979 Act included a clause related to Conscientious Objection which stated: 'Nothing in this Act shall be construed as obliging any person to take part in the provision of a family planning service, the giving of prescriptions or authorisations for the purposes of this Act, or the sale, importation into the State, manufacture, advertising or display of contraceptives'.[13] This meant that doctors and chemists could also refuse to provide contraception on moral grounds. Indeed, it appears from oral testimony, that some doctors continued to refuse to dispense the contraceptive pill for this reason.

[10] 'Contraception laws out!', *Socialist Republic: Paper of People's Democracy*, 3:5, (1980), p. 6. With thanks to Niall Meehan.

[11] 'Health (Family Planning) Bill, 1978', *Journal of the Irish Medical Association*, 12 January 1979, 72:1, p. 1.

[12] 'Letters to the editor', *Journal of the Irish Medical Association*, 16 February 1979, 72:2, p. 52.

[13] Health (Family Planning Act), 1979. Accessed: http://www.irishstatutebook.ie/eli/1979/act/20/enacted/en/print

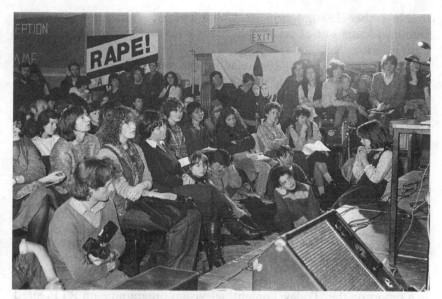

Figure 9.2 CAP anti-bill demo Junior Commons Room, Trinity College Dublin, November 1980.

Dr. Paddy Leahy, a Ballyfermot GP, was one of the few vocal voices from the medical profession to criticise the Family Planning Act. He denounced his fellow members of the medical profession for failing to speak out against the legislation and to discuss the issue at the Medical Union Conference, stating, 'Most of them are behaving like a crowd of overgrown altar boys. I never thought the day would come when I would be ashamed to be a member of the medical profession. But Irishwomen are now being degraded by pompous prigs sitting behind their desks with a few letters after their names and hiding behind the so-called conscience clause in this absurd Act'.[14] A well-attended meeting was held at TCD on 1 November 1980 under the banner of 'Contraception – Access for All', a new group set up by CAP and other campaigners (Figure 9.2). Speakers at the meeting included Senator Catherine McGuinness and Paddy Leahy. Leahy asserted, 'I shall continue to run my practice my way, I shall continue to give contraceptives to all and sundry who want them and need them'.[15] The profession was clearly divided, however.

[14] 'Defiant doctor prepared to go to jail', *Irish Times*, 31 October 1980, p. 6.
[15] 'Today Tonight', broadcast on RTÉ, 8 November 1980. Accessed : https://www.rte.ie/archives/2020/1029/1174622-family-planning-access

In November 1980, journalist Colm Toibin, discovered that three Dublin doctors out of six that he visited refused to provide him with contraception.[16]

For young people in 1980s Ireland there were limited ways of getting access to contraception and sexual health information. According to Jon O'Brien, who had been IFPA Youth Officer and later Education Officer, 'the chilling effect of the Irish solution to the Irish problem was that in the family planning clinics the feeling was, you couldn't just go in and get contraceptives, you had to be married. There was a fear that they would be judgemental'. Obtaining contraception was a challenge. O'Brien's testimony illuminates the rigmarole involved:

You know...what you had to do if you wanted to have sex, you had to go to the doctor. The doctor if he thought you needed them for *bona fide* family planning purposes would write you a prescription. The doctor was not supposed to give you the condoms. You'd then have to go to the pharmacist, the pharmacist then...if the pharmacist agreed with you and the pharmacist had them in stock, you'd get the condoms.

In a report on the 'Today Tonight' television programme on RTÉ, aired on 6 November 1980, reporter Joe Little found that three chemists he visited in Ranelagh did not stock contraceptives; one of the chemists stated explicitly that this was on conscientious grounds.[17] A survey begun by Minister for Health Michael Woods, and concluded by his successor Barry Desmond in 1983, found that only 300 of the 1,100 chemists in the country stocked and sold non-medical contraceptives.[18]

Family planning clinics continued to operate largely as normal, and they did not differentiate between married and single people. Cathie Chappell recalled the reaction of the LFPC to the Family Planning Act: 'I think we just laughed. It was ridiculous. I don't think it affected us at all really'. Brian Leonard (GFPC) stated, 'The law then changed to make condoms legal if you got a medical prescription, but only if you were married, of course. Which was one move. We weren't bothered by that nonsense, obviously. People came along wanting condoms, they got condoms.'

Yet for people living in rural areas, access continued to be challenging. In November 1984, the Tralee Women's Group announced plans to set up an information service in the town on all methods of contraception as well as other aspects of women's health. The spokesperson for the group,

---

[16] Jean Simms, 'Returning home', *Wimmin*, 1:1, (December 1981), p. 7.

[17] 'Today Tonight', broadcast on RTÉ, 8 November 1980.

[18] 'Family plan bill debate: no time now for a cop-out', *Irish Independent*, 7 February 1985, p. 8.

Marguerite Egan, pointed to the need for a service in Tralee, suggesting that in relation to contraceptives: 'You would think they were explosives the way they are treated'. Egan stated that women found out information through the grapevine about which doctors and chemists to go to in order to obtain contraception. Men and women who could afford to do so, travelled to Cork or Limerick to avail themselves of family planning services there, meaning that, in Egan's words, 'The people who can least afford to travel are the people who can least afford to have children'.[19] An article by Marianne Heron in the *Irish Independent* in 1984, also outlined the key failings of the act. She suggested that there were 'contraceptive blackspots' around the country, in particular in the Midlands, Sligo and Kerry, where people needed to travel to the nearest urban centre to obtain supplies, and that access to non-medical contraceptives was particularly poor in the Midlands, Cavan, the north-west, Wexford, Donegal and Kerry. She stated that 'in rural areas the great majority of pharmacists are not operating the law, presumably for reasons of conscience', pointing to Tralee, where only two out of nine chemists stocked non-medical contraceptives. In addition, 'the proportion of doctors not cooperating with the scheme is also higher in rural areas and rather than risk a rebuff, or possibly even a moral lecture, a number of people prefer to travel to the nearest family planning clinic or to try to obtain supplies through the post'. Contraception was also not available through the medical card scheme, meaning 'a growing number of people who want to use family planning cannot afford it', but some doctors navigated this issue by prescribing the pill as a cycle regulator to medical card holders.[20]

Essentially, all of this meant that well into the 1980s, and beyond, many Irish men and women were still having to travel for contraception or advice on family planning due to a failure on the part of chemists or doctors to provide these services locally, while those in lower income groups continued to be the most affected by the restrictions of the law.

There were some important challenges to the law. Some family planning clinics and student unions installed condom vending machines.[21] For example, the TCD SRC installed a condoms vending machine in 1979.[22] Brendan Smith, then president of the UCG Student union, made condoms available through the Student Union on Valentine's Day 1981, recalling, 'It was illegal to sell condoms but we were selling them every day, actually. And every so often, the college told us we

---

[19] 'Family planning centre for Tralee?', *Kerryman*, 23 November 1984, pp. 1 and 20.
[20] 'Why Irish solution to Irish problem has failed', *Irish Independent*, 29 June 1984, p. 6.
[21] Cloatre and Enright, 'Transformative illegality', p. 276.
[22] Conlon, *The Irish Student Movement*, p. 172.

couldn't do it, so we said fine. But we still did it, you know?' And, in 1982 Dr. Andrew Rynne deliberately sold condoms from his surgery over a weekend in order to directly challenge the law. Rynne was fined £300 at Naas district court in June 1983.[23]

In December 1982, when Barry Desmond was appointed Minister for Health, the government decided to amend the family planning legislation due to recognition that there were no official figures on the numbers of chemists who sold contraceptives, and that there 'was a strong group within the chemists' organisation that encouraged chemists not to sell them'. The amendment would remove the need for a prescription for non-medical contraceptives and also mean that they could be sold not only through chemists, but through family planning clinics, health centres, medical practitioners' surgeries and specified hospitals.[24] Yet, the amendment fell short of allowing contraceptives to be allowed on the medical card. Interviewed by the *Irish Times* in 1989, Jon O'Brien, then IFPA press officer, stated that in that in 1988, almost 12 per cent of first-time attendees at the IFPA clinics in Dublin 'did not have the financial means to exercise the right to control their fertility' and as a result, were treated for free.[25]

While it only resulted in a minor change to the law, the amendment to the 1979 act was controversial, and as mentioned in the previous chapter, letters to the government highlight individuals' concerns around young people and increased promiscuity. Others saw the legislation as an important way for the government to assert its separation from the Church. Tom Fahey from Tipperary, wrote to the Taoiseach in February 1985, to say 'please do not allow yourself and your government be pressurised by the Bishops on the contraceptive legislation', arguing that 'it is time that Dáil Éireann asserted its independence of the Church'.[26] Vivian and Mary Tarrant, also writing to the Taoiseach, said that they fully supported him in his 'courageous work for a new and better Ireland'.[27] Mona Farrell, wrote 'the family planning act must go through, because if the Church wins yet another battle against the people – predominantly against the women of Ireland – then democracy is gone and we will all again live in a society based on fear of the 'belt of the crozier'.'[28]

[23] Ferriter, *Occasions of Sin*, p. 425.   [24] Desmond, *Finally and in Conclusion*, p. 237.

[25] '"Irish solution" has little to offer on family planning', *Irish Times*, 5 June 1989, 2.

[26] Letter from Tom Fahey to the Taoiseach Garret FitzGerald, 11 February 1985. [NAI, 2015/88/611].

[27] Letter from Vivian and Mary Tarrant to the Taoiseach Garret FitzGerald, 17 February 1985. [NAI, 2015/88/611].

[28] Letter from Mona Farrell to the Taoiseach Garret FitzGerald, 15 February 1985. [NAI, 2015/88/611].

9.2 Access to Artificial Contraceptives: The Role of Chemists

Even after the 1985 amendment to the Family Planning Act, some Irish chemists still did not stock condoms. As Emilie Cloatre and Máiréad Enright have argued, while condoms were legally available from pharmacists under the 1985 law, they were rarely on display. The profession was generally conservative and many pharmacists were initially opposed to the sale of condoms. This meant that 'purchasing could be a furtive, secretive experience' and customers 'often associated a visit to the pharmacy with shaming, judgement and the risk of arbitrary refusal of service'.[29] In 1986, it was reported that less than one-quarter of pharmacies in Kerry stocked non-medical contraceptives, a total of 9 out of 40.[30] Moreover, a number of oral history respondents had issues in gaining access from their local chemist. Anne Roper, a health counsellor with the WWC, published a handbook on women's health called *Woman to Woman* in 1986 which included a list of chemists which were willing to advertise that they dispensed contraceptives. The Irish Medical Council refused to provide Roper with a list of 'sympathetic doctors' on 'ethical grounds'.[31] The handbook listed two chemists in Limerick, one in Meath, one in Louth, two in Castlebar, one in Birr, one in Athlone and one in Athenry, which were willing to advertise that they provided contraceptive supplies.[32]

However, many chemists were resistant to change. In an interview with Maurice O'Keeffe, Adare-based chemist, Lizzie O'Dea, recalled a group of Americans calling into the chemist shop she worked in and asking for contraceptives, and her boss telling them, 'Oh, you won't get those in Adare, you'll have to go to Dublin for those'. O'Dea felt that her boss 'was very devout. But by degrees she came round to it ... I'd say "Listen, for God's sake, we'll have to get them because people are coming in asking for them" so she relented and she stocked them after that. But 'twas a hard job, you know'.[33] The views of Michael Payne, a chemist based in Monkstown, Co. Dublin, are perhaps indicative of chemists' wider concerns. Payne wrote to the Taoiseach Liam Cosgrave in

---

[29] Cloatre and Enright, 'Transformative Illegality', p. 269.
[30] 'Nine Kerry chemists keep stocks', *Kerryman*, 7 February 1986, p. 24.
[31] 'Name doctors who advise on contraception, demands health writer', *Irish Independent*, 15 May 1986, p. 3.
[32] Anne Roper, *Woman to Woman: A Health Care Handbook and Directory for Women* (Dublin: Attic Press, 1986), p. 216.
[33] Life and Lore oral history recording by Maurice O'Keeffe with Elizabeth (Lizzie) O'Dea (b.1941). Accessed https://www.irishlifeandlore.com/product/elizabeth-lizzie-odea-b-1941/

1973 after reading reports in the press that the government intended to discuss the private bill relating to contraceptives. Payne stated that 'the Fine Gael representatives in this area gave a clear promise before the Election that the party would not support any change in the law on this matter. It would appear the Nation has now little other vision than Drink and the pursuit of Sex either in or outside marriage'.[34] Payne wrote again, this time to Taoiseach Garret FitzGerald in 1985, when there were ongoing debates about the liberalisation of the law around contraceptives, to state that FitzGerald was 'dedicated to imposing an alien morality on a Catholic people'.[35] Richard Woods, a chemist based in Mullingar, shared Payne's sentiments. He wrote to President Hillery in 1985 to 'delay the signing of the new contraceptive bill as debated in the Dáil last week, until an enquiry can be made to see if it is in accord with the letter and the spirit of the Constitution?' Woods wrote that he had 'never made such an appeal before but I am very worried about the effects that this law would have on the quality of life in this country'.[36]

A report on chemists and non-medical contraceptives in Tipperary in 1985 found that in Clonmel one chemist in the town stocked non-medical contraceptives, none of the three chemists in Cashel stocked them, and only one chemist in Tipperary town stocked them. Medical contraceptives such as the pill were not an issue because, as one chemist stated, 'they have uses other than contraceptive', but according to a Cashel pharmacist, in relation to non-medical contraceptives, 'there's no demand for them, we've had nobody in asking for them – maybe the odd tourist, but we've been able to direct them to Limerick (family planning clinic)'.[37] This testimony again, like others discussed above from chemists, suggests the persistence of the flawed view that the demand for contraception was not coming from Irish people.

It is evident that many men and women travelled to a family planning clinic to guarantee that they would secure contraception, rather than risk going to their local doctor or chemist. Brenda Moore-McCann, who worked as a doctor at FPS and later became its medical director recalled how the clinic attracted clients from outside the Dublin area:

---

[34] Letter from Michael Payne to Taoiseach Liam Cosgrave, 12 November 1973, [NAI, 2004/21/461].

[35] Letter from Michael Payne to Taoiseach Garret FitzGerald, 18 February 1985, [NAI, 2015/88/611].

[36] Letter from Richard Woods to President Patrick Hillery, undated but 1985, [NAI, 2015/77/94].

[37] 'What the women of South Tipp are saying about their TDs', *Irish Press*, 20 February 1985, p. 7.

In Family Planning Services, we were very well positioned, Ballsbridge in the basement of one of those big houses as you go down Pembroke Road. I think they are about three or four storey over basement and we were in the basement, so it was discreet. And we were quite near the RDS. I mention that because our patient numbers just jumped every Spring show. You had farmers and country people coming from all over the country to the Spring show and of course, they had the cover, 'I'm going to Dublin for the Spring show'. They could, with discretion go, because many of them were coming from small towns where they knew the doctor, they knew the pharmacist and they couldn't go in and ask for condoms.

Moore-McCann's statement here highlights the real difficulty and persistence of shame in relation to purchasing contraception, in the 1980s and beyond.

Other respondents expressed the embarrassment people felt around going into a chemist to ask for condoms. Jacinta (b.1954) for example, stated, 'But you'd be embarrassed. There's a lot of embarrassment in going to the chemist and they were judgemental as well, some of them'. Embarrassment about sex and asking for contraceptive advice was still an issue for people. A woman, who was planning to marry the following summer, writing to Mary Dowling's advice column in *Woman's Way* in 1984 for example, explained 'Our problem is contraception. The Cathal Brugha Street Family Planning Centre is the nearest to where I live in Dublin, but I would feel embarrassed walking in and I'm ignorant of the methods they offer'.[38] Alison (b.1953) who lived in a rural area in the north of the country, recalled:

I think you could've got condoms in... No, you could've got them in [rural area]. But people, people didn't. You tended to go somewhere where you were... Because [county] is a small rural community. Um, and you're not going to ask for that sort of thing over the counter in... Because it would've been only sold in chemists. You know, so you're not going to do that (laughs).

Instead, Alison and her husband bought condoms over the border.

Similarly, Ted (b.1951) who lived in a village in the west of Ireland, explained that when the Family Planning Act was introduced, 'many chemists wouldn't stock condoms, or wouldn't fill the prescription. We didn't use condoms, initially, as they were too hard to obtain'. His wife Maria (b.1957) recalled that obtaining condoms 'even into the '80s, it was difficult. Some chemists wouldn't stock them. [...] I remember being out of condoms one night. There was a weekend coming up, and Ted and I cycling round trying to get condoms. The family planning clinic was closed or something'.

[38] 'Getting things straight', *Woman's Way*, 16 November 1984, 53.

Gerry Curran, a member of the IFPA youth group, who would go on to be involved in the Virgin Condom case, similarly recalled:

A lot of pharmacies wouldn't sell them. Even into the '90s, there were pharmacies in Ireland that wouldn't sell them. I went into a pharmacy in Dundalk one day, because I was going to the local school to talk to them about contraception and I hadn't got a packet of condoms. I went in, 'Can I have a small packet of condoms?' 'We don't sell that sort of thing here'. That was the mid '90s. The girl who was working there gave me the eye, she said, 'Around the corner, they sell them at the chemist around the corner'.

Young Irish men and women were particularly penalised by this legislation. Writing in *Hot Press* in 1989, editor Niall Stokes remarked that the existing Irish law meant that 'those most in need of access to condoms – sexually active single people in their late teens and early twenties – inevitably finding them most difficult to obtain'.[39] Moreover, he added 'it is only the rare exceptions who are yet possessed of the audacity to step up to the chemists counter in a small town and ask for a couple of packets of Durex'.[40]

In addition, asking for condoms may have been particularly embarrassing in a small-town chemist. Colette (b.1946) and her husband, who had five children, began using condoms around 1991. She recalled, 'Our local chemist sold them, would only give them to you if you were married. They weren't on display in the shop'. She explained that customers had to ask for the condoms because they were kept under the counter. Ellen (b.1949) who lived in the rural south-east described one experience she had of buying condoms:

So I have six children all together, and sometimes we did use condoms for a while, but even at that, I wouldn't go into the local shop to buy them. And I remember going into a shop in [nearest city] one day, I thought they wouldn't know me in there and this woman came over, she was an older woman, and she came over all smiles and all lovely to me, and I said 'Can I have a packet of condoms please?' And her face changed straight away. She got very... she kind of threw them at me. But they weren't... it wasn't the thing to do.

She further explained, 'You just felt guilty, you'd feel bad about getting it. As I said, I wouldn't go in locally because you didn't want anybody to know what you were doing'.

9.3   1990s Activism

A condom counter was set up by the IFPA in the Virgin Megastore, Dublin on Friday, 13 February 1988 in order to challenge the law on

---

[39] 'Special Sex Aid Supplement', *Hot Press*, 9 March 1989, no page number.   [40] *Ibid.*

where condoms could be sold, with the hope that as in previous cases, the law would be changed as a result.[41] The proceeds of condom sales went to Richard Branson's Virgin Health Foundation to be spent on AIDS research. The IFPA youth group was responsible for selling the condoms. This group had been established in spring 1984 by Dr. Mary Short and Christine Donaghy, then IFPA Information and Education Officer, who realised that there was a 'need for a more direct and informal approach to young people ... we believed that we needed to involve young people in their own education'.[42] Over the course of its existence, members of the youth group, who were all young volunteers in their late teens and early twenties, ran a phone line called the Adolescent Confidential Telephone Line for support on sexual health matters, as well as a Young People's Family Planning Centre. They also provided advice through agony aunt columns in *Hot Press* and *Fresh* magazine and gave talks to local youth groups on sexual health.

By 1988, the IFPA was viewed as being in danger of being perceived as an outdated group among young adults; legislation around contraception was regarded as insufficient; and finally, the government's response to the AIDS crisis was believed to be inadequate. The IFPA recognised that it would be an ideal public relations opportunity if they were to sell condoms at the Virgin Megastore in Dublin and be prosecuted. Moreover, as Cloatre and Enright have argued, through this action, the IFPA could dismantle the structures around the selling of condoms, 'making open, visible, public sale the new norm'.[43] The IFPA chose to emphasise that they believed that it was the prophylactic rather than contraceptive use of condoms that they were most concerned about, especially in the era of AIDS.

The opening of the condom counter generated criticism from the chairperson of conservative group, Family Solidarity, Dick Hogan, who commented:

I think it is a very cheap shot. Many of the youngsters who buy records in that shop are as young as 12 or 13 years. I'd like to know how they intend to discriminate. Will they insist on checking birth certificates or will they just sell them to anyone?[44]

---

[41] Public relations case history: 'The Condom Controversy': Project 1, Year 2, P.R.I.I. Report by Jon O'Brien, Information/Press Officer, IFPA, 10 March 1990. [IFPA Archives].

[42] Jon O'Brien, *Young People & Family Planning: The Learning Experience of the Irish Family Planning Association, 1984–1990* (project report, c.1990), p. 4. Courtesy of Jon O'Brien.

[43] Cloatre and Enright, 'Transformative illegality', p. 268.

[44] 'Branson condoms plan attacked', *Evening Press*, 30 January 1988.

Similarly, in a letter to the *Irish Examiner* in 1988, secretary of the Responsible Society, John O'Reilly condemned the 'sales outlet for contraceptives in the Virgin Megastore where youngsters from eight upwards go to buy their record albums'. O'Reilly suggested that 'judging from its actions, the IFPA and its ilk worldwide has a code of morality all its own'.[45] These letters highlight continued fears about young people and sexuality. In an interview with *Hot Press* magazine in 1991, Bernadette Bonar of the Responsible Society stated 'I'm concerned with the youth who are being misled. There's already plenty of access to condoms, they're all over the place, in Family Planning Clinics and Pharmacies. Is that not enough?'[46]

While their actions were illegal, former IFPA youth group members expressed that they were not afraid of being arrested. John Callaghan stated:

We all knew that the optics of arresting a 19-year-old for selling condoms to a 17-year-old in the Virgin Megastore was nothing, it was toxic, that nobody wanted to touch it. So while we knew technically it was possible, I don't think any of us believed it was going to happen.

Gerry Curran explained the rationale behind the stunt, as well as the excitement he felt being involved in it:

It was certainly to raise awareness. It wasn't put there to be prosecuted, it was put there to first of all, provide for a very real need. 'Cause there was an extraordinarily real need for people to access contraception. It was put there to test the law, to see, did it extend to a licence of a pharmacy, or did it have to be sold in a physical pharmacy? It was certainly put there to test the law. It was certainly put there to highlight the issue of the ludicrous nature of the law. Now, when you look back now, it was always going to be the case that the state would intervene. That the guards would have to intervene from a complaint of the Attorney General, or whoever it was, was our moral overseer at the time, looking back on it now. At 20 odd years of age, I'm sure there was only a great sense of excitement. 'Oh, here we go. We're getting lagged.' No, it didn't bother us in the least.

In 1989, approximately 3,249 people availed of the condom counter service, with the annual report that year commenting that there was an increase during holiday periods 'suggesting that at these times people from rural areas tend to use the service while visiting Dublin'. 90% of condoms were sold to men, and 50% of clients were aged 18–25.[47] Jon O'Brien stated:

---

[45] 'Morality and contraception', *Irish Examiner*, 15 August 1988, p. 6.
[46] 'It's the end of the world as we know it', *Hot Press*, 21 March 1991, p. 7.
[47] *IFPA Annual Report, 1989*, pp. 7–8.

The interesting thing was young people did come along to buy them, but people came from all over the bloody country to buy them and they weren't all young people. Basically, older people were pissed off too.

IFPA youth group member, Joanne, explained that she was surprised at the popularity of the counter: 'And I was quite amazed actually because I was thinking at first, people won't be confident in a public place to be coming up to a counter, but we did get very busy'. She did recall, however:

there were some people who would go by and give a disdainful look or say, 'You really shouldn't be doing this'. And I know there was a set-up at one stage, I can't remember which group it was, sent in I think a 15-year-old to buy condoms, and of course, they were sold the condoms and all hell broke loose.

However, there were no arrests made and it was a full eighteen months before legal action was taken against the IFPA. According to Callaghan:

I guess what we'd shown is, there was no will on the part of the legal authorities or even the more conservative groups to challenge this. Really, by proving this and by doing it over a period of time it became apparent that the ban on the sale of condoms was hollow, that we could, that they could be sold pretty much anywhere.

Christine Donaghy recalled the moment when the Gardaí moved to prosecute and her real fears that she would go to prison:

The, I suppose a sergeant or, they were detective in their plain clothes who came in and questioned me and did I recognise these condoms, and were we selling condoms in the Virgin Megastore, and I said, 'yes, and they're on prescription, and they're agents of ours', or whatever. Anyway, it went to court, and the judge found us ... It was very serious at the time because I was the person who was representing the IFPA, so I was the person ... The barrister worked out that I was the one that would go to prison. I had a dog at the time and I lived on my own. I remember thinking, 'What the hell am I going to do?'

In the ensuing case, the IFPA was fined £400 for the condom counter activities. The court case to appeal the fine which occurred in 1991 attracted significant media attention and was reported internationally. The IFPA argued that they were not selling contraceptives, but prophylactics. While the court case was taking place, members of the Dublin AIDS Coalition to Unleash Power (ACT UP) organised a 'picket with a difference', dressed as condoms and handed out HIV/AIDS information and free condoms.[48] Among those who testified were Malcolm Potts, an American gynaecologist, and a young haemophiliac man who

---

[48] ACT-UP press statement, 14 February 1991 [IFPA Archive]. 'Condom-clad protesters greet Virgin boss at court', *Irish Press*, 15 February 1991, p. 3.

had HIV who testified that he had bought the condoms from the Virgin
Megastore as a prophylactic rather than a contraceptive, as he had
already had had vasectomy. Richard Branson, the owner of Virgin, also
testified that he believed that the condoms were being sold for their
prophylactic function. According to O'Brien:

It was hilarious, the journalists were falling around laughing. The judge was
banging the gavel telling everyone he'd clear the courtroom if we all didn't shut
up. Outside there was all the AIDS activists going bonkers. So it was all very
exciting … the judge informed us, in giving his decision, he informed us that he
had just taken Holy Communion that morning and he thought we were a filthy
bunch of people. He found us guilty, very guilty. He fined us and he told us that
they would keep increasing the fines and you know, every week or every day or
whatever, which would cost us a small fortune.

The appeal judge increased the fine to £500 and as the law stood, each
further condom sale could lead to a £5,000 fine, with an additional fine
of £250 for every day that condoms remained on sale.[49] An important
milestone in the case was when the rock band U2 agreed to pay the fine
on behalf of the IFPA and issued a press release supporting
the organisation.

Following this court case, there was a delay before the government
began to move to amend the 1985 legislation. In 1992, a short direct
action campaign, Condom Sense, was launched on Valentine's Day
1992. Condom Sense activists installed 140 condom vending machines
in pubs and nightclubs around Ireland in order to challenge the law on
the sale of condoms, arguing that they were essential for public health
during the AIDS crisis.[50] The campaign was initiated by Clare Watson
and Rachel Martin in Dublin, with regional groups in Cork and Galway.
In an interview with *Hot Press* magazine, Watson explained, 'We're just
fed up and very tired of what's happening or, more correctly, what's not
happening in regard to condom legislation', explaining that 'Our action
is a statement saying, "Look, we need these machines now"'. Martin felt
that vending machines were essential because 'they provide accessibility
and anonymity, they're open when chemists and health centres are
closed and people don't have to show their faces to the local chemist in
order to buy a packet'.[51]

Pete Smith, who had been involved in setting up the GFPC, university
lecturer Angela Savage, and Brendan Smith, who ran Setanta's night

[49] Ferriter, *Occasions of Sin*, p. 426.
[50] Cloatre and Enright, 'Transformative illegality', pp. 273–6.
[51] 'French letter day!', *Hot Press*, 13 February 1992, 16:2, p. 11.

club in Salthill, were the key members of the Galway branch of the Condom Sense campaign. Pete Smith recalled that Brendan Smith:

was the first person who said, 'Yes, you can come into my premises and put them up'. So, we went into his and we put two vending machines in the men's toilet and the women's toilet. And there was another pub in Tuam we did it, we put that in and were supplying.

As mentioned earlier, Brendan Smith had been vice-president of the UCG Student Union, which had sold condoms in 1981. He was also involved in supporting the establishment of GaySoc at the university in 1979 as well as women's groups. As a result of his previous activism, he was keen to get involved in the Condom Sense campaign. Smith explained his motivation was around 'empowering women, giving them the right to control their own pregnancy'.

Angela Savage, a lecturer in chemistry at UCG, had been involved in setting up the AIDS West campaign with Evelyn Stevens, one of the founders of the GFPC. Savage explained that Brendan Smith's night-club, Setanta's

was the only nightclub who would take at the end of the day, who would take the vending machines and so it was really just Pete and myself and Brendan and I would say in reality I would have done a huge amount of the work because the main work was going out every week and stocking the vending machines, so there was one in the ladies and one in the men's and I came up with the idea of installing them on Valentine's Day and Valentine's Day was a Thursday and *The Advertiser* comes out on a Thursday so it was front page in *The Advertiser*.

The activists were actively breaking the law and this came with risks. Savage recalled being told she had been read from the altar at the Galway Novena. She stated:

Now I wasn't – my name wasn't used but anybody who knew me knew exactly who it was but about installing you know vending machines and you know the usual promoting promiscuity and all the rest of it. So, that was kind of the climate there was of, you know, that you were accused of promoting promiscuity and breaking the law and all these sort of things but I knew that I couldn't be fired whereas for Brendan it was his livelihood, you know.

Yet, the campaign ended up being short-lived as a result of a quick change to the law, which came as something of a surprise to the campaigners. According to Pete Smith:

And in many ways it was strange because more or less as soon as we'd done it, they changed the law. So, there we are, really brave, breaking the law, the vanguard of revolution and the whole thing becomes legal.

As Cloatre and Enright have argued, 'Condom Sense's actions piled further pressure onto a system that the Virgin Megastore stall had already weakened. As such actions continued to demonstrate the inadequacies of both the law itself, and its enforcement, the legal system began to respond and adjust'.[52] In 1992, when the act was amended it specified that condoms could be sold to anyone over the age of 17 in most ordinary retail locations, including shops and pubs, however, the act retained an age limit as well as the prohibition on sale of condoms through vending machines. The following year, the age limit for purchase was sold as well as the ban on sale through vending machines.[53]

9.4   Shifts in Contraceptive Practices

The 1980s also witnessed some shifts in contraceptive practices. The morning after pill, for example, a post-coital form of contraception, was first introduced at the WWC in 1980.[54] By 1986, it appears to have been available at all Dublin family planning clinics.[55] However, the introduction of this was not without controversy, with considerable debate over whether the morning after pill was an abortifacient or not.[56] The 1980s also witnessed some resistance to artificial forms of contraception such as the pill and increasing concerns about its side effects. A report by the Irish Medical Association into the side effects of the contraceptive pill, published in 1978, was widely publicised and also helped to bolster fears around this issue.[57] Proponents of natural methods of family planning such as the Billings method, were vocal in outlining the potential dangers of the pill to women's health. Professor John Bonnar, who organised a WHO pilot study on the ovulation method in Ireland, believed that Irish doctors were too readily prescribing the pill to women. In a newspaper article in 1978, he explained his belief that doctors were the subject of 'very sophisticated advertising, saturation mailing, etc.' and that they were being 'bombarded with the benefits of this and the benefits of that. It is not surprising to find that they are prescribing the Pill'. Bonnar felt that doctors were resistant to teaching the ovulation method because women could employ this on their own without needing visits to the

---

[52] Cloatre and Enright, 'Transformative illegality', p. 276.   [53] *Ibid.*, pp. 276–7.
[54] 'Morning after pill', *Status*, December 1981, p. 32.
[55] 'Parents' problems', *Woman's Way*, 20 June 1986, p. 52.
[56] 'Is it contraception or abortion?', *Irish Times*, 22 December 1982, p. 10.
[57] 'Report of the Committee set up by the Executive of the Irish Medical Association to advise on the hazards and side-effects of ovulation suppressants', *Journal of the Irish Medical Association* (supplement), 71:2, (February 1978).

doctor's surgery.[58] In the same article, Mavis Keniry of NAOMI agreed with this perspective, suggesting that so many doctors prescribed the pill because it meant that women would have to keep returning.[59] Keniry also advocated the fact that the natural methods had a financial advantage and could 'be used for a couple's entire fertile life and does not require medication, or doctors'.[60] In an interview in 1978, Keniry explained that many of the women coming to NAOMI classes on the Billings method were doing so as a result of coming off the pill due to negative experiences.[61] During discussions with Minister for Health, Charles Haughey, around the introduction of the Family Planning Bill in 1978, Bonnar recalled feeling 'that natural family planning should also be looked at and doctors aware of it and all the rest of it and, not as a religious issue, but as something people would want'. The Family Planning Act in 1979 provided funding for natural family planning. As Hug has argued 'Haughey knew that his bill would have a greater chance of passing if it showed some goodwill towards the Catholic lobby, hence its sections about natural family planning'.[62] But it is also clear, given the success of lay groups such as NAOMI in the 1980s that there was also a demand for natural methods from some women, who were keen to avoid the side effects of artificial contraception, or wanted to adhere to Catholic teachings.

Women's magazines also featured articles outlining the potential side-effects of the pill. One article in *Woman's Way* in March 1979 interviewed several women who had come off the pill. The journalist, Shirley Johnson, found that most of the women interviewed 'had some instinctive feeling that nature should not be slighted' and expressed concerns that ovulation might 'cease altogether if suppressed for too long'. The women interviewed also reported side effects such as weight gain, low mood, energy and libido.[63] Natural methods of family planning such as the Billings method were put forward by advocates as being safer for a variety of reasons. One publication on natural family planning in 1984 advocated the method because of its lack of cost and that it allowed women to become aware of their cycle. The booklet also argued that the method promoted co-operation between the couple, and gave 'a couple dignity' as it meant that they did not need to be 'overdependent on their doctor, or an outside expert'. The booklet also claimed that when used correctly, it was 'effective and reliable', in 'keeping with a healthy

---

[58] 'The Bill and the doctors' dilemma', *Irish Independent*, 9 March 1978, p. 8.　　[59] *Ibid.*
[60] 'Plea for nature birth plan', *Irish Independent*, 17 February 1978, p. 7.
[61] 'The Bill and the doctors' dilemma', *Irish Independent*, 9 March 1978, p. 8.
[62] Hug, *The Politics of Sexual Morality*, p. 114.
[63] 'Why they came off the pill', *Woman's Way*, 23 March 1979, pp. 12–14.

non-polluting natural way of life' as well as Church teachings, and also allowed for 'more enjoyable and more natural sexual intercourse'.[64] A marriage guidance counsellor interviewed in 1982 explained that 'There's a far more enlightened attitude in many couples in their early twenties towards the whole subject. The possible side effects of the Pill are quite clear to them and many younger men are quite adamant that their wives should not be required to bear the health burden that something like the Pill can impose'.[65] The pill then, began to be seen as a less safe form of contraception, while this quote also highlights the fact that by the 1980s, men's role in sharing responsibility for family planning was beginning to be recognised. Such ideas were reflected in the oral history testimonies. Julie (b.1947) got married in 1982 and did not use the pill because 'I felt that, I just felt the side effects, the risk of... I didn't smoke, neither of us smoked, but I still felt that the risk of clots and things like that. Again I felt that there were so many things, if you were on antibiotics or anything like that, it could disrupt it'. Similarly, in the early 1990s, David (b.1948) decided he would have a vasectomy after he and his wife, Jean, had four children. Jean (b.1953) was taking the pill, and David expressed his concerns about the side effects, stating, 'So eventually I had a vasectomy after we had our fourth. Jean was on the pill, we didn't really want to be continuing for any side effects, any medical reasons that might occur. So I decided, we decided'.

There were also concerns about the IUD. As discussed in the previous chapter, conservative groups argued that the IUD acted as a type of abortifacient. But concerns around the IUD were also generated as a result of the press coverage of the Dalkon Shield case in the 1980s. In the United States, at least fifteen women who had been fitted with the Dalkon Shield IUD died and thousands of others experienced life-threatening infections, miscarriages, chronic pain and infertility as a result of 'wearing a device that was zealously marketed using false information.'[66] The Dalkon Shield was not officially recalled until 1984, although it was removed from use by the IFPA in July 1974.[67] As Holly Marley has noted, the Dalkon Shield became the centre of a 'a worldwide media spectacle. The influential press coverage, highlighting the painful insertions, removals and health consequences that women endured, consequently led to the reputation of the IUD being

---

[64] *How to Use Natural Family Planning* (Dublin: Veritas, 1984), p. 14.
[65] 'Why not the natural way?', *Woman's Way*, 23 April 1982, pp. 10–14.
[66] Takeshita, *The Global Biopolitics of the IUD*, p. 75.
[67] 'Hopes of payment soon for Dalkon victims', *Irish Times*, 15 December 1987, p. 4.

tarnished.'[68] In Ireland, the IFPA estimated that they had fitted 3,008 women with the Dalkon Shield.[69] By 1987 approximately 400 claims were being taken by Irish women against A.H. Robins.[70] It is unclear how many of these claims resulted in compensation for survivors.

9.5   Vasectomy

As Chapter 3 outlined, for the majority of men and women interviewed, it was primarily the woman in the relationship who took responsibility for family planning. However, from the 1980s, with the wider availability of vasectomy, some men, and particularly the younger men of the cohort, increasingly began to take responsibility. This form of sterilisation was used when the couple had decided they had completed their family. In comparison with tubal ligation, vasectomy was a straightforward and relatively short procedure, while tubal ligation was a more invasive procedure requiring a hospital stay.

The IFPA began to offer vasectomies from 1974. Initially, a female surgeon was flown in from England to perform the procedure, however, from 1975, Andrew Rynne, was taken on by the IFPA and performed vasectomies at the IFPA Synge Street clinic. In 1974, 25 vasectomies were carried out by the IFPA, rising to 131 in 1975.[71] In an oral history interview, Andrew Rynne described the stigma around the procedure in the 1970s:

Oh, well of course, the man coming in would almost be wearing a false mask or something really. He was worried. He'd phone us to make sure the coast was clear as it were, make sure we didn't have anyone else from Cahersiveen on the same day and they were coming from you know, from Kerry, from Donegal, from all over Ireland. We were the only show in town. And they were at that time, not unrealistically, concerned that they'd be bumping into people from their home town or anything, so we'd have to make sure they didn't. It was a false fear as it turned out.

Andrew Rynne was asked to publish a paper in *the Irish Medical Journal* on the vasectomies he had been doing at the IFPA Synge Street clinic. He found that the average age of men presenting for vasectomy at that time was 34.9 years and that they had an average of 3.8 children.[72]

[68] Holly Marley, 'A Deadly Depth Charge in Their Wombs'. A Study of the Dalkon Shield and the Culture of IUDs in Great Britain', unpublished MSc dissertation (University of Strathclyde, 2019), p.60.

[69] 'IUD damages', *Irish Times*, 11 July 1986, p. 9.

[70] 'Dalkon shield again', *Irish Times*, 9 November 1987, p. 15.

[71] *IFPA Annual Report, 1974*, p. 4 and *IFPA Annual Report, 1975*, p. 6,

[72] Rynne, *The Vasectomy Doctor*, p. 122.

Given the conservative attitudes towards vasectomy, Rynne had hidden the fact that he was engaged with this work from his parents, however, the article was picked up by the *Sunday World* which published an article with the headline 'Irish doctor sterilises 631 men in Dublin clinic'.[73] His father was particularly upset by the news and had the parish priest come round to talk to Rynne about the matter. Nevertheless, the publicity from the newspaper article meant that more men started to come to the IFPA clinic for the procedure.[74]

Male sterilisation became more common from the 1980s as more family planning clinics began to offer the service. A study of 1,000 cases of vasectomy conducted at FPS between September 1981 and April 1985 ascertained that 69% of clients (690) were aged 30–39 years; 23% were aged 40 years and over (230), and 8% (80) were less than 30 years. On average, clients were married for 11.3 years and had 3.4 children. The main reasons given for having a vasectomy were that the family was complete (976 cases) while 583 clients reported finding an alternative method of contraception unacceptable, 248 reported the 'advancing age of couple', 116 reported that they could not afford any more children. 112 clients stated that they could not cope with any more children, while 97 reported that their wife was in ill-health, 14 wanted to improve the sexual relationship, 3 reported the ill-health of the husband, and 4 reported 'other reasons'. Of these, clients, 26.7% were classed as 'skilled manual', 25.8% as 'white collar', 20.4% as 'lower professional'. Lower percentages came from the social categories of unskilled manual (7.4%), higher professional (5.8%), unclassified (9%), unskilled labour/ unemployed (3.3%) and farmers (2.6%).[75]

Consent was usually required from both the husband and wife for the procedure. Andrew Rynne explained that at the IFPA:

There was two places for the consent form to be signed by him and by her. It was strictly adhered to right into the 80s and 90s even, you know. It became the norm. But I tried to change it as best I could and I certainly, in my own private practice, never insisted on getting a consent from the partner or wife.

As Chapter 3 showed, none of the interviewees born in the 1930s used vasectomy as a form of birth control, likely due to its lack of availability in Ireland. However, the procedure became more common for respondents born in the 1940s and onwards. Five of the forty-five respondents born in the 1940s reported using vasectomy as a form of birth control after the

---

[73] *Ibid.*, p. 122.   [74] *Ibid.*, p. 123.
[75] Brenda Moore-McCann and David Orr, 'Vasectomy in Ireland – 1,000 cases', (Dr. Derek Freedman Papers, UCD).

completion of their family, and three mentioned tubal ligation (a total of 17% using sterilisation). Of the thirty-three respondents born in the 1950s, nine reported vasectomy and six reported tubal ligation (45%). The majority of respondents who attained tubal ligation, had this procedure in the UK or Northern Ireland.

Christine Donaghy, who was Education Officer at the IFPA in the early 1980s, felt that the wider availability of vasectomy was a positive thing in that it meant that men were able to take responsibility for family planning:

It was actually great because, imagine such, just for once, the men were forced because of that. It was them that had to choose to have vasectomies, rather than the women going through a procedure, which was more complicated and medically more dangerous than a vasectomy that we could do in 5 minutes in the Synge Street clinic. There was a far, far higher proportion of men vasectomized than women who had tubal ligations at that time. It was just an interesting sight.

Discussions around vasectomy were often linked to ideas of virility and masculinity. Edward (b.1950) who had a vasectomy, felt 'I think there's a lot of false sort of perceptions about it like. [...] Yeah, you know, it'll diminish your masculinity and all these things. I'd be reasonably practical about things you know. It didn't bother me'. Likewise, another man 'Colin' interviewed by *Woman's Way* in 1988, stated 'A lot of men think I was mad, or jeer me and there are all the old pub jokes that you can imagine, but I think it's about time men grew up about this and played their part'.[76]

Sarah Shropshire's innovative work on the history of vasectomy in Canada has shown how ideas around masculinity played an important role in public perceptions of the procedure. She has suggested that from the 1990s, definitions of masculinity which emphasised sexuality and virility were being replaced by an appreciation of caring, responsible behaviour. Vasectomy came to be seen, not only as acceptable but 'viewed as a marker of masculinity, a father's responsibility to sensibly adopt safe, modern techniques to secure the happiness and well-being of his family'.[77] Oral history testimony highlights that the decision to have a vasectomy was often centred around the husband's consideration

---

[76] 'The permanent contraceptive', *Woman's Way*, 18 March 1988, p. 5.
[77] Sarah Shropshire, 'What's a guy to do?: Contraceptive responsibility, confronting masculinity, and the history of vasectomy in Canada', *Canadian Bulletin of Medical History*, 31:2, (Fall 2014), 161–82, on p. 177.

for their wife's health. Ted (b.1951) had a vasectomy in the late 1980s at his local family planning clinic. He explained, 'Well, condoms weren't that effective and the pill didn't suit my wife and at that stage we definitely didn't want more children. So it seemed the best option'. Christopher (b.1946) decided to have a vasectomy because of the complications his wife had experienced during pregnancy and childbirth. He felt that undergoing another pregnancy was 'putting her life at risk' and that 'My thoughts in life is if you can avoid stress, avoid it, do whatever'. Margaret's (b.1954) husband decided to have a vasectomy after a heart attack in the early 1990s. She said, 'he realised he didn't want to leave me with young children...or the possibility of another child'. She explained, 'he says, "What can we do?" And I say, "Well, I can have my tubes cut, but that's an operation." "Oh", he says, "No, you've been through enough." So he went and had what he had done, it was done in 15 minutes in the Well Woman Centre in Dublin. And it was brilliant'. Margaret's testimony here highlights how her husband's decision to have a vasectomy was based on consideration for her health and well-being.

Additionally, in an era where access to contraception was still limited, even in the 1980s, vasectomy may have been a better alternative and helped to combat the strain that anguish about family planning placed on a marriage. Paula (b.1950) for example, told me that her husband had a vasectomy at their local family planning clinic after the birth of their second child, around 1983. She said 'He just said, "I'm not risking this condom business anymore in this ... two bit culture where we can't get access to condoms, not risking it anymore. I'm having a vasectomy"'. Vasectomy was also a preferable alternative when other forms of contraception were unsatisfactory. John X's account of vasectomy which appeared in *Woman's Way* in 1983 stated 'My wife tried the Pill and got headaches. I bought rubbers and contraceptive foam every so often, as we live near the border. My worldly-wise friends afterwards told me that was a mistake. Pregnancy was confirmed about half-way through the pack. We began to discuss vasectomy in earnest'. Pierce (b.1948) also felt that his decision to have a vasectomy reduced the anxiety he and his wife felt about family planning. He and his wife had tried the temperature method which had failed, his wife had found the coil unsatisfactory, and condoms were difficult to obtain. Pierce also expressed concerns that the pill, while possible to obtain, 'wasn't 100% proof'. After having four children, Pierce decided he would have a vasectomy 'And that, eh, relieved a lot of the stress attached to having a family without ... You know. Because most families that time had anything between, you know, six and ten'.

9.6   Tubal Ligation

Female sterilisation (tubal ligation) was difficult to obtain in Ireland from
the 1970s to the early 1990s. According to *Women's AIM* magazine in
1983, while vasectomy was available at some hospitals through the out-
patient department, female sterilisation, 'is almost unavailable in the
Republic of Ireland. The reason for this is that the majority of Irish
hospitals are administered by boards whose ethos is Roman Catholic'.[78]
Moreover, access to the procedure depended heavily on class. IFPA
doctor, Mary Short, interviewed by *Woman's Way* magazine in 1988,
stated, 'You'll get sterilisation here if you have money in your pocket,
but if you can't afford to pay for it, it's a very different story'.[79] Dr. Edgar
Ritchie provided tubal ligation through his gynaecological practice at the
Victoria Hospital in Cork, where he worked from 1970, which later
became part of the South Infirmary, as well as in some cases at the
Erinville Hospital. Dr. Ritchie explained that the although the South
Infirmary had a Catholic ethos 'thankfully the sterilisation was still provided in the Victoria part of the hospital. There was no problem over that'.
At the Erinville hospital, which was a voluntary hospital associated with
the UCC medical school, an ethics committee had to approve sterilisations, and these were often conducted at the time of caesearean section in
extenuating circumstances. According to Ritchie, 'thereafter it was mainly
then not so much in Erinville Hospital but in South Infirmary and Victoria
that people would come for sterilisation'. Demand for the procedure in
Cork was so high that the waiting list frequently had to be closed tempor-
arily. For example, in 1984, Dr. Ritchie reported that over 800 women
were on the waiting list for tubal ligation, and estimated that more than
40 women travelled to Northern Ireland or Britain each week to have the
operation.[80]

Like vasectomy, tubal ligation was an alternative for some women who
found other methods of contraception unsatisfactory and had completed
their families. Anne, interviewed by *Woman's Way* in 1988, had the
procedure aged 43, having had four children in rapid succession, and
'because she was sick of Irish family planning roulette'. Anne was unable
to take the pill due to health reasons, had experienced side effects from the
coil, and found condoms and the withdrawal method to be unsatisfactory.
As a result, she went to her GP and was referred to the Adelaide Hospital.

[78] 'Women's AIM opinion poll 1983', *Women's AIM: A Magazine of General Interest for
Women Published by Aim Group for Family Law Reform*, 13, Winter '83/'84, p. 11.
[79] 'The permanent contraceptive', *Woman's Way*, 18 March 1988, p. 10.
[80] *Evening Herald*, 24 February 1984, p. 1.

Following the procedure, Anne remarked 'Our sex life is much better because we're so relaxed about the whole thing'.[81]

Travel to the UK for tubal ligation is another example of what Mary Gilmartin and Sinéad Kennedy have described as 'reproductive mobility', meaning travel for the purposes of accessing reproductive services.[82] Having the procedure in the UK was often more financially viable. The family planning clinics and the WWC assisted women in making arrangements. In 1978, *Woman's Way* printed the story of 'Julie', who had travelled to Liverpool for tubal ligation. Following a traumatic childbirth experience and miscarriage, she went to a Dublin family planning clinic and arranged to travel to Liverpool for sterilisation at a cost of £90 which included her return boat fare and hotel accommodation.[83] Julie remarked on the high level of care and kindness she received from the nursing staff in Liverpool. After two nights, she got the boat back to Dublin, and had a check-up three weeks later at the family planning clinic where her clips were removed. The magazine reported on the positive impact of the procedure, stating 'Julie's whole life has been changed, her fears and anxieties wiped out and her emotional life made happier and more serene by a simple operation. Other women are making the same decision every day'.[84]

Sally (b.1956) also obtained the procedure in the UK. After her third pregnancy she had been advised not to have any more children. However, due to high blood pressure she was unable to take the contraceptive pill. She saved up for two years and organised a tubal ligation procedure in Liverpool through the WWC in the early 1990s. She explained the challenges she faced travelling to Liverpool to obtain a procedure she could not easily acquire in Ireland:

I didn't know, I'd never been there before. I was facing a medical procedure, I had paid for it in advance, the medical procedure, but I needed bed and breakfast. And I hadn't a clue whether I'd enough money or not, so it was all a lot and having to pretend coming back, getting the train and the boat. And I was violently ill, and trying to pretend to the children I'd just been away on a couple of days holiday, and I was extremely ill.

In 1983, *Woman's Way* magazine reported on the difficulties facing women who wanted to be sterilised. The magazine estimated that about

---

[81] 'The permanent contraceptive', *Woman's Way*, 18 March 1988, p. 6.
[82] Mary Gilmartin and Sinéad Kennedy, 'A double movement: the politics of reproductive mobility in Ireland', in Christabelle Sethna and Gayle Davis (eds.), *Abortion across Borders: Transnational Travel and Access to Abortion Services* (Baltimore: Johns Hopkins Press, 2019), pp. 123–43.
[83] 'Sterilisation: one woman's story', *Woman's Way*, 16 June 1978, p. 24.
[84] *Ibid.*, p. 26.

1,000 women a year travelled to Britain every year for the operation, and that this was only a moderate estimate. According to the magazine, as a result of the long waiting lists for the operation in Cork, many women preferred to go to England 'where there is no delay and where it costs less'. One GP interviewed by the magazine stated that consultants at the Dublin hospitals 'blame nurses and say they won't co-operate, but in my view that's an excuse to save the doctor the possibility of a clash with the archbishop who's on the hospital management board. I am often asked about sterilisation by patients and I hate having to say that nothing can be done for them in their own city.'[85] In 1983, the costs were estimated to be about £300 for the operation in Cork, with a reduced fee for medical card holders and women from the lower income groups, while in Northern Ireland, the fee was £300 in Belfast, and £95–£125 sterling plus travel costs in England.[86]

The procedure was controversial, however. In 1982, a consultant radiologist at Erinville Hospital, Dr. P. J. Galvin, claimed that it was illegal for the procedure to be conducted in health board hospitals.[87] The issue also illuminates the tensions between providing women with reproductive healthcare in Catholic run hospitals. Catholic teaching forbade sterilisation because of its impact on 'the integrity of the human body'. Pope Pius XII provided the most clear statement on sterilisation, arguing that it was immoral, even when done to prevent a future pregnancy which might not be sustained.[88] In 1985, during the sale of Calvary Hospital in Galway, then Bishop Eamonn Casey insisted that a ban on the procedure for family planning reasons should be included in an agreement governing the sale of the hospital.[89] Casey also wrote to all GPs in the Galway diocese at that time to remind them that sterilisation went against Christian teaching. He urged doctors not to involve themselves with such procedures. Michael Mylotte, the consultant gynaecologist at Galway University Hospital, had conducted tubal ligations there since 1984 for 'medical and social reasons', and at the time of Casey's letter, he argued against the 'interference by the clergy' in an issue which should have been a matter between patient and doctor. At the Galway hospital, unlike many of the Dublin hospitals, there was no ethics committee which made a decision on tubal ligation procedures.[90] However,

[85] 'The permanent contraceptive', *Woman's Way*, 26 August 1983, pp. 10–11.   [86] *Ibid.*
[87] 'Cork doctor seeks ban on sterilisation', *Irish Press*, 27 February 1982, p. 3.
[88] Maurice Reidy, 'Tubal ligation and medical indications', *Irish Theological Quarterly*, 1 June 1979, pp. 91–2.
[89] 'A 1985 agreement with Bishop on sterilisations is in force 9 years later', *Connacht Tribune*, 29 July 1994, p. 5.
[90] 'Sterilisation operations are available in Galway', *Connacht Tribune*, 24 January 1992, p. 21.

Professor Eamon O'Dwyer, chair of obstetrics and gynaecology at UCG, who expressed concerns about the number of sterilisations being carried out in Galway, had urged the Western Health Board to set up an ethics committee similar to those in the Dublin hospitals in 1985. This was turned down.[91]

By 1988, more hospitals were offering the procedure, including the Adelaide Hospital in Dublin, the Regional Hospital in Galway and Portlaoise General Hospital.[92] Yet, the availability of the procedure largely depended on the views of the consultant at the hospital and the hospital's ethos. For example, master of the Adelaide Hospital, Dr. George Henry was reported to have conducted 100 tubal ligations in 15 months during his time as master in the late 1970s, however, when this role was taken over by Professor John Bonnar, only about six tubal ligations were done per year. Bonnar stated that the operation 'would be done only for genuine medical reasons'.[93] And, at the Rotunda Hospital, under Henry's role as master, only fifteen sterilisations were carried out in 1984 and 1985.[94] Tubal ligation could also be paid for privately at great cost. In 1984 and 1985 respectively, two new private clinics, the Whitehorn Clinic in Celbridge, Co. Kildare, and Andrew Rynne's Clane Hospital, were opened to provide tubal ligation for women. The Whitehorn Clinic charged £250 for the procedure.[95] One doctor, John McManus, the Workers' Party spokesman on health, claimed that he knew of women who had gone to moneylenders in order to obtain the money for the procedure at the Celbridge clinic.[96]

The issue of class is crucial in relation to access to sterilisation as many public hospitals did not provide the procedure until the 1990s.[97] Master of the NMH, Peter Boylan argued in 1992 that the procedure was 'available in private hospitals and those who can afford it can usually get it without difficulty'.[98] The NMH did not end its strict regulations regarding sterilisation until 1992. Up until that point, sterilisation was only permitted in cases where another pregnancy would have posed a serious risk to the mother's life, or in cases where a woman was unable to give birth to a live child. The Coombe overturned its ban on the procedure in 1991. By 1994, the procedure was still difficult to obtain at public hospitals in the country; a report in the *Irish Medical Times* showed that

[91] *Sunday Press*, 25 August 1985, p. 6.
[92] 'The permanent contraceptive', *Woman's Way*, 18 March 1988, p. 6.
[93] *Sunday Press*, 25 August 1985, p. 6.   [94] *Ibid.*
[95] 'Women to pay £250 for sterilisation', *Irish Press*, 25 July 1984, p. 18.
[96] 'Women want to be sterile – doctor', *Irish Independent*, 22 April 1985, p. 5.
[97] 'Hospital lifts sterilisation ban', *Irish Independent*, 13 November 1992, p. 63.
[98] 'Hospital puts tubal ligation on agenda', *Irish Press*, 13 January 1992, p. 15.

seven public hospitals did not provide the procedure under any circumstances and five others only provided it by means of prior permission by
an ethics committee.[99] Contraceptive methods such as the pill and
sterilisation, but excluding condoms, were not available free to medical
card holders until 1995.[100]

9.7   Conclusion

By the mid-1990s, contraception was for the most part fully liberalised by
the law in Ireland. However, it had been slow to get to this point, and
there were lots of continuities in terms of access and activism. While the
1979 Family Planning Act made contraception available for *bona fide*
family planning purposes, it is clear that access remained restrictive well
into the 1980s. The less well-off, young people, and those living in rural
areas, were particularly affected by the legal restrictions. As in the 1970s,
through direct action activities played a crucial role in helping to change
the law. Debates around the liberalisation of the law reflected continuing
concerns about young people and promiscuity. As in the case of
condoms in the 1960s and 1970s, the UK market was predominantly
used for this form of contraception. Yet, this period also witnessed new
trends in relation to contraception, such as the introduction of post-coital
contraception for the first time and increased take up of vasectomy as
family planning became to be increasingly seen as a joint responsibility.
Contraception was not available to medical card holders until 1995, and
this only included female-centred methods such as the pill. Access
continued to be dependent on a sympathetic doctor or a chemist willing
to stock contraceptives. Moreover, women who wanted to undergo tubal
ligation were particularly affected.

---

[99] 'A 1985 agreement with Bishop on sterilisations is in force 9 years later', *Connacht Tribune*, 29 July 1994, p. 5.
[100] 'Health boards to provide sterilisation, contraception', *Irish Times*, 24 March 1995, p. 1.

Conclusion

This book has, for the first time, provided insights into the personal, lived experiences of men and women negotiating family planning and contraception in Ireland in the period from the 1920s to the 1990s, as well as illuminating the memories of activists who campaigned for and against the legalisation of contraception and the expansion of access to it. It is clear there are continuities across the history of the twentieth century: men and women writing to Marie Stopes for advice in the 1920s justified their need for contraception in similar ways to individuals trying to plan their families in late twentieth century. Moreover, the contraception question polarised activists, members of the medical profession, church hierarchies and government officials across the period.

Ultimately, this book has shown the impact that legal and religious restrictions can have on individuals' reproductive choices. It has highlighted the influence of Catholic Church teachings and legal structures on Irish life in the postcolonial period which meant that for many individuals, sex, contraception and related issues were clouded with feelings of stigma and shame. Ireland was not exceptional in this regard, as studies of contraception in other predominantly Catholic countries have shown, yet, the interplay between Church and State in Ireland which meant that Catholic teachings were enshrined in Irish law, and continued to influence Irish laws such as the Family Planning Act of 1979, had significant consequences in terms of access and attitudes to contraception. Yet, in spite of these constraints, many Irish men and women showed resistance. They found ways to access contraception and information about contraception through family planning clinics or by accessing the pill as a 'cycle regulator'. Others used natural methods, sometimes out of choice, and sometimes out of necessity. Many others exercised reproductive mobility.[1] This was done in a range of ways, from writing to Marie Stopes for information in the early twentieth century, to

[1] Gilmartin and Kennedy, 'A double movement: the politics of reproductive mobility in Ireland'.

obtaining contraceptives on the black market, or going over the border to chemists in Northern Ireland. Ironically, the UK and particularly England, which was negatively characterised by the State for its permissiveness throughout the twentieth century, provided the main market for contraceptives which were smuggled back in suitcases or sometimes successfully through the post, while many women also chose go to England for tubal ligations due to the lack of availability of the procedure in their own country.

A key theme in this book has been power. Power was wielded not only by Church representatives in relation to contraception, but by members of the medical profession and chemists, many of whom were responsible for restricting individuals' access to contraception, even after legalisation in 1979. Yet, there were exceptions, in the cases of sympathetic doctors, and in some instances, sympathetic priests, who were themselves struggling with the Church's stance on contraception in the wake of *Humanae Vitae*. Activists challenged this power, and in doing so, many took significant personal risks. They played a crucial role in opening up the debate on the contraception issue, challenging the law, and in the case of some family planning and feminist campaigners, providing contraception to individuals while the State dilly-dallied over the introduction of legislation. Yet, the issue of contraception was inexorably linked with abortion. Anti-contraception campaigners mobilised in the 1970s and their campaigns against contraception formed the foundation for the pro-life campaign in the 1980s. Their arguments reveal much about wider concerns within the Irish public about the tensions between a nationalistic vision of Ireland which had been honed-in the early twentieth century and concerns about modernity.

I hope that this book has also illustrated the power of oral history to illuminate individuals' lived experiences and attitudes, and it will inspire further studies which utilise this methodology. Oral history is a powerful tool for understanding 'hidden' histories, and there is much scope for future work which might explore the experiences of Irish people of colour, Travellers, and disabled people in relation to contraception and reproductive health more generally. Moreover, there is much scope for further studies of individuals' experiences of pregnancy, miscarriage, childbirth, as well as reproductive and sexual health in Ireland, and activism more widely.

Yet, while contraception is more widely available now, and there have been important legal changes in relation to sexual and reproductive rights in Ireland, there are many continuities between this history and more recent times in terms of provision and attitudes. A 2019 report by the Working Group on Access to Contraception has highlighted that there still remain issues with access to contraception in some parts of the country, and that cost can have an influence on individuals' choice of method. Notably, the report stated that embarrassment and stigma around contraception are still present, with research highlighting 'how young women have reported being afraid to reveal they are sexually active; embarrassed to be seen at a family planning clinic; or worried about confidentiality breaches. Embarrassment has also been reported in relation to talking to GPs, pharmacists and clinic staff about contraception and with regard to purchasing condoms, as well as asking partners to wear them and using them'.[2] In July 2022, the Health (Miscellaneous Provisions) (No.2) Act was signed into law, enabling the introduction of free contraception for women aged 17-25. While this is a positive step, arguably this law reflects the state's continuing anxieties over young women's sexuality and augments contraception as a woman's responsibility. Younger teenagers, women over the age of 25, men, and non-binary persons are not included in this legislation. Moreover, Ireland's abortion law, introduced in 2019 under the Health (Regulation of Termination of Pregnancy) Act (2018) also reflects continuities: the law stipulates that medical providers may object to providing abortions on conscientious grounds but that they must refer on; this means some women still have to travel for reproductive healthcare. Sex education remains a contentious issue. A report by the National Council for Curriculum and Assessment in 2019 on sex education in Irish schools found that for school-age students who were interviewed 'their recall of primary RSE was almost exclusively related to learning about the biological changes that happen during puberty. A small number of first-year students said they didn't receive any lessons in RSE'. Similarly, sex education in secondary schools, if provided, generally tended to focus on scientific facts.[3] Evidently, the stigma and shame combined with legal and moral restrictions relating to sexual morality in the early twentieth century have cast a long shadow. It is only through exploring the history of moral issues such as contraception that we can fully comprehend attitudes towards and experiences of sexuality and reproductive health in Ireland today.

[2] *Report of Working Group on Access to Contraception*, (2019), p.15.
[3] *NCCA Report on the Review of Relationships and Sexuality Education (RSE) in Primary and Postprimary Schools*, (2019), pp.15–17.

Appendix

Table 3.1 *Form of Family Planning Used by Respondents Born in 1930s*

Name	Gender	Year of birth	Year of marriage	Area lived in for most of childbearing years	Methods mentioned	Number of children
Bob	M	1931	1965	Rural	Billings	5
Eamonn	M	1933	1961	Small town	Billings	3
Jim	M	1933	1973 [married to respondent interviewed separately born in 1940s]	Small town	Pill, safe period, condoms	3
Ronan	M	1933	1961	Small town	Safe period	6
Audrey	F	1934	1957	Dublin	Billings	4
Anthony	M	1934	1967 [married to respondent interviewed separately born in 1940s]	Suburbs of city in the west of Ireland	Billings	4
Nuala	F	1935	1964	Dublin	None	4
Marian	F	1935	1961	Small town	Safe period, condoms, pill	3
Christina	F	1935	1959	Small town	Safe period	6
Deirdre	F	1936	1959	City in the west of Ireland	None, later had hysterectomy	6
Julia	F	1936	1965	Dublin	Temperature method	5
Clare	F	1936	1959	Small town	Safe period, temperature method, condoms	6

Name	Sex			Location	Contraception	Children
Gráinne	F	1937	1960	City in the west of Ireland	Safe period	8
Dennis	M	1937	1965	Suburbs of city in west of Ireland	Safe period	3
Tessie	F	1938	1959	Suburbs of Dublin	Safe period, withdrawal	4
Katherine	F	1938	1962	Small town	Safe period	7
Rosie	F	1938	1961	London	Fertility issues so did not practise family planning	0
Emer	Married couple interviewed together	1939	1961	Suburbs of city in west	None used	7
Tony		1939	1961	Suburbs of city in west	None used	7
Eugene	M	1939	1970	Rural	Safe period	4
Anrie	F	1939	1961	Rural	None used	11

Table 3.2 *Form of Family Planning Used by Respondents Born in 1940s*

Name	Gender	Year of birth	Year of marriage	Location	Methods mentioned	Number of children
Nora	F	1940	1967	Small city	Billings, pill	3
Evelyn	F	1940	1973 [husband born in 1930s and interviewed separately]	Small town	Pill, safe period, condoms before marriage	3
Con	M	1940	1967	Suburbs of city in west of Ireland	None mentioned	6
Colm	M	1940	1964	Rural	Safe period, wife had tubal ligation	5
Clodagh	F	1940	1962	Rural	Safe period, pill briefly, temperature	8
Siobhan	F	1942	1967	Dublin	Pill, rhythm method, Safe period, abstinence	4
Irene	F	1942	1964	Rural	Withdrawal	4
Jeremiah	M	1942	1974	Various	Pill, condoms	4
Maurice	M	1942	1971	Dublin and small town	Condoms, safe period, vasectomy	3
Stephen Christine	Married couple interviewed together	1943 1947	1969	Dublin suburbs	Abstinence but no active family planning	2
Eibhlin	F	1943	1975	Rural west	No method	5
Declan Mary Margaret	Married couple interviewed separately	1944 1945	1966	Suburbs of city	Safe period, breastfeeding	4
Úna	F	1944	1968	Small city	Coil	5 (3 of which adopted)

Name	Sex	Birth year	Marriage year	Location	Method	No.
Eileen	F	1944	1967 [husband born in 1930s and interviewed separately]	Suburbs of small city	Billings	4
Kate	F	1944	1966	Small town	Safe period	6
Mary Ellen	F	1944	1974	Rural	Safe period, later hysterectomy	3
Nellie	F	1944	1976	Rural	Safe period	3
Alice	F	1944	n/a	England	Condoms, withdrawal and later pill	1
Ellie	F	1944	1970	Dublin suburbs	Withdrawal, Temperature, coil	4
Brigid	F	1945	1973	Small city	Safe period	4
Ann	F	1945	1964	Rural	Pill, coil, hysterectomy	3
Bridget	F	1945	1972	Small town	Safe period, later hysterectomy	5
Helena	F	1945	1967	Small town	Billings	4
Teresa	F	1946	1970	England initially then Rural	Cap and IUD in England, then back in Ireland from 1975 Billings, withdrawal	4
Colette	F	1946	1970	Small city	Safe period, condoms	5
Lizzie	F	1946	1983	Small town	Withdrawal	1
Lily	F	1946	1972	Rural	Pill, safe period, tubal ligation	3
Christopher	M	1946	1967	Dublin	Condoms, vasectomy	2
Sarah	F	1947	1982	Small town	Billings	3
Myra	F	1947	1968	Small town	Billings/temperature, condoms, "minding ourselves"	3
Bernadette	F	1947	1972	Suburbs of small city	Safe period/temperature method	4

Table 3.2 (*cont.*)

Name	Gender	Year of birth	Year of marriage	Location	Methods mentioned	Number of children
Julie	F	1947	1982	Small town	Billings and diaphragm, condoms and vasectomy	4
Maud	F	1947	1969	England	Sterilisation in England	3
Aoife	F	1947	1970	Dublin	Pill	3
David	M	1948	1984 [wife born in 1950s, interviewed together]	Small town	Condoms over the border, pill, vasectomy	4
Marianne	F	1948	Late 70s	England then small town	Withdrawal	2
Pól	M	1948	1983	Suburbs of small city	None as married later	3
Virginia	F	1948	1973	England, moved back later	Condoms	0
Pierce	M	1948	1971	Dublin	Temperature method, Coil, condoms, pill, vasectomy	4
Ellen	F	1949	1973	Small town	Safe period, condoms	6
Cathy	F	1949	1973	Dublin	Pill	1
Áine	F	1949	1970s	Small town	Pill	4
Diane	F	1949	1969	Small town	Condoms, pill, withdrawal	2

330

Table 3.3 *Family Planning Practices of Respondents Born in 1950s*

Name	Gender	Year of birth	Year of marriage	Location during childbearing years	Methods mentioned	Number of children
Barbara	F	1950	1970	Small village	Safe period, condoms brought back from England	6
Elaine	F	1950	1972	Small city	Pill	4
Hannah	F	1950	1972	England then small town	Pill, Coil, hysterectomy	2
Judith	F	1950	1972	Dublin	Pill	1
Edward	M	1950	1976	Small city	Pill, condoms, vasectomy	2
Daithi	M	1950	1980	Small city	Vasectomy	3
Ted	Married couple interviewed separately	1951	1976	Small village	Withdrawal, condom, spermicidal jelly, pill, Billings, vasectomy	3
Maria		1957				
Hugh	M	1951	1974	Suburbs of small city	None/fertility issues	2
Sandra	F	1951	1974	Dublin	Pill	2
Carmel	Married couple interviewed together	1952	1973	Small town	Condoms, pill, vasectomy	3
Martin		1952				
Frances	F	1952	1976	Small town	Billings	2
Noel	M	1952	1975	Small city	Pill, condoms	2
Mark	M	1952	1975	Small city	Fertility issues	Adopted
Kenneth	M	1952	1977	Small city	Billings, pill, condoms, vasectomy	2
Jean	F	1953 [husband interviewed separately, born in 1940s]	1984	Small town	Condoms over the border, pill, vasectomy	4

Table 3.3 (*cont.*)

Name	Gender	Year of birth	Year of marriage	Location during childbearing years	Methods mentioned	Number of children
Tom	Married couple interviewed together	1953	1975	Dublin suburbs	Breastfeeding, withdrawal, later condoms	7
Jacinta		1954				
Catherine	F	1953	1975	England	Pill, vasectomy	4
Mairead	F	1953	1991	Small town	Cap, pill	0
Alison	F	1953	1981	Rural	Pill and condoms, tubal ligation	2
Nicholas	M	1953	1980	Small city	Pill, wife had hysterectomy	3
Niall	M	1953	1980	Small city	Safe period, pill	3
Noreen	F	1954	1982	Small town	Tubal ligation in NI	3
Carol	F	1954	1977	Small town	Pill, Billings, tubal ligation	3
Margaret	Married couple interviewed separately	1954	1976	Small town	Billings, vasectomy	3
Charlie		1951				
Richard	M	1954	1987	Small city	Wife sterilisation	3
Paula	F	1955	1976	Small city	Condoms, husband had vasectomy	2
Mary Anne	F	1955	1977	England and Rural	Pill	2
Martina	F	1955	1973	Small town	Pill, tubal ligation	4
Sally	F	1956	1974	Dublin	Avoiding sex, condoms from England. Sterilisation in England.	3

Table 6.1 *Percentages of married and single clients at first visit to IFPA clinics, 1971–81*

	Clinic location	Married	Single
1971	Merrion Square	80.9%	19.1%
	Mountjoy Square	90.1%	9.9%
1972	Merrion Square	66.5%	33.5%
	Mountjoy Square	90%	10%
1973	Merrion Square	71.5%	28.5%
	Mountjoy Square	87%	13%
1974	Merrion Square	68%	32%
	Mountjoy Square	73%	27%
1975	Synge Street	51.86%	48.14%
	Mountjoy Square	69.97%	30.03%
1976	Synge Street	44.50%	55.50%
	Mountjoy Square	70.85%	29.15%
1977	Synge Street	50%	50%
	Mountjoy Square	57.16%	42.83%
1978	Synge Street	53.34%	46.66%
	Mountjoy Square	59.12%	40.88%
1979	Not recorded in 1979 report		
1980	Synge Street	Not recorded	Not recorded
	Cathal Brugha St	52%	47%
1981	Synge Street	54%	46%
	Cathal Brugha St	43%	48%

Table 6.2 *Number of Children in the Family at First Visit to IFPA clinics in 1971, 1972 and 1975*[1]

		0	1	2	3	4	5	6	+
1971	**Merrion Sq**	28.8%	15.8%	15.8%	12.2%	7.9%	7.9%	4.0%	7.5%
	Mountjoy Sq	21.0%	12.9%	21.0%	16.6%	11.2%	6.6%	4.7%	6.6%
1972	**Merrion Sq**	30.0%	15.0%	15.0%	11.0%	9.0%	10.0%	4.0%	6.0%
	Mountjoy Sq	21.0%	12.0%	21.0%	16.0%	11.0%	6.0%	5.0%	8.0%
1973-1974	Percentages not recorded in 1973 and 1974 annual reports.[2]								
1975	**Synge Street**	54.48%	12.40%	13.22%	8.00%	6.02%	2.88%	1.29%	1.71%
	Mountjoy Sq	36.16%	16.58%	16,78%	11.79%	8.18%	4.70%	2.74%	3.07%

Not recorded thereafter

[1] Fertility Guidance Company, *Annual Report for 1971.* [IFPA Archives], p. 4.
[2] The 1974 report records numbers but there appear to be errors.

Table 6.3 *Method Chosen at First Visit at IFPA Clinics, 1971–80*[1]

	Clinic location	Oral	IUD	Cap	Condom	Temperature method	Advice	Vasectomy	Tubal ligation
1971	Merrion Sq	47.1%	15.2%	23.5%	2.1%	3.5%	8.6%		
	Mountjoy Sq	48.0%	14.9%	20.2%	6.4%	2.0%	8.5%		
1972	Merrion Sq	45.0%	25.0%	12.0%	6.0%	2.0%	10.0%		
	Mountjoy Sq	37.0%	40.0%	9.0%	6.5%	1.5%	6.0%		
1973	Merrion Sq	57.2%	18.4%	10.5%	3.3%	1.2%	9.3%		
	Mountjoy Sq	37.3%	42.3%	7.3%	6.6%	0.9%	5.6%		
1974	Synge Street (formerly Merrion Square)	66.0%	14.0%	7.0%	6.0%	1.0%	6.0%		
	Mountjoy Sq	48.3%	27.4%	6.0%	6.6%	1.0%	8.5%	No % but noted that 25 carried out in clinic	
1975	Synge Street	69.47%	11.66%	5.15%	5.74%	0.75%	5.03%	2.20%	
	Mountjoy Square	59.28%	19.24%	3.82%	8.38%	1.10%	9.18%	n/a	
1976	Synge Street	68.25%	9.51%	7.24%	4.76%	1.00%	9.24%	Not given	
	Mountjoy Square	59.16%	17.35%	6.28%	6.67%	0.65%	9.89%	n/a	

335

Table 6.3 (*cont.*)

	Clinic location	Oral	IUD	Cap	Condom	Temperature method	Advice	Vasectomy	Tubal ligation
1977	Synge Street	58.0%	10.05%	10.00%	4.0%	0.50%	11.0%	6.00%	
	Mountjoy Square	51.29%	18.93%	7.88%	5.27%	0.79%	15.73%	n/a	.001%
1978	Synge Street	50.87%	11.08%	11.51%	3.28%	0.24%	13.83%	6.84%	
	Mountjoy Square	44.06%	23.03%	9.04%	2.82%	0.50%	17.31%	n/a	0.02%[2]
1979	Figures not recorded in Annual Report for this year								
1980	Synge Street	50.47%	9.36%	10.77%	2.71%	(and Billings) 0.95%	13.63%	8.10%	
	Cathal Brugha Street	49.73%	19.91%	9.86%	2.31%	1.52%	7.81%	3.02%[3]	

[1] Fertility Guidance Company, *Annual Report for 1971*, p. 4. *and F.G.C. Annual Report 1972*, p. 4.

[2] In this year, 3.04% were listed as visiting Mountjoy Square and 2.36% at Synge Street for psychosexual problems, and 0.18% visiting Mountjoy Square for 'menopausal'.

[3] In 1980, 1.10% and 3.24% visited Cathal Brugha Street and Synge Street respectively for 'psycho-sexual problems', with 0.89% and 0.15% visiting the two clinics for infertility. 1.15% visited Cathal Brugha St clinic and 0.57% visited the Synge Street for advice on the menopause [IIFPA Annual Report, 1980].

Bibliography

Oral History Interviews

Áine (b.1949), 18 December 2019.
Alice (b.1944), 31 October 2019.
Alison (b.1953), 23 November 2019.
Ann (b.1945), 18 September 2019.
Annie (b.1939), 10 December 2019.
Anthony (b.1934), 9 May 2019.
Aoife (b.1947), 18 December 2019.
Audrey (b.1934), 12 December 2018.
Barbara (b.1950), 4 June 2019.
Bernadette (b.1947), 19 September 2019.
Bob (b.1931), 22 July 2019.
Bridget (b.1945), 7 October 2019.
Brigid (b.1945), 5 June 2019.
Carmel (b.1952) and Martin (b.1952), 12 June 2019.
Carol (b.1954), 23 November 2019.
Catherine (b.1953), 10 October 2019.
Cathy (b.1949), 9 October 2019.
Charlie (b.1951), 26 November 2019.
Christina (b.1935), 26 November 2019.
Christine (b.1947) and Stephen (b.1943), 1 February 2019.
Christopher (b.1946), 3 December 2019.
Clare (b.1936), 22 July 2019.
Clodagh (b.1940), 17 December 2019.
Colette (b.1946), 21 March 2019.
Colm (b.1940), 10 December 2019.
Con (b.1940), 24 July 2019.
Daithi (b.1950), 6 December 2019.
David (b.1948) and Jean (b.1953), 13 June 2019.
Declan (b.1944), 4 June 2019.
Deirdre (b.1936), 1 July 2019.
Denise (b.1961), 25 November 2019.
Dennis (b.1937), 10 May 2019.
Diane (b.1949), 7 March 2019.
Eamonn (b.1933), 5 March 2019.

Edward (b.1950), 3 December 2019.
Eibhlin (b.1943), 12 December 2019.
Eileen (b.1944), 9 May 2019.
Elaine (b.1950), 1 July 2019.
Ellen (b.1949), 19 September 2019.
Ellie (b.1944), 25 November 2019.
Emer (b.1939) and Tony (b.1939), 8 May 2019.
Eugene (b.1939), 13 December 2019.
Evelyn (b.1940), 4 March 2019.
Frances (b.1952), 12 June 2019.
Gráinne (b.1937), 9 May 2019.
Hannah (b.1950), 31 October 2019.
Helena (b.1945), 26 November 2019.
Hugh (b.1951), 3 December 2019.
Imelda (b.1935), 13 December 2018.
Irene (b.1942), 17 September 2019.
Jacinta (b.1954) and Tom, (b.1954), 8 October 2019.
Jeremiah (b.1942), 23 November 2019.
Jim (b.1933), 4 March 2019.
Judith (b.1950), 26 November 2019.
Julia (b.1936), 31 January 2019.
Julie (b.1947), 7 October 2019.
Kate (b.1944), 18 September 2019.
Katherine (b.1948), 24 November 2019.
Kenneth (b.1952), 11 December 2019.
Lily (b.1946), 22 November 2019.
Lizzie (b.1946), 31 October 2019.
Maggie (b.1943), 19 September 2019.
Mairead (b.1953), 22 November 2019.
Margaret (b.1954), 26 November 2019.
Maria (b.1957), 2 April 2018.
Marian (b.1935), 8 May 2019.
Marianne (b.1948), 1 November 2019.
Martina (b.1955), 10 October 2019.
Mark (b.1952), 6 December 2019.
Mary Anne (b.1955), 9 October 2019.
Mary Ellen (b.1944), 30 October 2019.
Mary Margaret (b.1945), 4 June 2019.
Maud (b.1947), 1 November 2019.
Maurice (b.1942), 12 December 2019.
Myra (b.1947), 17 September 019.
Nellie (b.1944), 30 October 2019.
Nicholas (b.1953), 4 December 2019.
Niall (b.1953), 6 December 2019.
Noel (b.1952), 5 December 2019.
Nora (b.1940), 7 June 2019.
Noreen (b.1954), 4 March 2019.

Nuala (b.1935), 1 February 2019.
Paula (b.1955), 22 March 2019.
Pierce (b.1948), 11 December 2019.
Pol (b.1948), 4 November 2019.
Richard (b.1954), 5 December 2019.
Ronan (b.1933), 13 December 2019.
Rosie (b.1938), 10 December 2019.
Sally (b.1956), 14 June 2019.
Sarah (b.1947), 6 March 2019.
Sandra (b.1951), 12 December 2019.
Siobhan (b.1942), 1 February 2019.
Ted (b.1951), 4 January 2018.
Teresa (b.1946), 4 June 2019.
Tessie (b.1938), 22 February 2019.
Úna (b.1944), 5 June 2019.
Virginia (b.1948), 25 November 2019.
Winnie (b.1938), 24 November 2019.

Activists, Campaigners, and Medical Professionals

Bernadette Bonar, 28 September 2017.
Prof. John Bonnar, 5 January 2017.
John Callaghan, 6 August 2017.
Cathie Chappell, 27 August 2020 (Zoom).
Evelyn Conlon, 9 January 2017.
Anne Connolly, 12 October 2017 (phone) and 9 September 2019 (in person).
Frank Crummey, 5 January 2017.
Dr. Philip Cullen, 27 November 2020 (Zoom).
Gerry Curran, 20 October 2017.
Margaret de Courcey, 6 January 2017.
Christine Donaghy, 6 January 2017.
Philomena Donnelly, 30 September 2017.
Mary Fahy, 25 January 2021 (phone).
Mary Freehill, 2 January 2017.
Ferga Grant, 18 September 2020 (phone).
Prof. Dermot Hourihane, 4 January 2017.
Joanne, 11 November 2017.
Mairin Johnston, 13 January 2017.
Prof. Brian Leonard, 24 July 2019.
Dorothea Melvin, 25 September 2020 (Zoom).
Nell McCafferty, 11 January 2017.
Ger Moane, 3 January 2017.
Dr. Brenda Moore-McCann, 13 January 2017.
Barbara Murray, 3 January 2017.
Joanne O'Brien, 31 January 2017 (Skype).
Jon O'Brien, 22 February 2017 (phone).

Taragh O'Kelly, 8 January 2017.
John O'Reilly, 10 January 2017 and 18 October 2017.
Dr. Eimer Philbin-Bowman, 12 January 2017.
Yvonne Pim, 12 January 2017.
Betty Purcell, 16 January 2017.
Ruth Riddick, 5 February 2017.
Dr. Edgar Ritchie, 2 September 2020 (phone).
Dr. Andrew Rynne, 11 May 2021 (Zoom).
Prof. Angela Savage, 31 August 2020 (Zoom).
Brendan Smith, 12 August 2020 (Zoom).
Prof. Pete Smith, 5 November 2020 (Zoom).
Dr. Evelyn Stevens, 6 November 2020. (Zoom).
Anne Speed, 16 November 2017.
Ruth Torode, 11 January 2017.
Finn Van Gelderen, 20 October 2017.
Miriam Watchorn, 7 November 2018.

Other Respondents

Father Bernárd Lynch, 8 January 2020.
Father Paddy Gleeson, 5 August 2020 (Zoom interview).
GP based in the west of Ireland, 17 August 2020 (phone).

Oral Histories from Repositories

Life and Lore oral history interview with Father James Good by
    Maurice O'Keeffe with. recorded as part of series on Cork city,
    2002–2003. Accessed via: www.irishlifeandlore.com/product/father-
    james-good/
Life and Lore oral history recording by Maurice O'Keeffe with
    Elizabeth (Lizzie) O'Dea (b.1941) www.irishlifeandlore.com/prod
    uct/elizabeth-lizzie-odea-b-1941/

Manuscript Sources

Dáil Éireann and Seanad Éireann Debates

Criminal Law Amendment Bill, 1934: Report Stage. Seanad Éireann
    debate, 6 February 1935.
Family Planning Bill, 1973: Second Stage (resumed), Seanad Éireann
    debate, 21 February 1974, Vol. 77, No.3.
Family Planning Bill, 1973: Second Stage (resumed), Seanad Éireann
    debate, 27 March 1974.
Questions: Availability of Contraceptives, Dáil Éireann debate, 24
    October 1978.

Health (Family Planning) Bill, 1978: Committee Stage, Dáil Éireann Debate, 9 May 1979.
Health (Family Planning) (Amendment) Bill, 1985: Second Stage (Resumed), 20 February 1985.

Dublin Diocesan Archives

John Charles McQuaid Papers.

IFPA Archives (Now Deposited at RCPI Heritage Centre)

IFPA Annual reports
Public relations case history: 'The Condom Controversy': Project 1, Year 2, P.R.I.I. Report by Jon O'Brien, Information/Press Officer, Irish Family Planning Association, 10 March 1990.

National Archives of Ireland

Contraceptives: resolutions and miscellaneous correspondence relating to legislation, Department of the Taoiseach, March–October 1971 [2002/8/459].
Contraceptives: resolutions and miscellaneous correspondence relating to legislation, Department of the Taoiseach, February 1972–January 1973, [2003/16/453].
Contraceptives: resolutions and miscellaneous correspondence relating to legislation, Department of the Taoiseach, October–December, 1973 [2004/21/461].
Contraceptives: resolutions and miscellaneous correspondence relating to legislation, Department of the Taoiseach, January 1974–February 1974, [2005/7/345].
Family planning: legislation, including Private Member's Bills, Department of the Taoiseach, November 1984–February 1985 [2015/88/611].
Family Planning (Amendment) Bill: miscellaneous letters received, Office of the Secretary to the President, 1985 [2015/77/94].

National Library of Ireland

Bruce Arnold Papers [MS 41,428].

University College Cork

Roisin Conroy/Attic Press Collection.

Wellcome Collection

Family Planning Association archive, early records [A21/7].
Letters to Marie Stopes concerning *Married Love*. [PP/MCS].

Contemporary Publications

Contemporary Literature

Clarke, Austin, *Old-Fashioned Pilgrimage and Other Poems* (Dublin: Dolmen Press, 1967).
Conlon, Evelyn, *Telling: New and Selected Stories* (Newtownards: Blackstaff Press, 2000).

Contemporary Publications

Bolt, Margaret, 'Who's who around the country: no.1 Family Planning Services', *Family Planning News*, 1: 1, August 1975.
Books Prohibited in the Irish Free State under the Censorship of Publications Act, 1929 (as on 30 April 1936) (Dublin: Eason & Son Ltd., 1936).
Bowman, Eimer Philbin, 'Sexual and contraceptive attitudes and behaviour of single attenders at a Dublin family planning clinic', *Journal of Biosocial Science*, 9: 4, (October 1977), pp. 429–45.
Cleary, James A., 'Is sex instruction needed in Ireland?', *Irish Theological Quarterly*, 1 October 1951.
Clinical Report of the Rotunda Hospital, 1st January 1962 to 31st December 1962 (Dublin: Cahill & Co. Ltd, 1963).
Clinical Report of the Rotunda Hospital, 1st January 1966 to 31st December 1966 (Dublin: Cahill & Co. Ltd, 1967).
'Contraception laws out!', *Socialist Republic: Paper of People's Democracy*, 3: 5, (1980).
'The Dublin clinic that defies convention', *This Week in Ireland*, 7 November 1969, p. 23. Courtesy of Susan Solomons.
Family Planning: A Guide for Parents and Prospective Parents (Dublin: Fertility Guidance Co., 1971).
Fertility Guidance Clinic leaflet, c.1970. Courtesy of Susan Solomons.
Finnegan, T. A., *The Boy's Own: A Practical Booklet for Teenage Boys* (Dublin: The Catholic Truth Society of Ireland, 1954).
    The Girl's Own: Questions Young Women Ask (Dublin: The Catholic Truth Society of Ireland, 1966).
Gift of Life (Dublin: Order of Knights of St. Columbanus, 1978).
Gleeson, Fr Paddy, *Helping Engaged Couples: A Guide for Priests* (Veritas Publications, 1978).
Horgan, John, 'Sugaring the pill', *Fortnight*, 6, (December 4, 1970).
Humphreys, Alexander J., *New Dubliners: Urbanization and the Irish Family* (London: Routledge and Kegan Paul Ltd, 1966).

Irish Family League, *Is Contraception the Answer?* (Dublin: Irish Family League, 1974).

Whither Ireland? A Study (August 1974) of Recent Trends. Contraception and Associated Issues (Irish Family League, Cahill and Co Printing, Dublin).

Alert: Oral Contraceptive (Dublin: Irish Family League, undated but *c*.1975).

Why You Should Oppose Contraception (Dublin: Irish Family League, 1976).

Irish Family Planning Association, *Facts on Contraception: An Answer to 'The Irish Family League'* (undated but likely 1974).

Johnston, Mairin, *Dublin Belles: Conversations with Dublin Women* (Dublin: Attic Press, 1988).

Letter to prospective FGC members, dated 1969. Courtesy of Susan Solomon.

McCarthy, J., 'Preparation for marriage', *Irish Theological Quarterly*, 18: 2, (1 April 1951), pp. 189–91.

Macnamara, Angela, *Living and Loving* (Dublin: Veritas Publications, 1969).

Mackey, Aidan, *What Is Love? A Guide to Right Attitudes to Love and Sex for Children and Younger Adolescents* (Dublin: Catholic Truth Society of Ireland, 1965).

McCafferty, Nell, *A woman to Blame: The Kerry Babies Case* (Dublin: Attic Press, 1985).

Memorandum and Articles of Association: The Galway Family Planning Association Limited, dated 7 January 1977. Courtesy of Dr. Evelyn Stevens.

Murray, Barbara, unpublished booklet on Irishwomen United, September, 1995, (MS in the possession of Barbara Murray).

O'Brien, Jon, *Young People & Family Planning: The Learning Experience of the Irish Family Planning Association, 1984–1990*, (Project Report, *c*.1990).

O'Kelly, Emer, *The Permissive Society in Ireland?* (Cork: Mercier Press, 1974).

O'Reilly, Emily, *Masterminds of the Right* (Dublin: Attic Press, 1988)

Response: Newsletter of the Irish Branch of the Responsible Society.

Riches, Valerie, 'The Responsible Society', *Journal of the Institute of Health Education*, 11:4, (1973), pp. 20–25.

Rohan, Dorine, *Marriage Irish Style* (Cork: Mercier Press, 1969).

Roper, Anne, *Woman to Woman: A Health Care Handbook and Directory for Women* (Dublin: Attic Press, 1986).

Solomons, Michael, *Life Cycle: Facts for Adults* (Dublin: Allen Figgis, 1963).

'Dublin's first family planning clinic', *Psychomatic Medicine in Obstetrics and Gynaecology*, 3rd International Congress, London, 1971 (Karger, Basel, 1972), pp.524–6, Courtesy of Susan Solomons.

Sweetman, Rosita, *On Our Backs: Sexual Attitudes in a Changing Ireland* (London: Pan Books, 1979).

Feminist Publications

Banshee: Journal of Irishwomen United
Fownes Street Journal
Wicca
Wimmin

Memoirs

Crummey, Frank, *Crummey v Ireland: Thorn in the side of the Establishment* (Dublin: Londubh Books, 2010).

Desmond, Barry, *Finally and in Conclusion: A Political Memoir* (Dublin: New Island, 2000).

Fennell, Nuala, *Political Woman: A Memoir* (Dublin: Currach Press, 2009).

Kenny, Mary, *Something of Myself and Others* (Dublin: Liberties Press, 2013).

Levine, June, *Sisters: The Personal Story of an Irish Feminist* (Cork: Attic Press, new edition, 2009).

McCafferty, Nell, *Nell* (Dublin: Penguin Ireland, 2004).

Mullarney, Máire, *What About Me? A Woman for Whom 'One Damn Cause' Led to Another* (Dublin: Town House, 1992).

O'Faolain, Nuala, *Are You Somebody? The Life and Times of Nuala O'Faolain* (London: Hodder and Stoughton, 1997 edition).

Robinson, Mary, *Everybody Matters: A Memoir* (London: Hodder & Stoughton, 2012).

Rynne, Andrew, *The Vasectomy Doctor: A Memoir* (Cork: Mercier Press, 2005).

Solomons, Michael, *Pro Life? The Irish Question* (Dublin: The Lilliput Press, 1992).

Newspapers and Magazines

Birth Control News
Connaught Telegraph
Connacht Tribune
Cork Examiner
Evening Echo
Freeman's Journal
Honesty
Hot Press
International Planned Parenthood News
Irish Examiner
Irish Independent
Irish Journal of Medical Science
Irish Press
Irish Times
Journal of the Irish Medical Association
Kerryman
Kerry News
Limerick Leader
Munster Express
Nikki
Observer
Sligo Champion
Sunday Independent
The Tablet

Westmeath Independent
Western People
Women's AIM: a magazine of general interest for women published by AIM group for Family Law Reform
Woman's Choice Weekly
Woman's Way

Secondary Sources

Abrams, Lynn, *Oral History Theory*, 2nd ed. (Abingdon: Routledge, 2016).

Adams, Michael, *Censorship: The Irish Experience* (Tuscaloosa: University of Alabama Press, 1968).

Ahmed, Sara, *The Cultural Politics of Emotion* (Edinburgh: Edinburgh University Press, 2014).

Anderson, Kathryn and Jack, Dana C., 'Learning to listen: interview techniques and analyses' in Sherna Berger Gluck and Daphne Patai (eds.), *Women's Words: The Feminist Practice of Oral History* (London: Routledge, 1991), pp. 11–26.

Angelides, Steven, 'The "second sexual revolution", moral panic, and the evasion of teenage sexual subjectivity', *Women's History Review*, 21:5, (November 2012), pp. 831–47.

Barry, Ursula, 'The movement, change and reaction: the struggle over reproductive rights in Ireland' in Ailbhe Smyth (ed.), *The Abortion Papers* (Dublin: Attic Press, 1992), pp. 107–118.

Beatty, Aidan, 'Irish modernity and the politics of contraception, 1979–1993', *New Hibernia Review*, 17:3, (Autumn, 2013), pp. 100–118.

Beiner, Guy, and Bryson, Anna, 'Listening to the past and talking to each other: problems and possibilities facing oral history in Ireland', *Irish Economic and Social History*, 30, (2003), pp. 71–8.

Black, Lawrence, 'There was something about Mary: The National Viewers' and Listeners' Association and Social Movement History' in Nick Crowson, Matthew Hilton and James McKay (eds.), *NGOs in Contemporary Britain: Non-state Actors in Society and Politics since 1945* (Cambridge, UK: Palgrave, 2009), pp.182–200.

Bourbonnais, Nicole C., *Birth Control in the Decolonizing Caribbean: Reproductive Politics and Practice on Four Islands, 1930–1970* (Cambridge, UK: Cambridge University Press, 2016).

Bourke, Joanna, 'Fear and anxiety: writing about emotion in modern history', *History Workshop Journal*, 55:1, (Spring, 2003), pp. 111–33.

Buckley, Sarah-Anne, *The Cruelty Man: Child Welfare, the NSPCC and the State in Ireland, 1889–1956* (Manchester: Manchester University Press, 2013).

Clear, Caitriona, *Women's Voices in Ireland: Women's Magazines in the 1950s and 1960s* (London: Bloomsbury, 2016).

'The decline of breastfeeding in 20th century Ireland' in Alan Hayes and Diane Urquhart (eds.), *Irish Women's History* (Dublin: Irish Academic Press, 2004), pp. 187–98.

Cloatre, Emilie and Enright, Máiréad, '"On the perimeter of the lawful": enduring illegality in the Irish Family Planning Movement, 1972–1985', *Journal of Law and Society*, 44:4, (December, 2017), pp. 471–500.

'Commentary on *McGee v Attorney General*' in Máiréad Enright, Julie McCandless and Aoife O'Donoghue, *Northern/Irish Feminist Judgments: Judges' Troubles and the Gendered Politics of Identity* (Oxford: Hart Publishing, 2017), pp. 95–116.

Cloatre, Emilie and Enright, Mairead, 'Transformative illegality: how condoms "became legal" in Ireland, 1991–1993', *Feminist Legal Studies*, 26, (2018), pp. 261–84.

Connell, R. W. , *Gender and Power: Society, the Person and Sexual Politics* (Cambridge: Polity Press, 1987).

Connolly, Linda, *The Irish Women's Movement: From Revolution to Devolution* (Basingstoke: Palgrave Macmillan, 2002).

'Sexual violence in the Irish Civil War: a forgotten war crime?', *Women's History Review*, 30:1, (2021), pp. 126–43.

Connelly, Matthew, *Fatal Misconception: The Struggle to Control World Population* (Cambridge, MA: Harvard University Press, 2008).

Cook, Hera, *The Long Sexual Revolution: English Women, Sex, and Contraception: 1800–1975* (Oxford: Oxford University Press, 2004).

Crane, Jennifer, *Child Protection in England, 1960–2000: Expertise, Experience and Emotion* (Basingstoke: Palgrave, 2018).

Crosetti, Anne-Sophie, 'The 'converted unbelievers': catholics in family planning in French-speaking Belgium (1947–73)', *Medical History*, 64:2, (April 2020), pp. 267–86.

Crowley, Una and Kitchin, Rob, 'Producing "decent girls": governmentality and the moral geographies of sexual conduct in Ireland, (1922–1937), *Gender, Place and Culture*, 15:4, (August 2008), pp. 355–72.

Cunningham, John, '"Spreading VD all over Connacht": reproductive rights and wrongs in 1970s Galway', *History Ireland*, 19:2, (March/April 2011).

d'Alton, Ian, "No country"? Protestant "belongings" in independent Ireland, 1922–49' in Ian d'Alton and Ida Milne (eds.), *Protestant and Irish: The Minority's Search for Place in Independent Ireland*, (Cork, Ireland: Cork University Press, 2019), pp. 19–33.

de Londras, Fiona, 'Constitutionalizing fetal rights: a salutary tale from Ireland', *Michigan Journal of Gender & Law*, 22:2, (2015), pp. 243–89.

Dale, Jennifer and Foster, Peggy, *Feminists and State Welfare* (London, 2012).

Daly, Mary E., *The Slow Failure: Population Decline and Independent Ireland, 1920–1973* (Wisconsin: University of Wisconsin Press, 2003).

Sixties Ireland: Reshaping the Economy, State and Society, 1957–1973 (Cambridge, UK: Cambridge University Press, 2016).

'Marriage, fertility and women's lives in twentieth-century Ireland (c. 1900–c. 1970)', *Women's History Review*, 15:4, (2006), pp. 571–85.

Davis, Angela, 'Generation and memories of sex and reproduction in mid-twentieth-century Britain', *The Oral History Review*, 45:2, pp. 249–64.

(2008) '"Oh no, nothing, we didn't learn anything": sex education and the preparation of girls for motherhood, c.1930–1970, *History of Education*, 37:5, pp. 661–7.

Debenham, Clare, *Marie Stopes' Sexual Revolution and the Birth Control Movement* (Basingstoke: Palgrave, 2018).

Dee, Olivia, *The Anti-Abortion Campaign in England, 1966–1989* (New York: Routledge, 2019).

Delay, Cara, *Irish Women and the Creation of Modern Catholicism, 1850–1950* (Manchester: Manchester University Press, 2019).

'Pills, potions, and purgatives: women and abortion methods in Ireland, 1900–1950', *Women's History Review*, 28:3 (2019), pp. 479–99.

'Kitchens and kettles: Domestic spaces, ordinary things, and female networks in Irish abortion history, 1922–1949'. *Journal of Women's History*, 30:4, (Winter, 2018), pp. 11–34.

'From the backstreet to Britain: women and abortion travel in modern ireland' in Charlotte Beyer, Janet MacLennan, Dorsía Smith Silva, and Marjorie Tesser (eds.), *Travellin' Mama: Mothers, Mothering, and Travel* (Ontario: Demeter Press, 2019).

'Wrong for womankind and the nation: anti-abortion discourses in Ireland, 1967–1992'. *Journal of Modern European History*, 17:3 (2019), pp. 312–25.

Delay, Cara and Liger, Annika, 'Bad mothers and dirty lousers: Representing abortionists in postindependence Ireland'. *Journal of Social History*, 54:1, (Fall 2020), pp. 286–305.

Diver, Cara, *Marital Violence in Post-Independence Ireland, 1922–96: 'A Living Tomb For Women'* (Manchester University Press, 2019).

Doyle-O'Neill, Finola, *The Gaybo Revolution: How Gay Byrne Challenged Irish Society* (Dublin: Orpen Press, 2015).

Drucker, Donna, *Contraception: A Concise History* (Cambridge, MA: MIT Press, 2020).

Duffy, Deirdre, 'From feminist anarchy to decolonisation: understanding abortion health activism before and after the repeal of the 8th amendment', *Feminist Review*, 124 (2020), pp. 69–85.

Earner-Byrne, Lindsey, *Mother and Child: Maternity and Child Welfare in Ireland, 1920s–1960s* (Manchester: Manchester University Press, 2007).

'Moral prescription: the Irish medical profession, the Roman Catholic Church and the prohibition of birth control in twentieth-century Ireland' in Catherine Cox and Maria Luddy (eds.), *Cultures of Care in Irish Medical History, 1750–1950* (Basingstoke: Palgrave, 2010), pp. 207–28.

'The boat to England: an analysis of the official reactions to the emigration of single expectant Irishwomen to Britain, 1922–1972', *Irish Economic and Social History*, 30, (2003), pp. 52–70.

'The rape of Mary M.: a microhistory of sexual violence and moral redemption in 1920s Ireland'. *Journal of the History of Sexuality*, 24:1, (January 2015), pp. 75–98.

Earner-Byrne, Lindsey and Urquhart, Diane, *The Irish Abortion Journey, 1920–2018* (Basingstoke: Palgrave, 2019).

Earner-Byrne, Lindsey and Urquhart, Diane, 'Gender roles in Ireland since 1740' in Eugenio F. Biagini and Mary E. Daly (eds.), *The Cambridge Social History of Modern Ireland* (Cambridge, UK: Cambridge University Press, 2017), pp. 312–26.

Farrell, Elaine, *A Most Diabolical Deed: Infanticide and Irish Society, 1850–1900* (Manchester: Manchester University Press, 2013).

Ferriter, Diarmaid, *Occasions of Sin: Sex and Society in Modern Ireland* (London: Profile Books, 2009).

Ambiguous Republic, Ireland in the 1970s (London, Profile Books, 2012).

Fischer, Clara, 'Gender, nation, and the politics of shame: Magdalen laundries and the institutionalization of feminine transgression in modern Ireland'. *Signs: Journal of Women in Culture and Society*, 41:4, (2016), pp. 821–43.

Fisher, Kate, *Birth Control, Sex and Marriage in Britain, 1918–1960*, (Oxford University Press, 2006).

Fisher, Kate and Szreter, Simon, *Sex Before the Sexual Revolution: Intimate Life in England, 1918–1963* (Cambridge, UK: Cambridge University Press, 2010).

Foley, Deirdre, '"Too many children?" family planning and *humanae vitae* in Dublin, 1960–72'. *Irish Economic and Social History*, 43:1, (December, 2019), pp. 142–60.

Freidenfelds, Lara, *The Modern Period: Menstruation in Twentieth-Century America* (Baltimore: Johns Hopkins Press, 2009).

Fuller, Louise, *Irish Catholicism since 1950: The Undoing of a Culture* (Dublin: Gill & Macmillan, 2002).

Geiringer, David, *The Pope and the Pill: Sex, Catholicism and Women in Post-War England* (Manchester, UK: Manchester University Press, 2019).

Gervais, Diane and Gauvreau, Danielle, 'Women, priests, and physicians: family limitation in Quebec, 1940–1970', *Journal of Interdisciplinary History*, 34:2 (2003), pp. 293–314.

Gialanella Valiulis, Maryann, 'Virtuous mothers and dutiful wives: the politics of sexuality in the Irish Free State', in M. G. Valiulus, (ed.), *Gender and Power* (Dublin: Irish Academic Press, 2008), pp. 100–114.

Gilmartin, Mary and Kennedy, Sinéad, 'A double movement: the politics of reproductive mobility in Ireland', in Christabelle Sethna and Gayle Davis (eds.), *Abortion Across Borders: Transnational Travel and Access to Abortion Services* (Baltimore: Johns Hopkins Press, 2019), pp. 123–43.

Girvin, Brian, 'Contraception, moral panic and social change in Ireland, 1969–79'. *Irish Political Studies*, 23:4, (December, 2008), pp. 555–76.

'An Irish solution to an Irish problem: Catholicism, Contraception and Change, 1922–1979'. *Contemporary European History*, 27:1, (2018), pp. 1–22.

Guldi, Jo and Armitage, David, *The History Manifesto* (Cambridge, UK: Cambridge University Press, 2014).

Hall, Lesley, *Sex, Gender and Social Change in Britain since 1880* (Basingstoke: Palgrave, 2012).

'The archives of birth control in Britain', *Journal of the Society of Archivists*, 16:2, (1995), pp. 207–218.

Harris, Alana, (ed.), *The Schism of '68: Catholics, Contraception and Humanae Vitae in Europe, 1945–1975*, (London: Palgrave McMillan, 2018).

Harris, Alana, 'A magna carta for marriage: Love, catholic masculinities and the *humanae vitae* contraception crisis in 1968 Britain', *Cultural and Social History*, 17:3, (2020), pp. 407–29.

Harford, Judith and Redmond, Jennifer, '"I am amazed at how easily we accepted it": the marriage ban, teaching and ideologies of womanhood in post-Independence Ireland', *Gender and Education*, (2019).

Hesketh, Tom, *The Second Partitioning of Ireland: The Abortion Referendum of 1983* (Dublin: Brandsma Books, 1990).

Hilevych, Yuliya, 'Abortion and gender relationships in Ukraine, 1955–1970', *The History of the Family* (2015), 20:1, pp. 86–105.

Hilliard, Betty, 'The Catholic Church and married women's sexuality: Habitus change in late 20th Century Ireland', *Irish Journal of Sociology*, 12:2, (2003), pp. 28–49.

Hilton, Matthew, McKay, James, Crowson, Nicholas, and Mouhot, Jean-François, *The Politics of Expertise: How NGOs shaped Britain* (Oxford: Oxford University Press, 2013).

Holmes, Katie, 'Does it matter if she cried? Recording emotion and the Australian generations oral history project', *The Oral History Review*, 44:1, (2017), pp. 56–76.

Holohan, Carole, *Reframing Irish Youth in the Sixties* (Liverpool: Liverpool University Press, 2018).

Hug, Chrystel, *The Politics of Sexual Morality in Ireland* (Basingstoke: Palgrave Macmillan, 1999).

Ignaciuk, Agata, 'Paradox of the pill: oral contraceptives in Spain and Poland (1960s–1970s) in Ann-Katrin Gembries, Theresia Theuke and Isabel Heinemann (eds.), *Children by Choice?* (Berlin: De Gruyter, 2018), pp.95–111.

Ignaciuk, Agata, 'Love in the time of El Generalisimo: debates about the pill in Spain before and after Humanae Vitae', in Harris (ed.), *The Schism of '68* (Basingstoke: Palgrave, 2018), pp. 229–50.

Ignaciuk, Agata and Kuźma-Markowska, Sylwia, 'Family planning advice in state-socialist Poland, 1950s–80s: Local and transnational exchanges', *Medical History*, 64:2, (April 2020), pp. 240–66.

Ignaciuk, Agata, Ortiz-Gómez, Teresa, and Rodríguez-Ocaña, Esteban, 'Doctors, women and the circulation of knowledge of oral contraceptives in Spain, 1960s–1970s' in Teresa Ortiz-Gomez, María Jesús Santesmases (eds.), *Gendered Drugs and Medicine: Historical and Socio-cultural Perspectives* (Farnham: Ashgate, 2014), pp. 133–52.

Inglis, Tom, *Moral Monopoly: The Catholic Church in Modern Irish Society* (Dublin: Gill and Macmillan, 1987).

Jasper, James M., *The Emotions of Protest* (Chicago: University of Chicago Press, 2018).

Jones, Claire L., *The Business of Birth Control: Contraception and Commerce in Britain before the Sexual Revolution* (Manchester: Manchester University Press, 2020).

Jones, Greta, 'Marie Stopes in Ireland: The mother's clinic in Belfast, 1936–47', *Social History of Medicine*, 5:2, (August 1992), pp. 255–77.

Jutte, Robert, *Contraception: A History* (Hoboken: Wiley Publishing, 2008).

Kearns, Kevin C., *Working Class Heroines: The Extraordinary Women of Dublin's Tenements* (Dublin: Gill Books, 2018).

Kelly, Laura, 'Debates on family planning and the contraceptive pill in Irish magazine *Woman's Way, 1963–1973*', (*Women's History Review*, online 2021).

Kennedy, Finola, *Cottage to Creche: Family Change in Ireland* (Dublin: Institute of Public Administration, 2001).

Kessler, Trisha Oakley, 'In search of Jewish footprints in the West of Ireland', *Jewish Culture and History*, 19:2, pp. 191–208.

Kiely, Elizabeth, 'Lessons in sexual citizenship: The politics of Irish school based sexuality education' in Máire Leane and Elizabeth Kiely (eds.), *Sexualities and Irish Society* (Dublin: Orpen Press), pp.297–320.

Kiely, Elizabeth and Leane, Máire, *Irish Women at Work 1930–1960: An Oral History* (Dublin: Irish Academic Press, 2012).

Kilgannon, David, '"Responsible, effective and caring": Gay health action, AIDS activism and sexual health in the Republic of Ireland, 1985–1989', *Irish Economic and Social History*, (online, August 2021).

Klausen, Susanne M., *Race, Maternity, and the Politics of Birth Control on South Africa* (Houndmills, UK: Palgrave MacMillan, 2004).

Kline, Wendy, *Bodies of Knowledge: Sexuality, Reproduction, and Women's Health in the Second Wave* (University of Chicago Press, 2010).

Kościańska, Agnieszka, 'Humanae Vitae, Birth Control and the Forgotten History of the Catholic Church in Poland', in Alana Harris (ed.), *The Schism of'68: Catholicism, Contraception and Humanae Vitae in Europe, 1945–1975* (Palgrave, 2018), pp.187–208.

Langhamer, Claire, '"Who the hell are ordinary people?" Ordinariness as a category of historical analysis', *Transactions of the Royal Historical Society*, 28, (2018), pp. 175–195.

López, Raúl Necochea, *A History of Family Planning in Twentieth-Century Peru* (Chapel Hill, NC: University of North Carolina Press, 2014).

Leane, Maire, 'Embodied sexualities: Exploring accounts of Irish women's sexual knowledge and sexual experiences, 1920–1970', in M. Leane and E. Kiely (eds.) *Sexualities and Irish Society: A Reader* (Dublin: Orpen Press, 2014), pp. 29–56.

Luddy, Maria, *Prostitution and Irish Society, 1800–1940* (Cambridge, UK: Cambridge University Press, 2007).

'Unmarried mothers in Ireland, 1880–1973', *Women's History Review*, 20:1, (2011), pp. 109–126.

'Sex and the single girl in 1920s and 1930s Ireland', *The Irish Review*, 35, (Summer, 2007), pp. 79–91.

Lyder, Hazel, '"Silence and Secrecy": Exploring Female Sexuality During Childhood in 1930s and 1940s Dublin', *Irish Journal of Feminist Studies* 5:1&2 (2003), pp. 77–88.

Marques, Tiago Pires, 'The Politics of Catholic Medicine: "The Pill" and Humanae Vitae in Portugal', in Harris (ed.), *The Schism of'68* (Basingstoke: Palgrave, 2018), pp.161–186.

McAuliffe, Mary, '"To change society": Irishwomen United and political activism, 1975–1979' in Mary McAuliffe and Clara Fischer (eds). *Irish Feminisms; Past, Present and Future* (Dublin: Arlen House, 2014).

McAvoy, Sandra, "'A perpetual nightmare": Women, fertility control, the Irish State, and the 1935 Ban on Contraceptives', in Margaret O hOgartaigh and Margaret Preston (eds.), *Gender and Medicine in Ireland, 1700–1950* (New York: Syracuse University Press, 2014), pp.189–202.

'The regulation of sexuality in the Irish Free State, 1929–1935' in E. Malcolm and G. Jones (eds.), *Medicine, Disease and the State in Ireland, 1650–1940* (Cork: Cork University Press, 1999), pp.253–66.

'Its effect on public morality is vicious in the extreme: defining birth control as obscene and unethical, 1926–32' in Elaine Farrell (ed.), *She Said She Was in the Family Way: Pregnancy and Infancy in Modern Ireland* (London: Institute of Historical Research, 2012), pp.35–52.

McCormick, Leanne, "'The scarlet woman in person": the establishment of a Family Planning Service in Northern Ireland, 1950–1974' in *Social History of Medicine,* 21:2, (August 2008), pp. 345–60.

Regulating Sexuality: Women in Twentieth-Century Northern Ireland (Manchester: Manchester University Press, 2009).

"'No sense of wrongdoing": Abortion in Belfast 1917–1967, *Journal of Social History,* 49:1, (Fall, 2015), pp. 125–148.

McCray Beier, Lucinda, "'We were as green as grass": learning about sex and reproduction in three working-class Lancashire communities, 1900–1970', *Social History of Medicine,* 16:3, (2003), pp. 461–80.

McDonagh, Patrick, *Gay and Lesbian Activism in the Republic of Ireland,* 1973–93 (London: Bloomsbury, 2021).

McKenna, Yvonne, *Made Holy: Irish Women Religious at Home and Abroad* (Dublin: Irish Academic Press, 2006).

Marks, Lara, *Sexual Chemistry: A History of the Contraceptive Pill* (New Haven, CT: Yale University Press, 2010).

Milne, Ida, *Stacking the Coffins: Influenza, War and Revolution in Ireland, 1918–19* (Manchester: Manchester University Press, 2018).

Mold, Alex, *Making the Patient-Consumer: Patient Organisations and Health Consumerism in Britain* (Manchester: Manchester University Press, 2016).

'Patient groups and the construction of the patient-consumer in Britain: an historical overview' *Journal of Social Policy,* 39:4, (October 2010), pp. 505–21.

Mosse, George L. , *Nationalism and Sexuality: Respectability and Abnormal Sexuality in Modern Europe* (New York: Howard Fertig, 1985).

Muldowney, Mary, *The Second World War and Irish Women: An Oral History* (Dublin: Irish Academic Press, 2007).

'We were conscious of the sort of people we mixed with: The state, social attitudes and the family in mid twentieth century Ireland', *The History of the Family,* 13:4, (2008), pp. 402–15.

'Breaking the silence: pro-choice activism in Ireland since 1983', in Jennifer Redmond, Sonja Tiernan, Sandra McAvoy and Sonja Tiernan (eds.), *Sexual politics in Ireland* (Dublin: Irish Academic Press, 2015), pp. 127–53.

Murphy, Eileen M., 'Children's burial grounds in Ireland (Cillíní) and parental emotions toward infant death', *International Journal of Historical Archaeology ,* 15:3 (September 2011), pp. 409–28.

Murray, Peter, 'The best news Ireland ever got? Humanae vitae's reception on the Pope's green island', in A. Harris (ed.), *The Schism of '68: Catholicism, Contraception and Humanae Vitae in Europe, 1945–75* (Basingstoke: Palgrave, 2018), pp. 275–301.

Nolan, Ann, 'The transformation of school-based sex education policy in the context of AIDS in Ireland', *Irish Educational Studies*, 37:3, (2018), pp. 295–309.

Ó Gráda, Cormac Ó. and Duffy, Niall, 'The fertility transition in Ireland and Scotland, c.1880–1930', in S.J. Connolly, R.A. Houston and R.J. Morris (eds.), *Conflict, Identity and Economic Development: Ireland and Scotland, 1600–1939* (Preston: Carnegie Publishing, 1995), pp. 89–102.

O'Toole, Eleanor, *Youth and Popular Culture in 1950s Ireland* (Bloomsbury, 2018).

Ortiz-Gómez, Teresa and Ignaciuk, Agata, 'The fight for family planning in Spain during late Francoism and the transition to democracy, 1965–1979', *Journal of Women's History*, 30:2, (Summer, 2018).

'"Pregnancy and labour cause more deaths than oral contraceptives": the debate on the pill in the Spanish press in the 1960s and 1970s', *Public Understanding of Science*, 24:6 (2015), pp. 658–71.

Panichelli-Batalla, Stephanie, 'Laughter in oral histories of displacement: "One goes on a mission to solve their problems"', *The Oral History Review*, 47:1, pp. 73–92.

Pašeta, Senia, 'Censorship and Its Critics in the Irish Free State 1922–1932', *Past and Present*, 181, (November 2003), pp. 193–218.

Pavard, Bibia, 'Du *Birth Control* au Planning familial (1955–1960): un transfert militant', *Histoire@Politique. Politique, culture, société*, n° 18, septembre–décembre 2012 [online: www.histoire-politique. fr].

Portelli, Alessandro, 'What makes oral history different', in Robert Perks and Alistair Thomson (eds.), *The Oral History Reader* (Abingdon-on-Thames: Routledge, 2003 edition).

Prescott, Heather Munro, *The Morning After; A History of Emergency Contraception in the United States* (New Brunswick, NJ: Rutgers University Press, 2011).

Quinlan, Carmel, *Genteel Revolutionaries: Anna and Thomas Haslam and the Irish Women's Movement* (Cork: Cork University Press, 2002).

Rattigan, Cliona, *What Else Could I Do?: Single Mothers and Infanticide, Ireland 1900–1950* (Dublin: Irish Academic Press, 2011).

Redmond, Jennifer, *Moving histories: Irish women's emigration to Britain from Independence to Republic* (Liverpool: Liverpool University Press, 2020).

'The politics of emigrant bodies: Irish women's sexual practice in question', in Jennifer Redmond, Sonja Tiernan, Sandra McAvoy, and Mary McAuliffe, (eds.), *Sexual Politics in Modern Ireland* (Dublin: Irish Academic Press, 2015), pp. 73–89.

Roberts, Dorothy, *Killing the Black Body: Race, Reproduction and the Meaning of Liberty* (London: Penguin, 1998).

Robinson, Emily, Schofield, Camilla, Sutcliffe-Braithwaite, Florence, and Thomlinson, Natalie, 'Telling stories about post-war Britain: popular individualism and the "crisis" of the 1970s', *Twentieth Century British History*, 28:2, (2017), pp. 268–304.

Rossiter, Ann, *Ireland's Hidden Diaspora: The Abortion Trail and the Making of a London-Irish Underground, 1980–2000* (London: IASC Publishing, 2009).

Rusterholz, Caroline, *Women's Medicine: Sex, Family Planning and British Female Doctors In Transnational Perspective* (Manchester: Manchester University Press, 2020).

'Reproductive behavior and contraceptive practices in comparative perspective, Switzerland (1955–1970)', *The History of the Family*, 20:1, (2015), pp. 41–68.

Ryan, Paul, *Asking Angela Macnamara: An Intimate History of Irish Lives* (Dublin: Irish Academic Press, 2012).

Sangster, Joanne, 'Telling our stories: feminist debates and the use of oral history', *Women's History Review*, 3:1, (1994).

Schweppe, J., (ed.), *The Unborn Child, Article 40.3.3 and Abortion in Ireland: Twenty Five Years of Protection?* (Dublin: Liffey Press, 2008).

Sethna, Christabelle and Hewitt, Steve, 'Clandestine operations: The Vancouver Women's Caucus, the abortion caravan, and the RCMP', *The Canadian Historical Review*, 90:3, (September 2009), 463–495.

Shropshire, Sarah, 'What's a guy to do?: Contraceptive responsibility, confronting masculinity, and the history of vasectomy in Canada', *Canadian Bulletin of Medical History*, 31:2, (Fall, 2014), pp. 161–82.

Siegel Watkins, Elizabeth, *On the Pill: A Social History of Oral Contraceptives 1950–1970* (Baltimore: Johns Hopkins University Press, 1998).

Silies, Eva-Maria, 'Taking the pill after the "sexual revolution": female contraceptive decisions in England and West Germany in the 1970s', *European Review of History: Revue européenne d'histoire*, 22:1, (2015), pp. 41–59.

Skeggs, Beverley, *Formations of Class & Gender: Becoming Respectable* (London: SAGE Publications, 1997).

Smith, James M., 'The politics of sexual knowledge: The origins of Ireland's containment culture and the Carrigan Report (1931)', *Journal of the History of Sexuality*, 13:2, (April 2004), pp. 208–33.

Ireland's Magdalen Laundries and the Nation's Architecture of Containment (Notre Dame: University of Notre Dame Press, 2007).

Smyth, Ailbhe, 'The Women's Movement in the Republic of Ireland, 1970–1990', in Ailbhe Smyth (ed.). *Irish Women's Studies Reader* (Dublin: Attic Press, 1993), pp. 245–69.

Smyth, Lisa, *Abortion and Nation: The Politics of Reproduction in Contemporary Ireland* (Farnham: Ashgate, 2005).

Srigley, K., Zembrzycki, S., and Iacovetta, F., *Beyond Women's Words: Feminisms and the Practices of Oral History in the Twenty-First Century*, (London: Routledge, 2018).

Summerfield, Penny, 'Culture and composure: creating narratives of the gendered self in oral history interviews', *Cultural and Social History*, 1:1, (2004), pp. 65–93.

Szreter, Simon, *Fertility, Class and Gender in Britain, 1860–1940* (Cambridge: Cambridge University Press, 1996).

Takeshita, Chikako, *The Global Biopolitics of the IUD: How Science constructs Contraceptive Users and Women's Bodies* (Cambridge, MA: MIT Press, 2011).

Tebbutt, Melanie, *Making Youth: A History of Youth in Modern Britain* (Basingstoke: Palgrave, 2016).

Tentler, Leslie W., *Catholics and Contraception: An American History* (Ithaca: Cornell University Press, 2008).

Thane, Pat and Evans, Tanya, *Sinners? Scroungers? Saints? Unmarried Motherhood in Twentieth-Century England* (Oxford: Oxford University Press, 2012).

Thompson, Paul, *The Voice of the Past: Oral History*, 3rd edition (Oxford: Oxford University Press, 2000).

Tone, Andrea, *Devices and Desires: A History of Contraceptives in America* (New York: Farrar Straus Girroux, 2001).

'Medicalizing reproduction: the pill and home pregnancy tests', *Journal of Sex Research*, 49:4, (2012), pp. 319–27.

'Black market birth control: contraceptive entrepreneurship and criminality in the Gilded Age', *The Journal of American History*, 87:2, (September 2000), pp. 435–59.

Vickers, Emma, 'Unexpected trauma in oral interviewing', *The Oral History Review*, 46:1, (2019), pp. 134–41.

Weeks, Jeffrey, *Sex, Politics and Society: The Regulation of Sexuality Since 1800*, 4th edition (Abingdon: Routledge, 2018).

Young, Iris Marion, 'Menstrual Meditations', in *On Female Body Experience: 'Throwing Like a Girl' and Other Essays* (Oxford: Oxford University Press, 2005).

Yung, Judy, 'Giving voice to Chinese American Women', *Frontiers: A Journal of Women's Studies*, 19:3, (1998), pp. 130–56.

Modern Reports

Clann Project Report (http://clannproject.org/)

Leanne McCormick, Sean O'Connell, Olivia Dee and John Privilege, *Mother and Baby Homes and Magdalene Laundries in Northern Ireland, 1922–1990, Report for the Inter Departmental Working Group on Mother and Baby Homes, Magdalene Laundries and Historical Clerical Child Abuse*, (January 2021).

NCCA *Report on the Review of Relationships and Sexuality Education (RSE) in primary and postprimary schools*, (2019).

Report by Commission of Investigation into the handling by Church and State authorities of allegations and suspicions of child sexual abuse against clerics of the Catholic Diocese of Cloyne (2011).

Report of Working Group on Access to Contraception, (2019).

Unpublished Dissertations

Conlon, Steve, *The Irish student movement as an agent of social change: a case study analysis of the role students played in the liberalisation of sex and sexuality in public policy*, (PhD thesis, Dublin City University, 2016).

Coon, Ruth, *The Impact of The Northern Ireland Troubles on Healthcare Provision and Medical Practice*, (PhD thesis, Ulster University, 2021).

Grimes, Lorraine, *Migration and Assistance: Irish unmarried mothers in Britain, 1926–1973*, (PhD thesis, NUI Galway, 2020).

Marley, Holly, *'A Deadly Depth Charge in their Wombs'. A Study of the Dalkon Shield and the Culture of IUDs in Great Britain*, (MSc thesis, University of Strathclyde, 2019).

Schoonheim, Marloes Marrigje, *Mixing ovaries and rosaries Catholic religion and reproduction in the Netherlands, 1870–1970*, (PhD thesis, Radboud Universiteit Nijmegen, 2005).

Meehan, Grainne, *Flourishing at the margins: an exploration of deaf and hard-of-hearing women's stories of their intimate lives in Ireland*, (PhD thesis, NUI Maynooth, 2019).

Index

Printed in the United States
by Baker & Taylor Publisher Services